AF680794

Environment and Health

CONGRESSIONAL QUARTERLY INC.
1414 22ND STREET, N.W.
WASHINGTON, D.C. 20037

Congressional Quarterly Inc.

Congressional Quarterly Inc., an editorial research service and publishing company, serves clients in the fields of news, education, business and government. It combines specific coverage of Congress, government and politics by Congressional Quarterly with the more general subject range of an affiliated service, Editorial Research Reports.

Congressional Quarterly was founded in 1945 by Henrietta and Nelson Poynter. Its basic periodical publication was and still is the CQ *Weekly Report,* mailed to clients every Saturday. A cumulative index is published quarterly.

CQ also publishes a variety of books. The CQ *Almanac,* a compendium of legislation for one session of Congress, is published every spring. *Congress and the Nation* is published every four years as a record of government for one presidential term. Other books include paperbacks on public affairs and textbooks for college political science classes.

The public affairs books are designed as timely reports to keep journalists, scholars and the public abreast of developing issues, events and trends.

They include such recent titles as *Health Policy,* the second edition of *Energy Policy* and the fifth edition of *The Middle East.* College textbooks, prepared by outside scholars and published under the CQ Press imprint, include such recent titles as *Congress and Its Members; Congress Reconsidered, Second Edition;* and *The Politics of Shared Power.*

In addition, CQ publishes *The Congressional Monitor,* a daily report on present and future activities of congressional committees. This service is supplemented by *The Congressional Record Scanner,* an abstract of each day's *Congressional Record,* and *Congress in Print,* a weekly listing of committee publications.

CQ Direct Research is a consulting service that performs contract research and maintains a reference library and query desk for clients.

Editorial Research Reports covers subjects beyond the specialized scope of Congressional Quarterly. It publishes reference material on foreign affairs, business, education, cultural affairs, national security, science and other topics of news interest. Service to clients includes a 6,000-word report four times a month, bound and indexed semi-annually. Editorial Research Reports publishes paperback books in its field of coverage. Founded in 1923, the service merged with Congressional Quarterly in 1956.

Copyright © 1981 Congressional Quarterly Inc.

All rights reserved. No part of this publication may be reproduced or transmitted in any form or by any means, electronic or mechanical, including photocopy, recording, or any information storage and retrieval system, without permission in writing from the publisher.

Printed in the United States of America

Library of Congress Cataloging in Publication Data

Main entry under title:

Environment and health.

Bibliography:
Includes index.
1. Environmental health — United States. I. Congressional Quarterly, inc.
RA566.3.E58 363.7'00973 81-15155
ISBN 0-87187-224-2 AACR2

363.7
En 89

Editor: Mary McNeil
Supervisory Editors: John L. Moore, Jean L. Woy
Major Contributors: Sari Horwitz, Michael Glennon, Martha V. Gottron
Contributors: Harrison Donnelly, Bill Keller, Kathy Koch, Carolyn Goldinger, Marc Leepson, Ann Pelham, Andy Plattner, Sandra Stencel, Bill Sweet, Margaret C. Thompson, Elizabeth Wehr, Elder Witt
Design: Mary McNeil
Cover: Richard Pottern
Graphics: Bob Redding, Cheryl Rowe

Book Department

David R. Tarr *Director*
Jean L. Woy *Deputy Director*
John L. Moore *Associate Editor*
Michael D. Wormser *Associate Editor*
Martha V. Gottron *Senior Editor*
Barbara R. de Boinville *Assistant Editor*
Lynda McNeil *Assistant Editor*
Margaret C. Thompson *Assistant Editor*
Susan Sullivan *Assistant Political Science Editor*
Michael Glennon *Editor/Writer*
Diane C. Hill *Editor/Writer*
Sari Horwitz *Editor/Writer*
Nancy Lammers *Editor/Writer*
Mary McNeil *Editor/Writer*
Claire L. Tury *Indexer*
Carolyn Goldinger *Researcher/Editorial Assistant*
Patricia M. Russotto *Researcher*
Patricia Ann O'Connor *Contributing Editor*
Elder Witt *Contributing Editor*

Congressional Quarterly Inc.

Eugene Patterson *Editor and President*
Wayne P. Kelley *Publisher*
Peter A. Harkness *Executive Editor*
Robert C. Hur *General Manager*
I.D. Fuller *Production Manager*
Maceo Mayo *Assistant Production Manager*
Sydney E. Garriss *Computer Services*

Contents

Editor's Note. The contamination of our basic elements, from the air we breathe to the water we drink, has begun to have severe consequences for our well being. *Environment and Health* focuses on the relationship between those tainted resources and a wide range of illnesses that afflict mankind. In particular, the book examines the comparatively new hazardous waste disposal problem that has contributed a strong sense of urgency to cleanup efforts. Added to this discussion is a chapter on the battle over nuclear safety and the dangers of radiation exposure. Political and legal problems arising from environmentally related disease — such as victim compensation, cost-benefit analysis and the protection of the worker — are discussed in later chapters. The book also examines the controversy over decreased federal spending in the area of pollution control. Scientists and environmentalists, concerned over the increasing incidence of disease caused by exposure to dangerous substances, are worried that a new cost-conscious Congress will be reluctant to pass legislation that, although expensive, will help protect the public health. As noted in the final chapter, the Reagan administration's early efforts to cut government red tape have begun to dramatically change the regulatory process. The book also contains a chronology of environment and health legislation from 1970 to 1980, selected documents on environment and health affairs, a bibliography and an index. *Environment and Health* is one of CQ's public affairs books that are designed as timely reports to keep journalists, scholars and the public abreast of issues, events and trends.

1

The Unhealthy Environment

We travel together, passengers on a little spaceship, dependent on its vulnerable reserves of air and soil; all committed for our safety to its security and peace; preserved from annihilation only by the care, the work, and, I will say, the love we give our fragile craft.

Adlai E. Stevenson

As the last quarter of the 20th century began, brooding clouds were gathering that threatened that fragile craft with new and unknown dangers to the health of Americans and citizens of other countries, particularly the industrialized nations. Gradually at first and then with a rush, men and women began to realize that the technological world they had created throughout the century might become their graveyard, or at least a huge international hospital ward.

It was not the threat of a nuclear holocaust that propelled these clouds, but a growing realization that all the basic substances humans take for granted may have been defiled by mankind in the search, ironically, for a better, healthier and more prosperous life. The human race was polluting the environment in dozens of different ways. Some of the dangers were clear and present, such as toxic chemicals dumped onto the ground and disease-causing particles pushed into the air. Other dangers were suspected or potential, such as additives to preserve or color food, or nuclear power plants that could release deadly radiation if they ran amok.

The extent of the danger was not a settled subject. Environmentalists saw ominous threats in the technological development of the modern world, and predicted dire health consequences for generations to come. Advocates of that development, although admitting that some problems existed, had two basic responses: first, health problems were far less than feared and in many cases were nonexistent; and second, the costs of providing complete safety had to be considered in light of overall benefits to society from the activities being criticized, such as nuclear power and pesticide spraying.

The scientific evidence was helpful but far from definitive. Even scientists themselves often disagreed, with reputable experts available to all parties in any health safety argument. But there was increasing knowledge about the dangers, which strongly suggested that humans were at least potentially vulnerable to serious health problems from activities undertaken and controllable by humans.

Those dangers seemed to be everywhere. The food people ate, the air they breathed, the water they drank — all might be carrying substances that could lead, someday, maybe 15 years or more in the future, to cancer, emphysema or some other debilitating disease. Large tracts of land were being contaminated by waste chemicals, dangerous sewage discharges and polluted rainfall. Even many workplaces carried threats to health, particularly at industrial sites. But the immediate danger was not so easy to see and, with the scientific evidence at least somewhat in dispute, the issue left a person feeling as if he had wandered into the Twilight Zone.

There was a pervasive danger that touched virtually everything basic to everyday life. An individual sensed that a threat to health was real and possibly quite close, but not always readily apparent, and in any event it was not clear what should be done about it. The complexities, grounded in sometimes incomprehensible and often conflicting scientific explanations, together with the huge financial investment in the production of many substances, magnified the political problem of seeking solutions.

Horror at Love Canal

The symbolic event of the new environmental health danger was known by the oddly incongruous name of Love Canal.

Love Canal was a tiny subdivision in Niagara Falls, N.Y., that in 1978 became a stark and chilling byword for the dark side of the chemical revolution. In the 20th century, chemical and engineering ingenuity had brought Americans thousands of new products — from pesticides that improve agricultural productivity to plastic spoons that ease the chores of a Sunday picnic.

These advancements brought with them unwanted consequences: waste products and byproducts of chemical production that needed to be handled and disposed of with great care, and often were not; accidental spills of toxic substances into the environment; the introduction into food and drink of substances thought to be harmless but later proven otherwise.

Love Canal was the site of a long-forgotten chemical

dump — a graveyard for toxic wastes. More than 200 families were evacuated from the area because dozens of chemicals had seeped into their basements, into a creek and even into the land on which a school was built. The community became a virtual ghost town after President Carter in 1978 declared it the first man-made environmental disaster.

But Love Canal was not an isolated case. In the last few years of the 1970s, horror stories about thousands of oozing chemical dumps began appearing on the front pages of daily newspapers throughout the country. Water supplies were found undrinkable as underground wells that had been pure for centuries suddenly were found contaminated by chemicals.

In 1979 the House Commerce Oversight Subcommittee reported that some 700 million tons of toxic wastes had been dumped since 1950 at 3,383 sites around the country. The federal Environmental Protection Agency (EPA) predicted that 126 billion pounds of toxic chemical wastes would be produced in 1980 — and that only 10 percent of it would be safely discarded. The same year the Congressional Research Service produced a survey of the natural resource losses caused by 219 chemical contamination incidents in 41 states.

The evidence of defilement was accummulating, and it prompted one U.S. senator, Robert T. Stafford, R-Vt., to speak of the "dark and bloody ground" caused by chemical pollution.

Environmental Movement Changes

The environmental movement did not spring from the Love Canal grave. The protection of natural resources had long been an American concern, dating from efforts in the 1880s to protect land, mostly in the West, from unregulated and rapacious use. This element in the environmental movement continued well into the modern day and was reflected in the emphasis given to preserving wilderness areas and wild rivers and creation of parks for recreational use.

In the 1960s and 1970s, in part because of a number of widely publicized environmental controversies such as pesticide poisoning of wildlife and a huge oil spill along California's Santa Barbara coast, the older "conservation movement" began to embrace broader issues of public health and safety. New groups sprang up, expanding the litany of causes and the repertoire of tactics.

The 1980s began with much tougher environmental conditions than the activists of a decade earlier foresaw. Energy shortages, rampant inflation and economic recessions brought in a new era of thinking about environmental issues. Although polls showed that the public still favored cleaning up the environment, people were beginning to ask: How clean? How fast? At what cost?

Broadening Horizons

The reorientation of the environmental movement took place as the link between environmental issues and human health became clearer, with increasing reports of pollution dangers springing up, literally, in the country's backyards. No longer was it enough to protect surface water and pristine air from contamination. More and more, hidden and dormant wastes that contaminated the earth and re-entered the water cycle were becoming an ecological nightmare.

From the concern about preventing and cleaning up pollution came the corollary: persons who had suffered health damage from environmental pollution should be compensated. Victims' compensation quickly swelled into a major issue, particularly for producers facing enormous liability payments for damages allegedly caused by their products.

One of the most publicized controversies grew from American spraying of the defoliant Agent Orange during the Vietnam War. Veterans said later that their exposure to the chemical caused birth defects in their children. Other groups blamed other substances for their maladies. Damage suits were filed for injuries attributed to work-related hazards such as black-lung disease, asbestos contamination, cotton dust inhalation and radiation exposure. By attempting to push environmental law beyond disease prevention into the area of compensation, veterans and other self-identified victim groups ventured into a legal and scientific quagmire that environmental groups and their congressional allies had avoided.

By the early 1980s no clear-cut body of law supporting victims' compensation had developed. But scientific knowledge, mainly in the area of cancer research, continued to accumulate showing a potential link between a person's poor health and exposure to certain substances during work. For example, according to a 1979 report on health from the U.S. surgeon general, plastics workers exposed to the chemical vinyl chloride were known to have a 200 times greater risk of developing lung cancer than the general population.

The Need for Energy

With the 1970s energy crisis and subsequent increases in oil prices came another dimension to the health and environment movement: The United States made a political commitment to free itself from dependence on foreign oil.

A variety of problems emerged. The United States had always been blessed with abundant coal reserves, but that source of energy was largely displaced after World War II by clean-burning and cheap oil and gas. Scientists and environmentalists now feared that extensive use of coal would exacerbate a newly emerging problem — the increasing acidity of rain and snow. Sulfur dioxide emissions from coal-fired power plants were suspected as the culprits causing the acidity to increase.

Environmentalists feared that development of synthetic fuels, mostly from coal, would have to be carried out in the arid West, placing impossible demands on water supplies and increasing air pollution and strip mining. In addition, burning synthetic fuels could increase the atmosphere's carbon monoxide content, which some scientists predicted could cause major changes in worldwide weather patterns.

Nuclear energy, theoretically a source of limitless electric power, produced its own particular health and environment challenges. Beyond the basic question of nuclear plant safety there remained the problem of designing sites to contain highly radioactive wastes. The public also faced many other contentious issues, such as the rights of the states to refuse nuclear dumps, the application of federal environmental restrictions to the building of new plants and the question of federal vs. private responsibility for the burned fuel being generated by private nuclear plants.

Environmental and Energy Knowledge Questions

Question	Correct	Partly Correct	Incorrect	Don't Know
1. What happened at Three Mile Island? (Ans: Nuclear power accident, close to meltdown)	74%	3%	4%	19%
2. Do we produce enough oil or do we have to import oil? (Ans: Have to import)	63	NA	29	7
3. Are nuclear power plants built near bodies of water because it is used as a power source, for waste deposit or for cooling? (Ans: Cooling)	52	NA	27	21
4. Which is the major source of air pollution: factories, automobiles or incinerators? (Ans.: Automobiles)	45	NA	46	9
5. Is cancer caused in rats by every, most or only some chemicals if fed in large doses? (Ans: Only some)	42	NA	45	12
6. What are synthetic fuels? (Ans: Gas or oil made from coal, oil shale or tar sands)	37	5	15	42
7. Is it possible for a nuclear power plant to explode and cause a mushroom-shaped cloud like the one at Hiroshima? (Ans: No)	31	NA	52	16
8. What is acid rain? (Ans: Polluted rain that harms lakes, land and water; that is like vinegar, etc.)	26	6	9	58
9. What happened at Love Canal, near Niagara Falls? (Ans: Chemical or toxic waste dump, place where chemical wastes harmed people or made them move, etc.)	22	4	8	65

Source: Council on Environmental Quality

Resources for the Future, a non-profit research organization in Washington, D.C., conducted a national public opinion survey on environmental issues in 1980 for the Council on Environmental Quality. The test results shown here dealt with environmental and energy topics considered to be relatively well known. Compared to a similar test given by the same organization in 1970, the results show that the public in 1980 is only slightly more knowledgeable about environmental issues than it was a decade ago.

The Cost-Benefit Issue

Probably the most emotional aspect of the environment-health relationship arises from the difficulty of placing a dollar figure on the worth of human well-being, or even a human life. Posed in those terms by opponents of strict environmental controls, the issue created a dilemma that contributed little to rational discussion. But the money question increasingly entered the public debate about health dangers from pollution.

A new and apparently growing public concern about cost-conscious treatment of environmental health protection was best illustrated by President Reagan's attempts, on coming to office in 1981, to restrict the power of federal agencies and ease the impact of their regulations. Business interests had pushed vigorously in Washington for some measure of cost-to-benefit that would force federal agencies to figure the worth of compliance before adopting regulations. Regulatory advocates, however, received strong backing from the Supreme Court, which ruled in 1981 that regulators are not required to temper worker protections against hazardous and poisonous substances to make their costs reasonable to industry.

The court's decision, which settled one of the most debated regulatory decisions of the decade, stemmed from EPA efforts to protect textile workers against cotton dust inhalation, a cause of brown-lung disease. In the decision, Justice William J. Brennan Jr. wrote that the health of workers outweighs "all other considerations" and that "Any standard based on a balancing of costs and benefits . . . would be inconsistent with the law."

Rep. Paul G. Rogers, D-Fla. (1955-79), a major figure in health and environment legislation, had warned in 1978 against uncritical application of strict cost-benefit analysis to health policy. The result, he said, could be a decision that "if getting sick is cheaper, then maybe we should not try to prevent illness."

Warnings also came from government and labor officials concerned with health, who said that economic techniques did not mesh neatly with traditional medical values of saving lives and alleviating pain.

EPA AND OSHA: THE TOP REGULATORS

At the federal level, the job of protecting the public against environment- and work-related hazards fell to a number of agencies, some new and some old. The established agencies included the 75-year-old Food and Drug Administration, which dealt with long-recognized dangers from substances in the food we eat and the medicine we buy. Other regulators included the Federal Trade Commission, the Consumer Product Safety Commission and the Nuclear Regulatory Commission. *(See box, p. 130-131)*

But among the newer agencies two in particular had become leaders in the environment/health field: the Environmental Protection Agency (EPA) and the Occupational Safety and Health Administration (OSHA), both created in 1970.

EPA: Consolidated Effort

The Environmental Protection Agency was established at a time when the nation was becoming increasingly concerned about pollution, declining air and water quality and general deterioration of human ecology. To help carry out the mandate of the National Environmental Policy Act of 1970 (NEPA), President Nixon submitted to Congress a plan to consolidate the federal government's widespread environmental protection efforts into a single agency. There was little congressional opposition and on Dec. 2, 1970, Nixon created the independent EPA by executive order.

Enthusiasm for environmental legislation continued throughout the early 1970s. Congress passed several laws designed to limit or halt the entry of pollutants into the environment, including the Water Quality Improvement Act; the Clean Air Amendments of 1970; the Resource Conservation and Recovery Act; the Federal Environmental Pesticide Control Act of 1972; the Noise Control Act; the Marine Protection, Research and Sanctuaries Act and the Water Pollution Control Act Amendments of 1972.

By the mid-1970s the environmental fervor in Congress began to cool. With much of their program already on the books, environmentalists let up some of the pressure that had stimulated the congressional activity. And the energy shortages following the 1973 Arab oil embargo slowed the rush of environmental programs as legislators sought to balance the benefits of sometimes costly anti-pollution programs against the need for a stable and productive economy.

Despite this trend, EPA's responsibilities expanded in certain areas. The Safe Drinking Water Act of 1974 set standards for chemical and bacteriological pollutants in water systems. During 1977 clean water standards were redefined and deadlines extended one year to 1984.

The Toxic Substances Control Act of 1976 gave EPA the responsibility for studying the risks attached to toxic substances and protecting the public from them. The Resource Conservation and Recovery Act of 1976 was intended to ensure that hazardous and non-hazardous wastes were disposed of in environmentally sound ways. Additional responsibilities in the hazardous waste area were given to the EPA in 1980 with the passage of controversial "superfund" legislation in the waning days of the 96th Congress.

During its first decade EPA grew to become both the largest federal regulatory agency and also one of the most controversial. Under Douglas Costle during the Carter administration, EPA attempted to deal with the concerns of industry while continuing to protect the environment. Costle served as chairman of the U.S. Regulatory Council, an organization Carter established in 1978 to ensure better coordination of federal regulatory activities.

Criticism of EPA came from many sources. One critic, Louis J. Cordia, accused the agency of neglecting to consider the effects of differing elements on the environment. "The EPA must give greater consideration to the 'total human environment — the health, food, energy, jobs, housing, recreation, safety and education of the nation," Cordia wrote. "The question has to be answered seriously: can we afford to try to protect 100 percent of the people 100 percent of the time from every conceivable risk? Can we assume that such total protection is possible? No statute requires this absolutism, but the EPA regulates toward a goal which assumes an affirmative answer."

EPA edged closer to a cost-benefit approach to regulation during the Carter administration, and was likely to move further in that direction under Reagan. In March 1981 Reagan asked for a 42 percent reduction in Carter's proposal for environmental funds. The new president sought $7.9 billion for fiscal 1982, $5.7 billion less than the $13.6 billion Carter had requested. The Reagan request included an 18 percent cut in EPA's pollution research funds, or $68.8 million less than the $375 million authorized for fiscal 1981. President Reagan also asked Congress to rescind $56.3 million in EPA's research funds for the current fiscal year, but there had been no action on that request by September 1981.

Criticism of EPA also focused on its standards, particularly those dealing with auto emissions. Automobile manufacturers, representing the largest U.S. industry, argued that they were unable to meet EPA emission standards and still produce reasonably priced cars. To the dismay of environmentalists, the emission deadlines were extended several times after their enactment in 1970. In April 1981 the Reagan administration proposed to go even further and eliminate an EPA requirement that all cars meet emission standards to protect air quality in high-altitude areas. The change would require Congress to amend the Clean Air Act but would save consumers $1.3 billion, according to the administration.

Another administration move that had environmentalists up in arms was proposed in July 1981, when EPA Administrator Anne Gorsuch recommended that the government use the Army Corps of Engineers to clean up the country's toxic waste dumps. Gorsuch told a House Energy subcommittee that the corps could complete the job faster and more economically than private companies under contract. Critics complained that the idea was a "radical departure" from the intent of the superfund legislation and would delay implementation of the cleanup.

OSHA: Workplace Safety

OSHA was established as an agency within the Labor Department by the Occupational Safety and Health Act of 1970. It is directed by the assistant secretary of labor for occupational safety and health, currently Thorne G. Auchter.

OSHA quickly became a controversial agency and many businesses — especially small businesses — remained unrelenting in their criticism of it. Within one month of its creation, OSHA adopted some 4,400 standards from existing federal regulations, industry codes and the American National Standards Institute. Critics charged that the agency's standards were difficult to understand and frequently were unreasonably rigid. They also complained that penalties for first violations were often unfair and that the cost of compliance and paperwork could drive small companies out of business.

At the same time labor groups complained that the agency's enforcement activities were sporadic and weak, that its administration of the act was poor and that it had failed to significantly reduce workplace hazards.

The attacks from both sides continued despite efforts by Eula Bingham, who headed the agency under President Carter, to have OSHA adopt "common sense" priorities. Responding to complaints from small business owners, Congress in 1979 exempted most companies with fewer than 10 employees from annual OSHA inspections.

Hearings were held in April 1980 on a bill that would have further curbed OSHA's authority. The proposal would have exempted an estimated 90 percent of the nation's small businesses and 85 percent of all businesses from the yearly inspections. Inspectors would have been allowed access to a business whenever a serious accident occurred, when health and safety rates began to decline or when employee complaints could not be resolved without an inspection. The bill died before the end of the 96th Congress in 1980.

Court decisions also have clipped OSHA's wings. In May 1978 the court ruled that an employer has the right, based on the Fourth Amendment, to keep out an OSHA inspector who does not have a search warrant. And the court in 1980 invalidated OSHA's benzene exposure standard because it said there was insufficient evidence to show the standard was needed to protect workers.

On the other hand, the same court affirmed some of OSHA's regulatory actions and the act under which it operates. Before it upheld OSHA's standard-setting authority in the 1981 cotton dust decision, the Supreme Court ruled in 1980 that the Occupational Safety and Health Act protects workers from recrimination if they refuse to perform tasks they consider unsafe.

At least partly in response to business opposition, OSHA has changed some of its own rulings. For example, in 1981 the agency modified a cancer policy it had instituted a year earlier. The policy, instead of regulating specific substances, established criteria for classifying carcinogens and set forth procedures for future rulemakings on them. OSHA said the policy gave the worker better protection by speeding up the regulating of carcinogens. After business leaders objected that OSHA was forcing them to spend billions of dollars without showing that the improvements would save lives or prevent injuries, the agency struck a compromise by altering the policy.

OSHA was likely to undergo considerable changes under Auchter's conservative stewardship. Soon after taking office, Auchter made clear that he believed OSHA symbolized government over-regulation.

But even OSHA's strongest critics generally conceded that in its first 10 years the agency increased the country's awareness of occupational safety and health matters. The conservative Heritage Foundation told President Reagan that the statutory framework of the Occupational Safety and Health Act, although imperfect, was flexible enough to allow some deregulation without enacting new legislation.

Business Week magazine said in March 1981 that it was "increasingly clear" that OSHA's direction under Auchter "will be significantly different in both style and substance from that of his predecessor [Bingham]...." Bingham worked closely with union groups and under her leadership OSHA promulgated numerous new health standards — many calling for extensive engineering controls paid for by industry. With Auchter in charge, OSHA was working more closely with industry, trying to keep its safety costs to a minimum. "The question of the least costly approach has an awful lot of merit," Auchter said. "If we can come up with a method that incurs lower cost, then that makes the most sense, provided we can reach the objective."

ENVIRONMENTALISTS REGROUP FOR THE 1980s

The environmental movement faced an uphill battle in the wake of the 1980 elections. The lengthy record of legislation racked up by environmentalists in the 1970s appeared headed for intense scrutiny in Congress from fiscal conservatives who had campaigned on cutting big government.

Foremost among the environmental antagonists was President Reagan, who at one point in his campaign had drawn derision by saying that "93 percent of the oxides of nitrogen" come from trees and other vegetation. Reagan had confused nitrogen oxide, a regulated pollutant, with nitrous oxides, a harmless product of plant respiration.

Aside from the resultant jokes about "killer trees," the new president was a serious exponent of going slow on environmental regulation. Some of his closest personal friends and advisers were rich businessmen leery of "environmental extremists." The appointments of Interior Secretary James G. Watt, Office of Management and Budget Director David A. Stockman and Council of Economic Advisers Chairman Murray L. Weidenbaum, all advocates of diminished government regulation, sent shivers through the environmental movement.

The public apparently shared some of the administration's skepticism. William Tucker, in a May 1981 article in *Harper's*, summed up the new attitude: "The time has come to reform environmentalism. No one can seriously deny this. Perhaps nothing has been more symbolic of the era of Great Expectations than the notion that by writing draconian regulations about air and water pollution, and enforcing them with penalties just short of hanging, we could restore America to the Eden of 1620, before we had arrived to foul the land."

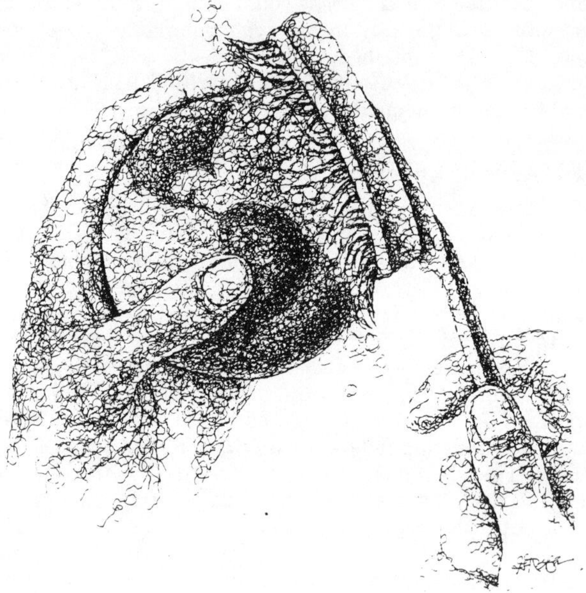

Fading Support?

In Congress, too, environmentalists lost several champions at a time when some of their legislative achievements were coming up for reauthorization. The Clean Air Act was slated to be the first major statute up for debate, followed by laws governing clean water, strip mining and a number of public land issues. In each case, a formidable business lobby was gearing up for a fight.

Environmentalists were afraid that Reagan, in implementing the laws already passed, particularly new ones like the superfund bill to help clean up toxic wastes, could do grave damage by doing not much at all. "Changing laws is difficult and slow," said Thomas L. Kimball, vice president of the National Wildlife Federation. "But regulations are another matter. An awful lot of discretionary power is given by law to the agencies. Within the framework of the law, you can make or break our environmental objectives."

But the environment movement still had a firm foundation of public support, according to a 1980 study conducted by Robert Mitchell for the Council on Environmental Quality. Comparing his own extensive poll with similar surveys taken through the 1970s, Mitchell found a decline, from the excitement of Earth Day 1970, in the public's willingness to sacrifice economic growth for a clean environment. But he also found a strong sentiment that continuing improvement in environmental quality "must be made regardless of cost."

Washington environmentalists conceded they had not done enough to frame arguments in dollars and cents, and would need to do so in the face of the rising anti-regulatory mood in Congress and the competition for scarce federal dollars. Cost-benefit analysis — the traditional tool of public works, military, transportation and environment planners — was being promoted as an antidote to "inflationary' regulation in other fields.

Return to Grass Roots

Another prospective change was a turning away from Washington. Many environmental activists and their allies in Congress conceded they had neglected their political base and had to rebuild popular support to enhance their lobbying credibility. "What we've got to do is not play confrontation games, not be purists," Rep. Morris K. Udall, D-Ariz., warned a symposium at the National Wildlife Federation. "Identify allies, play up the fact that conservation is a bipartisan issue."

Environmentalists considered themselves fortunate that their movement was well established on Capitol Hill long before the 1973-74 Arab oil embargo made energy a top national concern. The momentum they had developed with passage of major laws such as the National Environmental Policy Act of 1969, clean air legislation in 1970 and clean water measures in 1970 and 1972, helped push through other major legislation after the embargo. The trend continued up to the end of 1980, when Congress created the $1.6 billion superfund and enacted legislation to protect 104 million acres of Alaska from development.

After the 1980 election there was little agreement among environmentalists about the prospects for compromise with business. But a growing number of environmental leaders said they believed it was worth trying — not just because the election strengthened industry's hand, but because it could result in more effective environmental protection.

A sign of this new mood was the fact that at least two of Carter's in-house environmentalists went to work for industry. Joseph Browder, a veteran of the Audubon Society, Friends of the Earth and the Environmental Policy Center before Carter tapped him to handle public land issues in the Interior Department, opened a consulting business. James W. Moorman, a former Sierra Club Legal Defense Fund lawyer who headed the natural resources division of the Justice Department, joined a Washington law firm. Both said they hoped to help companies in their efforts to comply with environmental laws.

The environmental movement also drew a new element of urgency from the health hazards produced by misuse of the environment. While energy needs and cost-benefit analysis dictated moderation in the regulation of harmful side-effects of commercial production, the public appeared to realize that progress at the expense of good health is questionable progress at best.

2

Air: Is It Safe to Breathe?

When the Clean Air Act amendments were passed in 1977 environmental groups were pleased but not jubilant. In fact, when the smoke had cleared, most observers — including lobbyists involved in the fight — agreed that certain business interests, particularly automobiles and utilities, had won important battles while environmentalists had only a few sparse victories.

In 1981, with the Clean Air Act coming up for revision, environmentalists looked back on the 1977 amendments with a yearning for the good old days. With the Reagan administration hoping to weaken many provisions, the fight over renewal of the Act provided the first major indication of the president's ability to turn back the tide of environmental regulation.

Authorization for the Clean Air Act, the nation's most complex and far-reaching environmental law, was to expire Sept. 30, 1981. Chairmen of two congressional panels reviewing it doubted that the landmark Act would be rewritten in 1981 and Robert T. Stafford, R-Vt., chairman of the Senate Environment and Public Works Committee, predicted that the bill would not get to the Senate floor until February 1982. Debate on the issue was expected to be long and bloody, with decisions being made by a more cost-conscious Congress than the one that thrashed out the 1977 amendments.

At first, the Reagan administration saw renewal of the Act as a chance to pare down the federal role in air pollution control, restricting it to advising the states on clean air standards. Anne Gorsuch, administrator of the Environmental Protection Agency, disclosed this plan in a memo that Sen. Gary Hart, D-Colo., made public in July 1981. Hart said the proposal would have repealed 51 provisions of the 1977 legislation and relaxed 64 others.

Under existing law EPA was required to set standards to protect public health "allowing an adequate margin of safety." The memo said the administration was considering eliminating that requirement and allowing standards to be set according to "a degree of significant risk" to public health.

But at a news conference in August 1981 Gorsuch presented the administration's position in a simplified, nine-point plan that indicated Reagan had second thoughts about defending complex new legislation on such a controversial issue. Gorsuch said that the federal government would continue to maintain clean air standards with high enough margins of safety for asthmatics, infants and the elderly. The modified plan also called for continued federal enforcement of secondary standards to protect the environment, visibility and other values not directly related to health.

Environmentalists said that some of the "minor adjustments" proposed by the administration would radically undercut the basic foundation of the law. They feared that, because the law was so complicated, major changes could still easily slip by the uninitiated. Their fears were heightened by the fact that 179 members — a third of Congress — had been elected since 1977 and had not dealt with the baffling legislation.

A CHANGED POLITICAL CLIMATE

As Congress reworked the Clean Air Act, members had to decide whether to continue a decade-long commitment to protect all citizens equally from harmful air pollution — regardless of cost — or whether to accept more air pollution in the interests of economic development.

Members also had to consider:

- Whether children, pregnant women and old people — who were the most vulnerable to air pollution — should have the same right to protection under the law as other persons.
- Whether the nation should continue trying to protect citizens from temporary episodes of watery eyes and difficult breathing, or if it could only afford to protect them from permanent lung damage.
- Whether to continue protecting unspoiled areas from encroaching air pollution.
- Whether energy development was so important that strip mining and belching smokestacks had to be allowed in clear view of national parks.
- Whether the government was using valid scientific data in setting the air pollution standards.

While trying to consider what impact these decisions would have in the future, Congress was looking back to see how well the Clean Air Act had worked in its first 10 years of operation.

Purpose of the Act

The Act's fundamental purpose was to protect the public from dirty air. But to achieve that seemingly simple goal the law required American industry to spend billions of dollars each year and it affected nearly all U.S. industrial, energy production, transportation and real estate activities. Consequently, industry was ready with a raft of amendments that it said would merely "fine-tune" the Act to make it work better.

The National Commission on Air Quality, authorized by Congress in 1977 to provide information and proposals for revision of the Act, agreed that some changes should be made but it recommended against significant weakening of the 1977 standards. The commission, which released its report March 2, 1981, was composed of four members of Congress and nine private citizens appointed by President Carter.

Sen. Gary Hart, D-Colo., commission chairman, said the panel recommended "that Congress retain the current statutory formula for setting the national air quality standards. The standards should continue to be set at the level necessary to protect the health of the most susceptible people — the old and the infirm — with an adequate margin of safety. Only health considerations should go into the determination of the appropriate level of the standards."

The commission found that, on the whole, contrary to many industry claims, the Clean Air Act had not been an important obstacle to energy development and, in fact, allowed substantial increases in domestic energy production. Although the commission said costs should be considered in the development of air pollution control standards, it explicitly rejected setting regulations that were based on costs.

The commission did recommend that EPA review certain air quality standards. It said that the standard for controlling airborne particles might be improved and it requested a review of ozone standard and carbon monoxide standards to ensure they were adequate for long-term exposures. It recommended that Congress keep existing protections for important national parks and wilderness areas designated before 1977, all national parks and wilderness areas protected against visibility impairment in 1977 and national lands that could not, under the existing Act, be redesigned as Class III (wildlife refuges, national monuments, national recreation areas, national seashores, wild and scenic rivers and those national parks and wilderness areas designated after 1977). The report concluded that the "mobile sources" section had been the most effective part of the Clean Air Act, substantially reducing pollution from automobiles.

Three commissioners, however, expressed disagreement with the report in four major areas of controversy. *(Details p. 16)*

New Mood in Congress

Some of the architects of the 1977 Act were not around in 1981 to defend their handiwork. Sen. Edmund S. Muskie, D-Maine (1959-80), and Rep. Paul G. Rogers, D-Fla. (1955-81) — who led the fight to protect the Act in 1977 — had retired. Robert T. Stafford, R-Vt., the moderate chairman of the Environment Committee, was filling Muskie's shoes in the Republican Senate. Liberal Rep. Henry A. Waxman, D-Calif., headed the House Commerce Committee's Subcommittee on Health and Environment, formerly chaired by Rogers.

Stafford and Waxman both supported Muskie and Rogers in 1977. Neither would express opinions on the 1981 issues in advance, but they said they wanted to protect the Act's basic framework. Waxman said he was "apprehensive" about what Reagan would propose. "During the campaign he said some incredible things about the Clean Air Act," Waxman said. "I'm hoping their proposals will be moderate, and they realize that the Act is a very important piece of health legislation."

Stafford said the length of the debate would depend on the lobbyists. "If those on all sides of the issue decide to take off their gloves and make this a major contest, rather than a cooperative venture, then we are going to be in for a long and difficult journey," he said.

Whatever the outcome, it would be decided in a political context vastly different from the one that prevailed in 1977. A Republican administration dedicated to renewal of American industry would be overseeing the legislative review, which would take place against the backdrop of a troubled economy, amidst arguments that the Act causes unemployment and hampers energy development.

As for the general public, in a poll commissioned by the Council on Environmental Quality (CEQ), only 20 percent of the respondents agreed that "we must relax environmental standards in order to achieve economic growth," and 42 percent thought environmental problems "so important ... that continuing improvement must be made regardless of cost." But only 27 percent agreed that economic growth should be sacrificed to protect the environment, compared with 58 percent in 1978.

Political Alignments

In June 1980 Douglas Costle, then EPA administrator, expressed anxiety that the Clean Air Act might be "gutted" in 1981. He said the "inherent complexities of air pollution control make it easy for an opponent to propose language changes which — seemingly innocuous on their face — in fact weaken the law to a serious degree."

"Still more serious," he said, "is the fact that at no time since the late 1800s have private interests had so much influence in Congress as they do today. In 1974, there were 608 political action committees organized to channel funds to candidates. By December 1979 the number of such committees had jumped threefold, to nearly 2,000. Labor union representation had held relatively stable, at 240; trade associations had grown to 512 from 38; corporate political action committees, by contrast, had soared from 89 to 979."

Business Groups

Investor-owned utilities were relying on the Edison Electric Institute, their trade association, to promote their interests in the clean air fight. The institute was just one of the groups lobbying for industry.

In addition to many individual trade groups, four well-known business organizations — the Business Roundtable, the U.S. Chamber of Commerce, the National Association of Manufacturers (NAM) and the National Environmental

Development Association (NEDA) — had prepared detailed positions on clean air revisions. In addition to the lobbying efforts mounted by individual corporations and trade associations such as the American Petroleum Institute, four groups representing a variety of businesses launched programs to promote revision of clean air legislation. The organizations were:

National Environmental Development Association/Clean Air Project. Of the four groups, NEDA was likely to be the most influential voice. Among other things, the organization planned to recommend improving the scientific foundation for air standards, relaxing significant deterioration requirements, abolishing EPA's bans on construction of new pollutant sources in nonattainment areas (where air quality had not yet been brought up to federal standards).

Founded in 1973 to provide information on balancing environmental and economic needs, NEDA organized its air project (CAP) in March 1979. Participants included the 17 members of the Building and Construction Trades Department of the AFL-CIO and 34 corporations including Exxon, Dow Chemical, General Motors, Kaiser Aluminum, the Union Pacific and Weyerhaeuser. The steering committee, chaired by John Quarles, EPA's former general counsel, head of enforcement and deputy administrator, issued a report Nov. 18, 1980, recommending changes in the Clean Air Act.

Business Roundtable. The Roundtable has as members the chief executive officers of 200 large corporations. Its Environmental Task Force, headed by Union Pacific Chairman James H. Evans and William M. McDonald, Union Pacific senior vice president for law, singled out four clean air issues for detailed attention: 1) procedures for setting air quality standards, especially health standards; 2) prevention of significant deterioration; 3) procedures for permitting; and 4) analysis of regulatory costs.

U.S. Chamber of Commerce. The environmental committee of the chamber, which has roughly 100,000 individual and business members, was expected to recommend changes in clean air legislation to the board of directors in late 1981. Problems facing firms in non-attainment areas were a top priority, but prevention of deterioration, confusion and delays in the permitting process and unpredictable factors in environmental regulation also ranked high. The chamber expected to publish two pamphlets on clean air legislation in mid-December.

National Association of Manufacturers. NAM's 12,000 member companies account for roughly 75 percent of U.S. manufacturing capacity. NAM's recommendations were likely to be similar to those advanced by the Chamber of Commerce and the Roundtable.

Depending on their members' interests, the various associations emphasized different aspects of clean air legislation in their preparations for the revision. Because many of its members were small- and medium-sized businesses in the older and dirtier parts of the Northeast and Midwest, the chamber devoted a lot of attention to rules affecting non-attainment regions. It also worked to simplify regulations and reduce time-consuming paperwork, because, in the words of the chamber's environmental expert, small businesses "don't have the resources that big corporations have to cope with regulation."

Organizations representing big business, on the other hand, were working for fundamental revisions of regulations that affect corporate balance sheets. Typical of these big companies was Union Pacific, a leading participant in the Business Roundtable's clean air effort. No longer merely a railroad, Union Pacific became a holding company in 1969. Its mining subsidiary, Rocky Mountain Energy, owns vast coal, uranium and soda ash reserves in southern Wyoming, Utah and Colorado. Its multimillion-ton coal reserves in the Great Divide Basin in Wyoming may become a significant source of synthetic fuels, according to the company's 1979 annual report. An oil subsidiary, Champlin Petroleum, owns refineries in Texas, Oklahoma and Southern California and drills for oil all over the West. In 1979, for the first time in the company's history, more than half its earnings — 61 percent — came from energy and natural resources.

Compliance Status, Major Air Pollution Sources, 1980

Industry	Total Sources	Number in Compliance	Number Violating Emission Limits
Powerplants	700	559	67
Iron and steel	204	110	56
Primary smelters	28	13	8
Pulp and paper	475	417	24
Mun. incinerators	72	60	7
Petro. refineries	214	170	21
Alum. reduction	49	37	8
Portland cement	200	176	18
Sulfuric acid	262	246	10
Phosphate fertilizers	69	62	4
Coal cleaning	409	395	4
Grey iron	433	381	29
Asphalt concrete	2.862	2.752	39
Total	**5,977**	**5,378**	**160**

Source: Environmental Protection Agency

Environmental Groups

Arrayed against the industrial associations were a number of environmental, public health and "public interest" groups that hoped to see the clean air laws maintained in their essential features and, if possible, strengthened. The Sierra Club, the League of Women Voters, National Parks and Conservation, Friends of the Earth, the Natural Resources Defense Council and the Environmental Defense Fund were coordinating their efforts as members of the "Clean Air Coalition," founded in 1973. According to coordinator Betsy Agle, the coalition was preparing working papers on acid rain and toxic air pollutants.

Environmentalists have accused EPA of not acting quickly and energetically enough on toxic pollutants and the opinion was widely held that acid rain problems — which involve long-range transport of pollutants — would not likely be solved within the framework of a system that relied almost exclusively on states in enforcing rules compliance.

As the hearings approached, groups supporting stronger clean air legislation were far behind the industrial associations in their preparations. Many observers attributed the environmentalists' slow start to their shortage of

Steel Industry Position

Steel companies loomed large in industry's efforts to obtain some relaxation of the Clean Air Act. The steelmakers said they had spent 15 percent of their capital costs on pollution control since the Clean Air Act became law in 1970, and would spend another $7 billion in 10 years unless Congress changed the law.

Most emissions from a steel mill's furnace are caught by hoods that cover vessels holding molten metal. Particulates arising in the hot gases, mostly iron oxides, are removed by electrostatic precipitators and water scrubbers. Some emissions escape when molten iron is poured into the vessel of a basic oxygen furnace to make steel, or when other processes are being carried out. To catch these fugitive emissions, companies employ a giant vacuum cleaner system called a "bag house." The air inside a steel mill is passed through huge cloth bag filters that collect the particulates. The system is expensive to run and consumes a great deal of energy.

Steel executives argue that they have removed 95 percent of their particulate emissions and that it is unreasonably expensive to remove the remaining 5 percent. Opponents of this stance see the industry willing to spend much more money in other ways including wages. They question the industry's priorities.

money, the loss of several leading clean air experts to other jobs and to the groups' preoccupation with issues that had been more pressing in 1979-80, such as toxic dumping, Alaska lands, and nuclear regulation.

Environmental groups hoped for support from affected federal, state and local officials. According to S. William Becker, a Washington representative of the Association of Local Air Pollution Control Officials (ALAPCO) and the State and Territorial Air Pollution Program Administrators (STAPPA), local officials were seeking more discretion in implementing federal rules and they agreed with business groups that federal regulation needed to be faster and more efficient. But he said they also thought "a lot of these problems are administrative items that may be ironed out administratively without a complete revamping of the Clean Air Act."

Unions

Labor's position seemed to be divided. The United Steelworkers of America, for example, had not accepted as of September 1981 the argument that air regulations were largely responsible for the steel industry's problems, according to Jack Sheehan, a Steelworkers' official and member of the National Commission on Air Quality. "Our people are constantly pushed with this environmental blackmail, but we have resisted that and have not joined in the general attack on EPA," he said in an interview Oct. 29, 1980.

The United Auto Workers, on the other hand, had tended to support relaxation of emission standards while the United Mine Workers were opposing strict anti-sulfur regulations. The AFL-CIO's construction unions were participants in NEDA's drive to relax clean air standards.

Reagan Position

At the 1980 Democratic National Convention, Sen. Edward M. Kennedy, D-Mass., aroused peals of laughter when he quoted Ronald Reagan as saying that "80 percent of our air pollution comes from plants and trees." Most of the delegates no doubt assumed this was a statement Reagan would prefer to forget. But a few months later, on Oct. 7, 1980, Reagan defended his remark during a campaign stop at Steubenville, Ohio: "First of all, I didn't say 80 percent. I said 92 percent — pardon me, 93 percent. And I didn't say air pollution; I said oxides of nitrogen. And I am right. Growing and decaying vegetation in this land are responsible for 93 percent of the oxides of nitrogen." In the same speech, Reagan said he suspected that the eruption of Mount St. Helens had released more sulfur dioxide into the air in just a few months "than has been released in the last 10 years of automobile driving or things of that kind. . . ." Later that day, Reagan told an audience in Youngstown, Ohio, that air pollution "has been substantially controlled."

The same day that Reagan was promising Ohio audiences he would revise clean air laws in consultation with the coal and steel industries, the Los Angeles area was in the second week of the worst smog episode in recent memory. Carter administration officials lost no time in taking Reagan to task for his views. EPA Administrator Costle said that Reagan had confused nitrogen dioxide, a regulated pollutant, with nitrous oxides, harmless products of plant respiration. CEQ Chairman Gus Speth pointed out that soil bacteria — not trees — was the primary source of nitrous oxides. Calling Reagan's remarks "strange and bewildering," Speth said that human sources emit sulfur dioxide at a rate 40 times higher than that from Mount St. Helens, and he reminded Americans that power plants — not cars as Reagan had implied — were the principal source of sulfur pollutants.

Reagan's misstatements about air pollution and his record on air quality issues made Carter the favored presidential candidate of most environmental groups, once Kennedy and Gov. Edmund G. Brown Jr. of California were defeated in the Democratic primaries. The League of Conservation Voters, a Washington-based organization, gave Carter a "C+" on air quality issues and Reagan an "F."

During his campaign, Reagan often attributed the serious problems of the automobile and steel industries to excessive government regulation, and he indicated that the country's booming coal economy would be even stronger but for environmental rules. In speeches prepared for delivery at Steubenville and Youngstown, Ohio, the day he made his off-the-cuff remarks about trees and Mount St. Helens, Reagan said that "Mr. Carter's EPA appointees apparently don't know and don't care about coal. It's time we had a president who will see to it that EPA has leaders who understand how vital coal is to the nation and to Ohio's economy."

As governor of California, Reagan signed one of the

toughest air pollution control laws in the country. But before he signed it he insisted that it call for local, rather than state, control over stationary sources of pollution. As a result, the law was poorly enforced, according to later investigations by Democratic Gov. Brown's administration.

Reagan also fought the development of mass transit, despite the heavy auto pollution in California. This situation led later to EPA rejection of California's air pollution control plan during the Nixon administration.

Reagan opposed the state Legislature's attempt to require pollution devices on used cars. When the state Air Resources Board tried to implement the law, Reagan fired two of its members and replaced them with persons who agreed with him.

THE CLEAN AIR ACT AND ITS IMPLICATIONS

After the 1970 Clean Air Act required the Environmental Protection Agency to set national air quality standards for major pollutants, state and local governments had the task of bringing air into compliance with those standards by whatever procedures proved necessary and acceptable. At the same time, emissions of certain pollutants were required to be reduced at the source — be they emissions from automobiles, other modes of transportation, industrial facilities or power plants.

When it appeared most states would not meet the deadline, Congress in 1977 extended it to 1982 (and 1987 for areas with severe automobile-related pollution). The 1977 amendments relaxed several compliance deadlines but also tightened clean air legislation in several important respects. The amendments 1) established three categories of areas with air that is cleaner than required under national standards, 2) specified how much levels of sulfur and dioxides and particulates could increase in each category and 3) required the EPA to propose regulations for "prevention of significant deterioration (PSD)" — in levels of nitrogen oxide, hydrocarbons, carbon monoxide and photochemical oxidents.

The PSD provisions were designed partly to prevent the nation's air from deteriorating to a mediocre national average, and partly to prevent industries from relocating facilities from exceptionally dirty to clean areas. The amendments gave states until July 1, 1979, to complete their revised State Implementation Plans (SIP) for attainment of ambient air standards and required all plans to contain a permit program for major stationary sources of pollution. The amendments also provided for the establishment of a National Commission on Air Quality (NCAQ) that was given three years to complete its report.

Early Results

The Act has resulted in cleaner air, but progress has been slower than sponsors hoped, partly because some industries have resisted compliance, often in court, and partly because EPA has been slow in implementing the Act. In 1981 EPA estimated that 93 percent of industry was in compliance. The non-complying companies primarily were power plants, steel plants and heavy metal industries.

Significant improvements in the nation's air quality were not achieved until the late 1970s. As late as May 31, 1975, the original deadline for compliance with the 1970 Act, pollution levels were still higher than specified in two out of every three air quality regions.

Despite the improvements, the CEQ stressed that air pollution was still a problem. "In 1977, the air in two of the 41 urban areas for which reliable data were available still

Ranking of Cities, 1976-78

(PSI: Pollutant Standards Index)

Severity Level		PSI > 100	PSI > 200
More than 150 days	Los Angeles	242	118
	New York	224	51
	Pittsburgh	168	31
	San Bernardino Riverside-Ontario	167	88
100-150 days	Cleveland	145	35
	St. Louis	136	29
	Chicago	124	21
	Louisville	119	12
50-99 days	Washington, D.C.	97	8
	Phoenix	84	10
	Philadelphia	82	9
	Seattle	82	4
	Salt Lake City	81	18
	Birmingham	75	19
	Portland	75	3
	Houston	69	16
	Detroit	65	4
	Jersey City	65	4
	Baltimore	60	12
	San Diego	52	6
25-49 days	Cincinnati	45	2
	Dayton	45	2
	Gary-Hammond East Chicago	36	8
	Indianapolis	36	2
	Milwaukee	33	6
	Buffalo	31	5
	San Francisco	30	1
	Kansas City	29	6
	Memphis	28	2
	Sacramento	28	2
	Allentown	27	1
0-24 days	Toledo	24	2
	Dallas	22	1
	Tampa	12	1
	Akron	10	0
	Norfolk	9	0
	Syracuse	9	1
	Rochester	6	0
	Grand Rapids	5	0

Source: Council on Environmental Quality

registered in the 'unhealthful' range for more than two-thirds of the days of the year," the council said. "These two, the New York and Los Angeles urban areas, together contain almost 8 percent of the nation's population. Only 16 of the 41 urban areas had 'unhealthful' readings for fewer than 10 percent of the days during the year.... The pollutants that most frequently drove index readings into the 'unhealthful' range in the 41 urban areas were carbon monoxide and photochemical oxidents (ozone)."

Ambient air levels for one pollutant, nitrogen dioxide, showed little change during the years 1974-77. But violations for most of the other "criteria" pollutants — the pollutants for which EPA sets national air quality standards — decreased significantly in at least some areas. Violations of ozone standards generally dropped in the western parts of the United States, but not in the eastern and central parts. Despite improvements, the Los Angeles area continued to suffer more smog violations than any other part of the country. Carbon monoxide levels improved markedly almost everywhere, but most of all in the East, while levels of suspended particulates displayed no strong regional trends. Sulfur dioxide levels generally were not severe except where smelters were located.

Altogether ozone violations decreased 24 percent between 1974 and 1977, carbon monoxide violations, 43 percent; sulfur dioxide, 54 percent; and particulates, 2 percent. Even so, EPA statistics indicate that the total quantity of primary pollutant emissions dropped by less than 10 million metric tons between 1970 and 1977. With the total reaching 193.9 million metric tons in 1977, there was nearly a ton of pollutants for every person in the United States.

By 1979, however, the Council on Environmental Quality was reporting on the basis of combined data from 25 metropolitan areas that the "number of unhealthful days had declined by 15 percent between 1974 and 1977 while the number of very unhealthful days declined 32 percent." The CEQ attributed the decrease mainly to a reduction of auto pollution. Taking data from about 50 of the most polluted counties, the CEQ found that "violations of ambient air quality standards generally either stayed constant or decreased between 1974 and 1977. The greatest improvements were made in reducing violations of the carbon monoxide and sulfur dioxide standards."

1980s Goals

Although progress had been made, the 1981 NCAQ report said that millions of Americans still were breathing air that was dirtier than the national standards called for, and it said there were serious doubts that some regions would meet the 1982 and 1987 deadlines. At least four areas of the country — Los Angeles, Houston, New York and Boston — may never meet the national standards for carbon monoxide.

NCAQ also warned that dangerous levels of carbon monoxide, nitrogen dioxide and cancer-causing formaldehyde can accumulate in well-insulated buildings and homes. And EPA was concerned about the increase of potentially carcinogenic diesel emissions as auto manufacturers were beginning to switch to diesels to meet mileage requirements.

Environmentalists complained that a campaign was under way to weaken the Act just as the state plans for achieving clean air were being implemented. The plans were to have been approved by July 1, 1979. But by late 1981 only five had been fully approved, 15 had been conditionally approved and 25 had been partially approved. South Dakota's was rejected.

EPA said the process had been slowed because states with severe automobile pollution balked at imposing transportation control programs required in the Act. But state air pollution control agencies blamed the delay partly on the approval process, which they said was laborious. EPA also failed to meet the Act's December 1980 deadline for reviewing the national air quality standards to ensure they reflected the latest scientific findings. And it was behind schedule in controlling toxic air pollutants, dangerous fine particles and short-term exposure to nitrogen dioxide.

National Air Standards

Whether Congress should change EPA's way of setting national air quality standards was shaping up as the key issue of the 1982 debate. In the existing Clean Air Act, Congress gave EPA the authority to set standards to protect public health "allowing an adequate margin of safety" for vulnerable segments of society. The standards were the heart of the Clean Air Act because the rest of the law was designed to force the states to meet those standards within certain deadlines. Thus environmentalists feared significant changes could mean radical alterations in the Act's basic thrust.

A controversial report released in November 1980 by the Business Roundtable suggested that the standards, instead of allowing an "adequate margin of safety," should be set at levels to protect the public against "serious and irreversible threats to life and health." The National Coal Association and the Chemical Manufacturers Association recommended similar changes, which if enacted would mean that citizens would not be protected against temporary air pollution episodes causing attacks of asthma, angina or minor discomfort.

The Business Roundtable report, which projected that by 1987 the law will have cost industry $400 billion, recommended applying cost-benefit analyses in developing the standards. Many business groups had argued that the benefits of environmental control should outweigh or balance the costs of pollution control equipment. Existing law required the health standards to be set without regard to costs. However, it directed the states to consider costs when imposing emission limits on individual plants.

Opponents of the cost-benefit approach charged that it was extemely difficult to put accurate price tags on intangible benefits. The NCAQ report said that "unchallengeable estimates [of costs and benefits] are virtually impossible."

Environmentalists argued that the cost-benefit argument was a smokescreen for cutting the heart out of the Act. "Anybody who tells you they want to mandate that benefits outweigh costs wants to gut the Act," said Roy N. Gamse, EPA's deputy assistant administrator for planning and evaluation.

Business groups also challenged the validity of the scientific data used by EPA to establish the standards. They said the agency's findings were not subject to independent peer review because EPA appointed the scientific advisory board that reviewed the data. Environmentalists, on the other hand, feared that any outside board would be loaded with industry scientists.

How PSD Works

Because nearly every city or county already had met

The Clean Air Act in a Nutshell

The primary goal of the 1970 Clean Air Act and the 1977 amendments to the Act was to control the seven most common air pollutants — carbon monoxide, hydrocarbons, lead, nitrogen dioxide, ozone, particulates and sulfur dioxide.

The Act directed the Environmental Protection Agency (EPA) to determine maximum concentrations of each of those pollutants that should be allowed nationwide. The Act further directed EPA to set two types of these *national ambient air quality standards (NAAQS)* — primary and — secondary — without considering the cost of compliance. *Primary standards* were to protect human health with an added margin of safety for vulnerable segments of the population such as the elderly and infants. *Secondary standards* were to maintain visibility and prevent damage to crops, buildings, water and materials. The Act set Dec. 31, 1982, as the deadline for the nation to meet the primary standards. Five-year extensions were available for regions with severe automobile-related pollution. No specific deadline was set for meeting the secondary standards.

EPA Responsibilities

Besides issuing national air quality standards for the seven basic pollutants, EPA was to set maximum emission limits for plants and factories, called *new source performance standards (NSPS)*. These were to be set on an industry-by-industry basis for states to use as guidelines in imposing more specific emission restrictions on individual factories. The state limits could be the same as or stronger than EPA's new source standards, but could not be weaker.

EPA's guidelines were to cover any new or expanding plant that potentially could emit 100 tons or more of pollution a year. For these guidelines EPA was to take into account the costs, energy requirements and environmental effects the guidelines would have on industry. By 1981 EPA had issued new source standards for 34 industries ranging from coal-fired power plants to grain elevators.

For existing factories, EPA was to issue *control technique guidelines (CTG)*, which told states what types of pollution control equipment could be economically retrofitted on existing plants. By 1981 EPA had issued 23 such guidelines, mostly dealing with hydrocarbons.

State Responsibilities

States were directed to take into account the federally set emission standards for new factories and vehicles in developing *state implementation plans (SIPs)*, outlining how they intended to clean up the air within their borders by the 1982 deadline.

EPA was to approve state plans by July 1, 1979; plans not approved were to be revised by the state or EPA. Under the Act, the country was divided into 247 regional air basins, called *air quality control regions (AQCRs)*. Regions were classified into two categories. Regions that violated standards for one or more of the seven pollutants were designated *non-attainment areas* for those pollutants. States had to limit new construction of pollution sources until the air in these "dirty" areas met federal standards.

Regions that met the standards for specific pollutants were called *attainment areas* for those pollutants. States could not allow the air in these areas to deteriorate beyond certain levels and were to enforce a complex set of *prevention of significant deterioration (PSD)* rules. A region could be a non-attainment area for one pollutant and a PSD area for others. States were to impose emission cleanup requirements for factories depending on whether they were located in non-attainment or PSD areas.

Existing factories in non-attainment areas were required by states to retrofit their plants with pollution control equipment representing *reasonably available control technology (RACT)*. Companies wanting to expand or build new plants in these dirty-air areas were required to install equipment that limited pollution to the least amount emitted by any similar factory anywhere in the country. These *lowest achievable emission rate (LAER)* requirements were to be set by the states without regard to cost.

New plants could not be built in dirty-air areas unless pollution from existing factories or plants was reduced enough to more than compensate for the pollution expected from the new plant. That way, air quality would improve in the non-attainment regions.

Thus a company wanting to build in a non-attainment area not only had to install the best possible pollution control equipment, but also had to purchase *emission offsets* from existing companies. Companies could obtain offsets by buying new pollution control equipment for an existing polluter or buying and closing down an old plant.

States in non-attainment areas could have until 1987 to meet the carbon monoxide and ozone standards if they required annual inspection and maintenance of catalytic converters on cars. Federal sewer and highway construction funds could be withheld from states that failed to initiate such programs.

In PSD areas, the Act mandated that new plants install the *best available control technology (BACT)*, defined by states on a factory-by-factory basis. Companies wanting to build a new plant also had to conduct one-year computer modeling and monitoring tests to show that the proposed plant would not degrade the air quality beyond the specific levels, or *increments*, outlined in the Act.

the national standards for at least one pollutant, the part of the Clean Air Act that continued to affect most of the country concerned the PSD (prevention of significant deterioration) restrictions. Essentially, this program was designed to prevent the air in attainment areas (areas that had met the standards for specific pollutants) from deteriorating beyond certain pre-set ceilings, or "increments" to keep it cleaner than the national standards.

The Act established three classes of PSD areas ranging from Class I, having the cleanest air, to Class III, where the air was allowed to become the dirtiest.

Class I areas included national memorial parks and wilderness areas exceeding 5,000 acres, and all national parks of more than 6,000 acres. Almost no increases in pollution were allowed in the 158 Class I areas.

Class II areas were all other regions with air cleaner than the national standards. They could be redesignated as *Class III* — where more pollution is allowed — but as of late 1981 no state had sought to do that.

The law set maximum increments for particulates and sulfur dioxide in Class II and III areas. EPA was to issue increments for other pollutants by 1979, but did not meet that deadline. When issuing construction permits in PSD areas, states were to assign a portion of the pollution increments to the new industries on a first-come first-served basis. Once the increments were used up, no new construction could be allowed unless the area was redesignated as Class III.

Besides installing the best pollution control equipment and showing its pollution would not violate the increments, companies wanting to build near PSD areas had to show that their emissions would not impair visibility in nearby Class I national parks or wilderness areas. But since most of the West's oil, coal and oil shale reserves were located right next to such Class I areas, a major conflict was anticipated between the clean air law and the nation's goals of energy independence.

Although industry spokesmen admitted that the PSD program had not yet prevented energy development, they feared that both the visibility-protection requirements and PSD regulations would hamper synthetic and conventional fuels development. However, the NCAQ report found that the PSD program would not hamper energy development in the Southwest through 1995, even with three times as much electrical generating capacity, four times as much strip mining, 10 new coal-gasification plants and a 1.5-million-barrel-a-day shale oil industry. Many industry leaders wanted to eliminate the PSD increments, except for Class I areas, and weaken the visibility requirements.

Critics of the PSD provisions said the system was designed to limit economic growth in the South and West to protect industries in the Northeast and Midwest. Thus it was possible the PSD debate would turn into a Snow Belt-Sun Belt confrontation.

Industry also criticized EPA's Class I visibility protection regulations as overly obtrusive. They said the rules went beyond protecting national parks from pollution drifting into them from upwind companies, and forced companies to clean up smoke plumes visible from the parks. Such regulations could cause havoc in Southwest desert areas where visibility is sometimes 200 miles or more, said Blaine Fielding, director of air quality programs for the American Paper Institute.

Environmentalists countered that protecting vistas in national parks was as much a national priority as developing energy. The National Commission on Air Quality, following its final report, concluded that only the Class I PSD program had been successful in maintaining air quality. Class II and Class III programs, according to the commission, were causing delays in permitting new industries and that red tape involved in the process held up industrial progress to some extent. Business representatives joined the commission in maintaining that the location of industries in the West would be adversely affected if the standard was retained.

Permission to Pollute

An entirely different set of regulations applied to companies building factories in urban areas that had not met the national standards for the pollutants those firms would emit. The complicated system allowed companies to buy, sell, trade and "bank" permission to pollute.

As provided in the Clean Air Act, here is how the system would work if a company wanted to build a plant emitting sulfur dioxide in a city that already had unhealthy

Mobile Source Contributions to Pollution Levels, 1977

Vehicle	Particulates	Carbon Monoxide	Hydrocarbons	Nitrogen Oxides
Automobiles	3.85%	50.73(68) [a]	23.65(69) [a]	16.03(55) [a]
Light trucks	0.74	10.75(14) [a]	5.64(16) [a]	3.85(13) [a]
Heavy trucks	1.62	13.93(18) [a]	4.97(15) [a]	9.07(32) [a]
Motorcycles	0	0.64	0.74	0
Off-Highway	0.79	5.88	1.99	5.57
Rail	0.47	0.26	0.64	3.06
Air	0.54	0.73	0.78	0.48
Vessels	0.24	1.48	1.59	0.63
Total	8.38	83.52	39.86	38.7

[a] Figures in parentheses are relative percentages of total automobiles, light trucks, and heavy trucks.

Source: Environmental Protection Agency.

Tall stacks help add to the long-range transport of pollutants; the taller the stack, the higher the gases rise into the atmosphere and the farther they may be carried. The highest group of stacks includes at least a half-dozen electric utility stacks that are taller than 1,000 feet, the tallest nearly a quarter-mile high.

Number of Tall Stacks Constructed, 1970-79

Stack Height	*Electric Utilities*	*Smelters*	*Pulp and Paper*	*Steel*	*Oil, Gas, Chemical*	*Total*
≧800	34	2	—	—	—	36
700-799	37	1	—	—	—	38
600-699	45	1	1	—	—	47
500-599	55	0	—	—	3	57
400-499	55	0	2	—	4	61
300-399	34	1	12	2	11	60
200-299	23	3	34	4	65	129
Total	283	8	49	6	83	429

Source: Council on Environmental Quality

amounts of that pollutant. Besides installing equipment that emits the least possible amounts of sulfur dioxide, the company must obtain a reduction in sulfur dioxide emissions from other plants in that city.

These reductions must *more than offset* the amount of sulfur dioxide the new company will emit. That way, total sulfur dioxide levels will decrease, despite the addition of the new factory. Offsets are obtained by buying new pollution control equipment for an existing polluter, or by buying and closing down an existing plant that is too expensive to clean up. Or, an existing firm that has earned "pollution reduction credits" by installing cleanup equipment can sell its credits to the firm wanting to build or modernize.

Congress devised the "offset" system so economic growth could continue as the air was being cleaned up. By creating market incentives, Congress hoped companies would devise new ways to reduce pollution. But industry complained that in practice the system did not work because offsets often were unavailable.

As of late 1981 only 26 offsets had been purchased by new companies from existing firms. One reason they were so scarce was that the clean air law required existing polluters in non-attainment areas to retrofit their plants with "reasonably available" pollution control equipment by July 1, 1979. Since mandatory reductions did not qualify as offset, the law eliminated most potential offsets new industries could have obtained.

Another reason offsets were hard to find was that existing factories were allowed to reduce their pollution and "bank" their credits for use in later expansion. But a bigger criticism was that the offset system put new companies at the mercy of existing firms. The system, in effect, gave "squatters' rights" to the very companies that had polluted the region and created the need for offsets, say critics.

Because they controlled the price and availability of offsets, existing industries could keep competitors from moving into an area and literally control the future economic growth of their region, opponents charged. Industry wanted to eliminate offsets and extend the 1982 deadline for achieving national standards if emissions in a non-attainment area showed improvement over the long term.

Some industry groups also wanted to eliminate EPA's authority to impose construction bans in non-attainment areas that lacked approved state plans showing they can meet the 1982 attainment deadline. Industry complained that bans often applied to factories when automobile pollution was the real culprit.

Industrial Implications

Industrial facilities and combustion accounted for nearly all sulfur dioxide emissions, more than 80 percent of particulate emissions and more than half of nitrogen oxide emissions. Because of the pressure on them to reduce those emissions, on top of their other problems, it was possible that heavy industries would try to junk the State Implementation Plans (SIP) prepared so carefully since 1970.

Many of EPA's decisions on standards have been controversial either because industries considered them too onerous, or because environmentalists thought them too lax, or both. For example, when the agency relaxed the ozone standard in January 1979, questions were raised as to whether it had violated its mandate not to take the costs of compliance into account when setting standards. The diesel emission standards the agency set for cars and trucks in February 1980 impressed some environmentalists as a concession to the U.S. auto industry. But other environmentalists — concerned about U.S. dependence on oil from the volatile Middle East — thought that the standards were too tight and would hamper the development of highly fuel efficient diesel cars.

To control air quality, the Act gave the EPA and the states the power to review all proposed industrial construction and modernization to make sure major new facilities had the best possible pollution control equipment and would not cause air quality to deteriorate.

National Commission Urged Dropping . . .

The report of the National Commission on Air Quality, released March 2, 1981, contained 433 findings and 109 recommendations on how Congress should amend the Clean Air Act. The most controversial was a recommendation that Congress scrap the nationwide deadlines for cleaning up dirty-air cities. A proposed change in pollution control for clean-air cities was almost as controversial.

Those two revisions would represent a "serious weakening of the Clean Air Act," charged David Hawkins, an attorney for the National Clean Air Coalition, an environmental group that had vowed to "fight hard" to protect the law. He charged that the commission "chose to cut the heart out of . . . the act rather than complete the more difficult process of fine-tuning it."

The business community was expected to object just as strenuously to other recommendations, including those to continue setting national standards without considering cost, to control acid rain by reducing sulfur dioxide and to speed up the control of cancer-causing air pollutants and fine particles.

Sen. Gary Hart, D-Colo., who as NCAQ chairman had tried to get unanimous approval so that the report would carry more weight with Congress, said the recommendations reflected a "general consensus" on most issues. Some environmentalist members dissented from the report.

At a luncheon speech two days after he released it, Hart told a group of environmentalists he thought the dissenters had refused to sign it to maintain a bargaining position. He said those tactics would increase the polarization of industry and environmentalists, and could result in all of the act being opened up for attack.

But the dissenting members charged that in many cases the panel went "beyond compromise," overreacted to complexities in the act and chose to eliminate basic elements rather than improve them.

Dissenters objected to recommendations to:

- Eliminate the national deadlines.
- Change pollution regulations in clean-air areas.
- Eliminate requirements that new plants in dirty-air areas install the tightest possible emission controls.
- Mandate automatic approval of state air pollution control plans not reviewed by the Environmental Protection Agency (EPA) within 90 days of submittal.

Commission Findings

Major commission findings were that:

- The nation's air was "measurably better" and was continuing to improve. In six or seven years, probably only eight metropolitan areas would fail to meet the national standards.
- Improved air quality had brought benefits worth from $4.6 billion to $51.2 billion per year, while costs of installing, maintaining and operating pollution equipment were estimated to have been $16.6 billion in 1978.
- Air pollution controls had added about 0.2 percent to the annual inflation rate.
- Costs for air pollution control were likely to rise. One estimate was that about $37 billion (in 1978 dollars) would be spent in 1987 for construction, operation and maintenance of pollution controls.
- The Act has not been an important obstacle to energy development and "substantial increases in domestic energy production" could occur without changes being made.
- The law has not significantly inhibited economic growth.

"There is virtually no evidence ... that the Clean Air Act has actually prevented construction of new industrial facilities," said Hart. However, the commission did find that air pollution control requirements had contributed to — but not been the sole cause of — some plant closures.

That construction-permitting process came under fiery industry criticism for being overly slow and duplicative. Before building a new plant in a clean-air area, a company must obtain a permit from the state air pollution board requiring the best possible pollution control equipment for every emission source at that plant. In the case of a large petroleum refinery, the permit could regulate more than 150,000 minor emission sources, such as pumps, compressors and valves.

In certain dirtier areas, industry found the requirements even tougher to satisfy. Owners of new factories had to promise to install the best control equipment and clean up emissions at existing plants. In addition, all companies were required to gather data on existing air quality where they want to build and then use computer models to predict how the air would change as a result of the new facility. The company also had to monitor emissions after the plant was built to show they did not exceed projections.

The permit must be approved by several entities, including the county, regional and state air pollution boards, the regional EPA office and the Washington office of EPA. A study commissioned by the Business Roundtable found that the permitting process took three years or more and cost $250 million to $300 million per plant. Critics said the

... Deadlines for Cleaning Up Dirty Air

Recommendations

Hart said the commission proposed to retain provisions of the Act that work, streamline or eliminate those not working and expand the Act to meet new problems.

Standards. The commission recommended continuing the existing method of establishing national air quality standards to protect the health of vulnerable populations, with a margin of safety.

Rejecting suggestions of some industry groups that standards be based on cost-benefit analyses, the commission recommended that EPA analyze the costs and benefits of a proposed standard, but that the study should not be used to set the standard.

The commission also urged EPA to determine whether fine particles should be controlled, whether there should be a standard for long-term exposure to ozone and whether there should be a separate carbon monoxide standard for high altitude areas.

Deadlines. The panel recommended eliminating the 1982 and 1987 deadlines for states to comply with the national standards. Instead all new factories, no matter where located, would have to install the best possible pollution control equipment. Every three years EPA would review each state's progress in meeting the standards. States would set their own dates for compliance, but these would not be federally enforceable.

PSD. Although the commission found that the program to prevent the significant deterioration (PSD) of the air in regions that are cleaner than the national standards had not affected energy development, the report added the program had imposed more regulatory complexity on industry than could be justified by the benefits.

Thus the panel recommended that Congress:

- Retain requirements that all new plants install the best available pollution control technology.
- Eliminate the system that allows pollution to increase only up to certain preset "increments," except in national parks and wilderness areas where both air quality and visibility would be protected.
- Retain slightly less restrictive controls on 168 million acres of wildlife refuges, national monuments, national recreation areas, national seashores, wild and scenic rivers, and new national parks and wilderness areas.

Non-attainment Areas. For areas that had not attained the national standards, the commission recommended:

- Eliminating requirements that new industries achieve the lowest possible emission rate. Instead they would have to install slightly less stringent pollution control equipment (called "best available control technology"), the same equipment required on similar plants in clean-air regions.
- Requiring inspection and maintenance of automobile pollution control devices only in large cities where the peak 1981 ozone or carbon monoxide levels were 50 percent higher than the national standards.
- Allowing new industries to pay a fee rather than obtain emission "offsets" from existing polluters, if the state used the fees to reduce emissions at existing plants.

Mobile Sources. The commission recommended that Congress attempt to relax the current carbon monoxide emission standard from 3.4 grams per mile to 7 grams per mile. Hart said devices that achieve the 3.4 standard are unreliable and, if they fail, pollute more than devices that emit 7 grams.

Acid Rain. The commission recommended an immediate moratorium on state efforts to relax controls on the burning of high-sulfur coal in the Eastern United States, while requiring a "significant reduction" of sulfur dioxide emissions over the next 10 years.

Indoor Air. The panel recommended that Congress establish an interagency task force to study the health risks posed by indoor air pollution.

---

process had to be streamlined or it would impede industrial growth. The process could also impede industrial modernization and stymie the development of synthetic fuels in the West.

A new rule, proposed March 9, 1981, would allow polluters such as steel or oil companies to treat new furnace or refinery "smokestacks" as part of their existing allowable "bubble" (the overall amount of pollutants they can release.) Formerly, under the Carter administration, only old or existing exhaust stacks were included under the bubble. New stacks had to be fitted with the best air-cleaning equipment in use elsewhere. The EPA proposal was made by Vice President George Bush who was appointed in January 1981 as head of President Reagan's Task Force on Regulatory Relief

Environmentalists argued that the new policy would slow progress in cleaning up the air, and at best serve to maintain existing pollution standards. The control process was further complicated because regions are classified as attainment or non-attainment depending on whether they meet the national standards for a specific pollutant. Thus a city can be in an attainment area for one pollutant, but not for others.

As a result, in the same city a company could be

subject to one set of requirements if it emitted pollutants for which the area was violating the standards, and another set of regulations if it emitted pollutants for which the area was not in violation.

Many industries recommended that instead of the plant-by-plant, valve-by-valve review, EPA's industry-wide specifications should be imposed nationwide, regardless of where the plant was located.

Automobile Emissions

The major auto manufacturers had not issued position papers as of fall 1981 on what amendments they would like to see, but they were expected to seek relaxation of the standards and extension of the deadlines for cleaning up auto exhausts.

Autos were to have met the national standards by the 1981-model year. But EPA waived the carbon monoxide standard for 30 percent of the 1981 and 1982 model cars; and about 5 percent of the fleet — primarily diesel-powered cars — were exempted from the 1981 deadline for meeting the oxides of nitrogen standards. The agency rejected most such requests and the waivers it granted covered only about 28 percent of the vehicles scheduled for sale in 1981.

Although some environmentalists urged EPA to push states much harder to promote mass transit and adopt regional land-use planning as a means of reducing auto use, the Reagan administration was expected to be even less receptive to such ideas than was the Carter administration. Market force was likely to be the major factor in reducing auto emissions for some years to come. To the extent Americans continued to buy smaller, more fuel-efficient cars, emissions would be cut roughly in proportion to the drop in gasoline consumption. Some of the automobile engine technologies under development promised to deliver lower emission rates.

Emissions From Energy Sources*, 1978

Source	Total Suspended Particulates	Sulfur Dioxide	Nitrogen Oxides	Carbon Monoxide	Volatile Organic Compounds
Electric Utilities					
Coal	2,585	17,490	5,632	—	—
Fuel oil	154	1,892	1,353	—	—
Natural gas	11	0	946	—	—
Total	2,750	19,382	7,931	—	—
Industrial					
Coal	770	2,079	671	—	—
Fuel oil	99	1,265	363	—	—
Natural gas	44	0	3,949	—	—
Other fuels	308	165	429	—	—
Total	1,221	3,509	5,412	—	—
Commercial					
Coal	22	44	11	—	—
Fuel oil	66	990	297	—	—
Natural gas	11	0	154	—	—
Total	99	1,034	462	—	—
Residential					
Coal	22	66	0	—	—
Fuel oil	22	286	154	—	—
Natural gas	33	0	231	—	—
Total	77	352	385	—	—
Subtotal Stationary Sources	4,180	24,310	14,190	1,320	330
Transportation					
Highway vehicles	990	440	7,370	84,810	10,230
Other	440	440	2,970	9,240	1,540
Total	1,430	880	10,340	94,050	11,770
Total All Sectors	5,600	25,190	24,530	95,370	12,100

**Total may differ slightly from the sum of the source category totals because of independent rounding of data.*

Source: National Commission on Air Quality

According to the National Commission on Air Quality, reductions in particulate emissions in the industrial sector are a result of the installation of additional control equipment and the 20 percent reduction in coal use over the past 10 years. During that time, particulate emissions from industrial combustion sources declined by more than 50 percent.

Energy and Environmental Concerns

Although the United States has abundant supplies of coal, producing and using that coal could increasingly conflict with protection of the environment.

Coal and utility groups would be happy to see standards relaxed. In the Ohio Valley and especially in Ohio itself, where 21 aged coal-fired plants added up to the most concentrated source of sulfur pollutants in the country, utilities had fought hard for exemptions from clean air regulations. In many cases, they brought coal-fired plants into compliance with ambient air standards — which are enforced on the basis of local ground readings — by building tall stacks. The effect was to blow sulfur pollutants, a principal source of acid rain, over the eastern parts of the United States and Canada. Local producers of coal feared that strict clean air rules would give an unfair advantage to Western state producers of low-sulfur coal.

In the West — where coal-burning plants increasingly export electricity to California and the Midwest and where massive development of synthetic fuels based on coal and oil shale could threaten air quality in countless new ways — many energy corporations were planning projects that could be jeopardized by the especially strict clean air restrictions affecting national parks. Conflicts over clean air requirements already had arisen in connection with Montana's coalstrip power plants, which send electricity to the East, and several facilities in the Southwest, which send electricity to the West. One of the more ambitious synfuel projects, a brainchild of Exxon Corp., would involve the construction of 150 processing plants in the northwestern corner of Colorado. According to Exxon Chairman C. C. Garwin, the area would have to be declared a "national emergency zone" in which "normal rules do not apply."

One of the most important standards developed by EPA affected coal-fired power plants. Revised in May 1979 as mandated in the 1977 Clean Air Amendments, the revised standards required 70-90 percent of the sulfur to be removed from coal stack emissions, depending on the coal's sulfur content — a compromise between high-sulfur and low-sulfur coal states. Another important performance standard, the one for coal-fired industrial boilers, was scheduled for promulgation in 1981 or 1982.

Utilities complained about May 1979 EPA rules that limited emissions from power plants built after 1978. The utilities and the coal industry were gearing up to work for revisions easing these "new source performance standards" and other emission controls that, they said, hindered increased coal use. In addition, they were preparing to head off moves to tighten controls on pollution from existing plants and to reduce acid rainfall, which critics charged was caused principally by coal emissions.

The Clean Air Act controlled three emissions from coal-burning plants — sulfur dioxide, nitrogen oxides and particulates (or soot). Another emission, carbon dioxide, was not controlled, but was considered to have a detrimental effect on the environment.

The standard that evoked the greatest controversy concerned sulfur dioxide, a gas that causes respiratory difficulties and can mix with other air pollutants to cause coughs, colds, bronchitis, asthma and emphysema. The gas can be controlled by washing the coal before burning it or by using smokestack "scrubbers," devices that remove the sulfur before the gases are emitted from the stack.

A scrubber for a 500-megawatt power plant could cost $50 million, according to the Edison Electric Institute. But environmentalists argued that the price of uncontrolled sulfur emissions also was high. A University of Washington environmental economist found that an uncontrolled 500-megawatt coal-fired plant can cause environmental damage of from $7 million to $50 million a year. The figure included damage to lakes, buildings and vegetation, decreased visibility caused by acid rain and increased mortality allegedly caused by acid sulfates.

The new scrubber standards applied only to future power plants. Older plants still were controlled by individual state air pollution control plans, developed to enforce the Clean Air Act. Many of these — particularly in the Midwest — allowed utilities to build tall smokestacks to get around the local pollution limits. By discharging their pollutants high into the air, the companies could burn dirtier coal — without having to install pollution control devices — and still meet local health standards.

Existing plants spewed an average of up to 6.5 times as much pollution into the air as that allowed new plants.

Industry Incentives

The Environmental Protection Agency has instituted two methods of getting private industry to comply with emission standards. The first is called the "bubble concept." Instead of determining emission standards for every process within a factory, the agency would put an imaginary "bubble" over the plant and set allowable standards for the entire operation. This gives factory management a greater incentive to make changes in the basic plant operations rather than just adding pollution control devices.

The second approach is to grant "offsets" in areas where pollution standards are not being met. If a new factory wants to move into an overpolluted area, it must induce existing factories to reduce their pollution levels by more than the amount that the new factory will produce. Another variation allows a company having more than one factory in the same area to offset higher-than-standard emissions at one factory by lower-than-standard emissions at another.

To facilitate trading between two companies, the EPA encouraged the development of "banks" to buy, sell and broker pollution "credits." A company would be able to sell a credit for a certified pollution reduction to the bank, which in turn could sell that credit to a company that found pollution control economically unfeasible. The objective was to bring about an overall decrease in air pollution by making the buyers "pay" for more emission reductions than they can use. By 1981 three pilot pollution banks had been set up: Louisville, Kentucky; San Francisco, California; and Houston, Texas.

EPA estimated that by the year 2000 as much as 70 percent of the sulfur dioxide emitted would be coming from power plants built before 1970.

A potential problem was that many utilities might delay retiring their older plants because of the high cost of new scrubber-equipped plants. "A number of utilities may now be planning to artificially extend the life of their existing generating plants from a normal expected life of approximately 35 years to perhaps 50 or even 60 years," Robert Rauch, staff attorney for the Environmental Defense Fund, told the House Commerce Committee's Oversight Subcommittee in February 1980.

"If this occurs on a widespread scale, it will eliminate any chance of reducing present sulfur dioxide levels in the rest of this century," Rauch warned. "In short, controls on new power plants simply are not enough. The key is emissions from existing facilities."

He urged EPA to establish a sulfate standard, require early retirement of older plants or use several other tools available under the Clean Air Act.

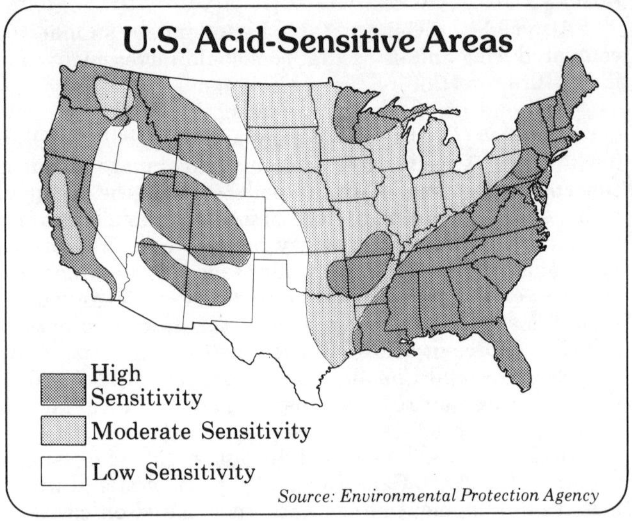

The main contributor to the natural acidity of rain is carbon dioxide. Carbon dioxide generates carbonic acid in the presence of water.

UNCLEAN AIR: ITS EFFECT ON HEALTH

There is a great deal of uncertainty about the effects of bad air on health. Most studies indicate that even though severe pollution episodes are unnerving, there is no convincing evidence that they cause disease. Victims of air pollution generally suffer from respiratory conditions such as asthma, chronic bronchitis and emphysema. Pollution, although it may not be the direct cause of a disease, can promote the frequency with which people, especially children, contract these short-term respiratory ailments. People who live in polluted areas suffer more often from chest infections than those who live in clean air areas.

Because labored breathing strains the heart, air pollution can contribute to death by coronary disease. Carbon monoxide can also promote cardiac deaths. When inhaled from cigarette smoke or heavy traffic it reduces the blood's capacity to provide oxygen to body tissues.

Seven substances found in polluted air are listed as hazardous under the Clean Air Act — asbestos, mercury, beryllium, vinyl chloride, benzene, radionuclides and arsenic. Others under consideration as being harmful to health are polycylic organic matter, cadmium, ethylene dichloride, perchloroethylene, acrylonitrie, methylene chloride, methyl chloroform, toluene and trichloroethylene. In this country, the five most common primary air pollutants in tons emitted annually are carbon monoxide, sulfur oxides, hydrocarbons, nitrogen oxides and particles. Their major sources are automobiles, industry, electric power plants, space heating and refuse disposal.

Sulfur oxides and particulate matter from industry account for more than half the health problems caused by air pollution, according to Erik Eckholm in *The Picture of Health,* even though they comprise only a fourth of all emissions. Automobiles generate only one-tenth to one-fourth of the health hazards, yet they create half of all the air pollution.

Nitrogen Oxides and Particulates

Direct exposure to nitrogen oxides is believed to increase the risks of acute respiratory disease and susceptibility to chronic respiratory infection. Nitrogen oxides can mix with other pollutants to form urban smog, which reduces visibility and can aggravate respiratory diseases such as bronchitis and pneumonia. Coughing, eye irritation, headaches and sore throats are common complaints during smog episodes.

EPA research indicated that nitrogen oxides could become one of the most troublesome air pollutants of the 1980s. In 1980 more than 20 million metric tons of nitrogen oxides were polluting the air annually. Half of that amount came from cars and trucks and half from coal- and oil-burning plants.

But by 1985 vehicles were expected to contribute only 30 percent of the total, with industry and utilities contributing 70 percent. If current trends continued, nitrogen oxide emissions could increase by 50 percent over the next 20 years, while sulfur dioxide emissions were expected to stabilize. The reason is that emission control technologies developed so far have provided only a 50 percent reduction in nitrogen oxide emissions, while sulfur dioxide controls can achieve 90 percent reductions.

One way of controlling nitrogen oxides is by fine-tuning the combustion process to make it more efficient, much like tuning a car. EPA and the coal industry were researching new methods of controlling nitrogen oxides.

Particulates are solid particles such as dust, soot or smoke that irritate the lungs. The smaller the particle, the more likely it is to lodge in the inner-most parts of the lung. Scientists are concerned that the smaller particles can carry traces of toxic metals released when coal is burned. Particulates can contain traces of up to 27 toxic metals — such as arsenic, cadmium, mercury and uranium. But it is not known whether these are emitted in large enough quantities to harm the lungs or the environment. They also contain small amounts of radioactivity.

Because of their light-scattering properties, these fine particles — those smaller than one, 1000th of an inch in diameter — also contribute to reduced visibility. About 99.5 percent of the larger particulates can be controlled, compared with only about 80 percent for fine particles.

Acid Rain and Dust

A British study published in 1911 connected acidic precipitation with coal combustion in the industrial city of Leeds. The discovery attracted little attention at the time, however, and it was not until well after World War II that scientists began a systematic study of the chemistry and effect of acid rain. By the early 1960s, a confluence of seemingly unrelated research in agriculture, atmospheric science and limnology — the study of lakes — established acid precipitation as a serious environmental problem.

While much still is unknown about the causes of acid rain, there is little argument that the major contributors are sulfates and nitrates. When these pollutants combine with moisture in the atmosphere, the droplets eventually form rain, snow or sleet high in acidity, sometimes as acidic as lemon juice or vinegar.

When the acid enters lakes, either in rainfall or as runoff through lakeside soils, entire ecosystems can be affected. The acid can cause fish egg cases to dissolve and can destroy lake food chains. Aquatic plant life slowly comes to a halt. Toxic metals, such as mercury, extracted from the lakeside soil by the acid runoff, can contaminate fish. Aluminum, broken down in the soil by the acid runoff, can destroy the gills of fish. Eventually, the lakes become deceptively crystal clear — totally devoid of life.

Although most media attention has concentrated on acid rain damage to fish and vegetation, scientists are becoming increasingly concerned about the direct health effects on humans of dry acid fallout. Not all sulfates and nitrates mix with rain, sleet or snow. Some, after traveling long distances, float back to Earth as "acid dust."

Acid sulfate particles can lodge in the lungs and contribute to chronic bronchitis, emphysema and asthma. Scientists fear the particles mix with other pollutants.

Dr. Leonard Hamilton, director of biomedical and environmental research at Brookhaven National Laboratory, said sulfates have a "corrosive" effect on lungs, bringing on or exacerbating respiratory illnesses. In another study, Drs. Robert Mendelsohn of the University of Washington and Guy Orcutt of Yale University found after analyzing more than two million death certificates that sulfates may account for up to 187,686 deaths a year in the United States. Even by conservative estimates, the authors said, sulfates account for more than 150,000 deaths annually.

The statistical evidence that links sulfates with mor-

According to the National Commission on Air Quality, government, under the Clean Air Act, must control potentially harmful pollutants in the air despite scientific uncertainty about the precise harm they cause and the levels of exposure that cause that harm. On this principle, the Act requires EPA to set quality standards to protect against pollution levels that "endanger public health, allowing an adequate margin of safety." This list shows major air pollutants and their impact on health.

Major Air Pollutants and Their Health Effects

Pollutant	Major Sources	Characteristics and Effects
Carbon Monoxide (CO)	Vehicle exhausts	Colorless, odorless poisonous gas. Replaces oxygen in red blood cells, causing dizziness, unconsciousness or death.
Hydrocarbons (HC)	Incomplete combustion of gasoline; evaporation of petroleum fuels, solvents and paints	Although some are poisonous, most are not. Reacts with NO_2 to form ozone, or smog.
Lead (Pb)	Anti-knock agents in gasoline	Accumulates in the bone and soft tissues. Affects blood-forming organs, kidneys and nervous system. Suspected of causing learning disabilities in young children.
Nitrogen Dioxide (NO_2)	Industrial processes, vehicle exhausts	Causes structural and chemical changes in the lungs. Lowers resistance to respiratory infections. Reacts in sunlight with hydrocarbons to produce smog. Contributes to acid rain.
Ozone (O_3)	Formed when HC and NO_2 react	Principal constituent of smog. Irritates mucous membranes, causing coughing, choking, impaired lung function. Aggravates chronic asthma and bronchitis.
Total Suspended Particulates (TSP)	Industrial plants, heating boilers, auto engines, dust	Larger visible types (soot, smoke or dust) can clog the lung sacs. Smaller invisible particles can pass into the bloodstream. Often carry carcinogens and toxic metals; impair visibility.
Sulfur Dioxide (SO_2)	Burning coal and oil, industrial processes	Corrosive, poisonous gas. Associated with coughs, colds, asthma and bronchitis. Contributes to acid rain.

Source: Environmental Protection Agency

tality is extremely controversial. After reviewing some of the criticisms, researchers at Congress' Office of Technology Assessment (OTA) concluded that there is evidence pollutants cause significant health damage.

"It is not entirely clear, however, that sulfates are the culprit, or the only culprit," said OTA's Alan Crane. He said that tiny particulates emitted from coal-burning plants, which are suspected of carrying the largest amounts of toxic metal residues, may be the biggest contributor to respiratory diseases.

Industry says not enough is known about acid rain to start regulating it. The National Coal Association cites an Energy Department study showing that oil-fired boilers produce three to 10 times as much acid-rain producing emissions as coal-fired units. The study estimated that cleaning up the 50 largest coal-fired power plants in the East would cost $10 billion to $15 billion.

According to the World Coal Study released in May 1980 it will be economic in the coming decades to burn much more coal both in the United States and worldwide while at the same time insisting on strict emission controls. The study said that while acid rain "is acute in some regions and may require early actions by nations in such regions," available technologies can effectively control long-distance airborne pollutants.

Representatives of utilities and coal interests argue, on the other hand, that expensive pollution controls should not be required until specific benefits are firmly demonstrated. Jack Kearney of the Edison Electric Institute has said that EPA should be required to show exactly how much effect each added piece of equipment would have on acid precipitation.

Legislative Outlook

Environmentalists hoped that Congress would put EPA on a "fast track" in controlling cancer-causing pollutants. Since 1970 EPA had issued regulations for only four, although dozens had been found to cause such diseases as leukemia and lung cancer. EPA was regulating asbestos, beryllium, mercury and vinyl chloride; it had proposed regulations for benzene, arsenic and radioactive pollutants.

As of late 1981 the agency was more than three years behind schedule in issuing regulations to control polycyclic aromatic hydrocarbons — created when coal and synthetic fuels are burned — and cadmium, which is emitted by nonferrous metal smelters. Other uncontrolled dangerous pollutants included coke oven emissions at steel plants, chlorinated solvents used in dry cleaning and acrylonitril released during plastics production.

Under proposed policies, when a substance is determined to be a clear carcinogen and that judgment holds up under review, with a population clearly at risk, then regulations would be issued based on best available technology. An assessment then would be made of how much it would cost to develop technology to clean up the substance altogether.

Environmentalists also wanted Congress to give EPA a one-year deadline to begin controlling fine particulates. Although larger particulates were controlled by EPA, the agency had not yet issued emission standards for fine particles. EPA had promised since 1973 to control these pollutants, but not until 1981 did it set up a 100-station monitoring network to study the problem.

OZONE CONTROVERSY: THE DEBATE CONTINUES

The ozone controversy burst into public debate in the mid-1970s with confusing and frightening suddenness. Americans were told that their use of aerosol spray cans and air conditioners, among other things, might be endangering the ozone layer that protects Earth from solar ultraviolet rays. If the ozone layer were depleted, it was said, the result would be more human skin cancer, damage to plant life and even global climatic changes. Cries to ban fluorocarbons — the allegedly guilty substances used primarily as propellants and refrigerants — were heard throughout the land.

Emissions of Major Pollutants, 1970-77 (millions of metric tons)

Year	Suspended Particles	Sulfur Oxides	Nitrogen Oxides	Hydro-carbons	Carbon Monoxide	Total
1970	22.2	29.8	19.6	29.5	102.2	203.3
1971	20.9	28.3	20.2	29.1	102.5	201.0
1972	19.6	29.6	21.6	29.6	103.8	204.2
1973	19.2	30.2	22.3	29.7	103.5	204.9
1974	17.0	28.4	21.7	28.6	99.7	195.4
1975	13.7	26.1	21.0	26.9	96.9	184.6
1976	13.2	27.2	22.8	28.7	102.9	193.8
1977	12.4	27.4	23.1	28.3	102.7	193.9

Source: Environmental Protection Agency.

Although it is impossible to say precisely what pollution levels would be if major control efforts had not been required during the 1970s, it is clear that for a number of pollutants the level of emissions would now be several times as great in many areas. This chart shows the decreasing rate of pollutant emissions from 1970 to 1977.

Indoor Pollution: Insulation Adds To Problem

Air-tight insulation can cause indoor pollution that is oftentimes as hazardous as pollution in the air outside. Most people spend 90 to 95 percent of each day inside so that their exposure to pollutants is mostly determined by the condition of air indoors. Increased insulation as a result of the 1978 National Energy Conservation Act requiring electric utilities to help customers insulate their homes has also succeeded in making many homes so airtight that indoor pollutants cannot escape.

Pollutants captured inside homes include carbon monoxide, carbon dioxide from gas stoves, human respiration, particulates from fireplaces and cigarettes, plywood, particle board and formaldehyde gas. The most deadly pollutant is radon, a gas produced by the decay of ranium and radium that is often found in rocks, soil, water and many building materials. Indoors, radon in close concentration attaches to dust particles and lodges in the lungs. Radon, according to the Environmental Protection Agency (EPA) is believed to be the second leading cause of lung cancer in this country.

Interestingly enough, the two specific air pollutants regulated in outdoor air, nitrogen dioxide and carbon monoxide are found in higher levels in inside rather than outside air. Gas cooking, for example, emits significant amounts of nitrogen dioxide and carbon monoxide into the air. One study indicates that levels of nitrogen dioxide during cooking were five times higher than the federal outdoor standard. The situation becomes more dramatic when studies show that 50 percent of American homes have gas stoves.

Studies have also shown that repeated indoor exposures to cigarette smoke impose air pollution burdens on nonsmokers that far exceed federal outdoor standards for total particulates.

When the National Energy Conservation Policy Act was passed in 1978, indoor pollution was not much of a concern. Research in the area is now being conducted at the Lawrence Berkeley Laboratory in California where the Energy Department spent more than a million dollars in 1980 to explore scientific aspects of the problem. The Consumer Product Safety Commission (CPSC), the Occupational Safety and Health Administration (OSHA) and the Housing and Urban Development Department (HUD) are all also studying the effects of indoor pollution. Most of these agencies disagree as to what degree increased energy conservation will increase the threat of indoor pollutants. EPA officials say that the conservation program could add an additional 10,000 to 20,000 deaths a year from exposure to radon. The Energy Department argues against that claim, saying that the benefits from the program in terms of lessened energy consumption must be weighed against any health risks. The Energy Department plans to go ahead with its conservation program until EPA can persuade it to do otherwise.

Examples of indoor pollution affecting office workers have also become known. Symptoms include dizziness, nausea, severe headaches and watery eyes. In offices, sealed windows and drop ceilings, synthetic furniture, copy machines and carpeting can all contribute to air pollutants.

Congress was urged to consider the indoor pollution problem when reauthorizing the Clean Air Act. Suggestions that the Act be amended to mandate EPA responsibility in the area were contained in an interagency research group report on indoor air quality, a National Academy of Sciences report on indoor air pollution and a report by the General Accounting Office. At least one congressional draft of the proposed 1981 legislation also contained that provision.

Before long, however, a catch appeared: it turned out that scientists disagreed as to the seriousness of the hazard. No one really knew how fast the ozone was being depleted, how long it would take before an imminent danger existed, or even if aerosol sprays and other consumer products were indeed the culprits. Findings and conclusions differed, and for every scientist who called for an immediate ban on fluorocarbons there was one who contended that more research was needed.

The focus of concern, the ozone layer, is a thin belt in the stratosphere about 10 to 20 miles about the Earth's surface. Ozone, a bluish gas that is a toxic pollutant on Earth, is a form of oxygen whose molecules consist of three atoms instead of two. It is highly unstable, ready to give up its extra atom at almost any time. There is about 100 times as much ozone in the upper atmosphere as there is on Earth, but at sea-level temperature and pressure the ozone layer would measure only about a tenth of an inch.

The fact that fluorocarbons might affect the ozone layer was not even suspected until 1974, when two University of California chemists began an academic investigation of what happens to fluorocarbons in the atmosphere. The two principal fluorocarbons, known as F-11 and F-12, are used primarily as propellants.

Growth of Fluorocarbon Usage

The fluorocarbon industry got its start in 1928, when a General Motors research director and a Frigidaire chief engineer (Frigidaire then was a division of GM) decided that the refrigeration industry needed a new refrigerant. Refrigeration then was based on materials such as ammonia, carbon dioxide and hydrocarbons, all of which had drawbacks. Thomas Midgley Jr., a GM chemist who had discovered earlier that tetraethyl lead was an effective anti-knock gasoline additive, tried using various fluorine compounds as refrigerants. Fluorocarbons worked. They were nonflammable, had low toxicity and low reactivity.

By 1976 aerosol sales and marketing represented a $3 billion annual business in the United States, with personal products such as hair sprays, deodorants and shaving cream accounting for 50 percent of the sales. In 1973 nearly three billion aerosols were made and sold — about 14 for every U.S. citizen.

Still, the aerosol spray problem is considered minor compared with the refrigeration issue. Mechanical refrigeration systems using fluorocarbons as the coolant include household refrigerators, fresh meat and vegetable storage systems, home and automobile air conditioners, commercial and residential freezers, building air conditioners, and transportation cold-storage systems. "Given the heavy dependence of virtually every link of the food chain upon refrigeration, an immediate ban on their use would be a recipe for mass food spoilage, shortages, price increases, and wrenching economic dislocations," Tom Alexander wrote in *Fortune*. Even if a suitable substitute were found, there still would be some release of fluorocarbons into the atmosphere from systems that had not been converted or old systems which had been discarded.

As for aerosols, alternatives include compressed gases such as nitrogen, carbon dioxide or nitrous oxide; soluble liquefied gases such as vinyl chloride, propane and butane; and mechanical devices such as finger pumps, squeeze bottles and roll-ons. However, these have various drawbacks including corrosiveness (carbon dioxide), large drops (nitrogen), toxicity (vinyl chloride), insufficient solubility (nitrous oxide) and flammability (propane and butane). Mechanical devices, industry spokesmen argue, have proved less desirable than aerosols in free market competition. Nevertheless, by 1981 many manufacturers had converted to pump sprays or "environmentally safe" aerosols that did not contain fluorocarbons.

Ozone Depletion and Skin Cancer

The connection between ultraviolet radiation and some forms of skin cancer is well established. It is widely believed that a 1 percent decrease in the ozone layer will produce about a 2 percent rise in skin cancer cases. Skin cancer can be treated and is seldom fatal, although there are about 8,000 cases per year of the dreaded melanoma, a form of skin cancer that is often fatal. Melanoma is not known to be caused by ultraviolet radiation, even though there is strong suspicion of a link. Increased ultraviolet radiation also can cause severe sunburn, eye damage and possible changes in Vitamin D balance in some individuals. And there is evidence that it might have a detrimental effect on livestock and wildlife.

As for climatic effects, there has been speculation that a thinning of the ozone layer could mean temperature and wind changes in the stratosphere since ozone acts as a heat source by absorbing ultraviolet, as well as infrared and visible, radiation. Such shifts in the stratosphere might lead to changes in growing seasons, the location of deserts and rain belts and even the levels of the oceans. Robert E. Dickinson, leader of a climate research project at the National Center for Atmospheric Research in Boulder, Colo., said in congressional testimony that possible human-caused changes in the ozone layer could change global mean temperatures by a few tenths of a degree Centigrade; a 1°C change would be regarded as a major shift in climate.

So the fluorocarbon-ozone controversy, like many other issues in recent years involving technology and the environment, tends to become more complicated the more it is studied. The scientific experts disagree, the industry spokesmen press for more time, the policy makers are confused and the public is exasperated. It seemed likely that some restriction on fluorocarbons would be put into effect in the 1980s, but the nature and timing of such action could not be foreseen. Meanwhile, if the ozone-depletion theories proved correct, there inevitably would be some thinning of the earth's protective ozone layer — however serious or insignificant the result.

PROSPECTS FOR REGULATORY CHANGE

Cleaning the air presents ever-changing regulatory problems to which there will never be any permanent solutions. As consumption habits, lifestyles and industrial processes are modified, the sources of pollution change as well, and regulators struggle to keep up.

As energy prices skyrocketed in the 1970s, to take just one example, it became fashionable and economical for Americans living in New England, the northern Midwestern states, the Northwest and even the Southeast to heat their homes with wood. In 1980 more than one-fifth of the households in northern New England burned wood for winter heating and roughly one million wood-burning stoves were sold nationwide.

Although burning wood strikes many people as a happy and wholesome activity, wood combustion emits annoying particulates that aggravate respiratory ailments. Even more serious, wood combustion produces polycyclic organic materials (POMS), which are known carcinogens. Some communities already have passed ordinances that limit installation of fireplaces in new buildings.

If wood burning continues to grow in popularity, federal action on wood emissions eventually may be necessary. Other changes in customs may present similar problems. In the immediate future, however, the country's greatest air quality problems will continue to arise from auto use and from industrial sources of pollution.

The Reagan administration was likely to call for subjecting all environmental regulations to rigorous cost-benefit analysis. In this approach, which the business community generally favors, the government makes public policy decisions the same way a company or a consumer would make a decision about what to buy. But this would pit administration economists against environmentalists, physicians and others reluctant to weigh health hazards against costs.

The Council on Environmental Quality has estimated that total public and private expenditures on air pollution control came to $19.3 billion in 1978 — close to half of the nation's spending on pollution abatement. Of that, expenditures resulting from federal legislation were estimated at $16.6 billion. A study commissioned by CEQ estimated the benefits of air pollution control, including improved public health, reduced cleaning expenses, better vegetation, less damage to materials and higher property values, at $21.4 billion in 1978. But the study said that the true benefits in 1978 could have been as low as $4.6 billion or as high as $51.2 billion, and it concluded that "the estimation of certain kinds of environmental benefits is still in need of much additional refinement."

On the other hand, Sen. Hart said when issuing the National Commission on Air Quality's report in March 1981 that although the Clean Air Act had "imposed substantial additional costs on industry and consumers. . . . air pollution control has not been a major obstacle to economic growth or an important factor in the shape of the national economy." Hart went on to estimate that the total costs for air pollution control had amounted to only .2 percent of the annual inflation rate. "But the rate of inflation," said Hart, "does not include directly the health and other benefits 'bought' by the pollution control expenditures."

"The commission concluded," continued Hart, "that it is fruitless to try to compare meaningfully the costs and benefits of air pollution control. There are too many uncertainties in the calculation of both sides of the situation, especially the benefit side."

Industry groups had not accepted estimates of the benefits resulting from air quality control, and many figures were certain to be bandied about in the debate over clean air legislation. In the end, the future of such regulations could well depend on how strongly people felt about the air they breathe and on whether they were willing to make sacrifices to make it cleaner, rather than on elaborate cost-benefit analysis.

3

The Land: Seeping Poisons

We look back on the Middle Ages, and we say, "No wonder they had bubonic plague — they used to throw their garbage in the streets." Now I just hope that in the year 2025 my grandchildren don't look back on this generation and say, "No wonder they had problems — look at all the chemicals just carelessly introduced into the environment, uncontrolled."

Douglas Costle, former administrator
Environmental Protection Agency

The typical American wakes up in the morning to the sound of an alarm clock made from plastic developed in a chemical process. He brushes his teeth with toothpaste containing various chemicals, and washes with manufactured soap. For breakfast, he drinks milk poured from a plastic container, fries eggs in a chemically coated non-stick pan and then washes the pan with a man-made detergent. Many parts of his modern kitchen are pre-formed in a plastics factory and his floor is covered with glued-on fabricated sheets of vinyl. For lunch he wraps a sandwich in a disposable plastic bag and in the evening may listen to records made from yet another chemical process.

Americans, in their everyday lives, are inundated with products connected with more than 70,000 chemicals manufactured commercially in this country alone.

The federal Environmental Protection Agency estimated that as many as 1,000 new chemical compounds are added to that number each year.

Increasingly, Americans are questioning whether these compounds — either in their usable form or as wastes generated by the chemical processes — are a threat to human health. How to use the compounds and to dispose of the wastes safely has become an overwhelming problem that promises to persist throughout the 1980s.

The chemical industry was a principal participant in and beneficiary of the post-World War II economic and technological boom in the United States, which one governmental task force termed "a new chemical era." The industry rapidly developed a variety of new chemicals for use in fuels, synthetic fibers, plastics, building materials, fertilizers, pesticides, food additives, detergents, drugs and other products.

The entire chemical industry, including manufacturers of substances such as plastics, drugs and paints, sold about $113 billion worth of products in 1977, an 11 percent increase over the previous year. By comparison, the industry sold only $13.7 billion worth of chemicals in 1947.

This enormous growth in the industry has produced increasing concern, expressed most vigorously by environmentalists and health officials, that many chemical substances are finding their way into humans and creating serious health hazards.

Scientists and doctors are not certain what effects many of these chemicals have on human health. But the potential dangers have been seen in a number of areas, particularly cancer research. In addition, poisonous substances such as PCBs, dioxins, benzene and vinyl chlorides have been linked to arteriosclerosis, heart disease, hypertension, emphysema, bronchitis and kidney disease. To make matters worse, contaminants may remain dormant within the body for long periods, causing health problems as much as 15 to 40 years after initial exposure to a substance.

Wastes are generated not only by disposal of such common items as plastic cups, packaging, utensils and the like, but also from more hazardous materials generated from products basic to everyday needs: paints, pesticides, solvents and industrial cleaners. About 60 percent of these wastes are generated by the chemical industry. Leather tanners, electroplaters, paper mills and textile firms make up the rest, with smaller amounts coming from research labs, painters, electricians and gas stations.

Uncontrolled dumpsites, where chemicals have leached into nearby soil and drinking water sources, are proliferating across the country. Following increasing reports about environmental damage from these dumpsites and from chemical, petroleum and other spills, Congress in late 1980 passed legislation to cover the cost of cleaning up the damage. The legislation established a $1.6 billion "superfund" to help cover the cost of dumpsite cleanup. Victims of dumping do not receive compensation under the law, a controversial issue that Congress may debate later. The federal government's principal environmental arm, the Environmental Protection Agency (EPA), must decide how to implement the superfund and to prosecute violators of dumping regulations.

How the EPA will proceed during the 1980s was expected to be fundamentally influenced by President Reagan's commitment to reduce federal spending and regulation of private enterprises. On taking office in 1981, the Reagan administration began drastic budget reductions for most agencies including the EPA. Advocates of vigorous federal government involvement in environmental issues were much concerned that extensive reductions in EPA's budget would prevent that agency from having significant influence on waste site cleanup and control.

EPA already had launched new efforts to reduce the serious health hazards that were widely believed to result from contamination of the land. The agency established a new "cradle to grave" policy that required chemical manufacturers to keep careful inventory of wastes from point of creation to point of disposal. Although steps were taken to guard against future illegal dumping of chemical wastes, cleanup of sites already in existence was seen as a major task that would not be easily accomplished.

By the beginning of the 1980s, the problem of land pollution caused by negligent dumping of industrial by-products had gained the urgency once given in the 1970s to the cleanup of the nation's air and water.

TOXIC WASTES: A SLEEPING GIANT

In Woburn, Mass., a small working-class community north of Boston, residents in September 1980 feared a chemical disaster was in the making. Radioactive wastes, arsenic, chromium and other deadly chemicals had produced foul tasting water and concentrations of explosive swamp gas within the town's boundaries.

According to state health statistics, Woburn had the highest cancer rate of any town its size in the state. Residents blamed an 800-acre industrial tract on the eastern edge of town for the problem. The property was passed along for years by various chemical companies until 1971 when Consolidated Chemical Industries sold it to a local land developer.

The developer's bulldozers uncovered long-forgotten piles of animal carcasses, used by Consolidated Chemical to produce glue from animal hide and bone. A rotten-egg smell enveloped the area. Residents complained of eye-burning fumes and strange skin rashes. Property values slumped, and bottled water sales boomed. Cleanup costs were estimated at $2 million, but local officials didn't know where to get the funds. As of September 1981, EPA was still conducting tests to determine the extent of ground water contamination in the area.

Filling the Superdome

The contamination in Woburn, Mass., was but one of many incidents around the country where chemical dumpsites have caused serious health damage. The Woburn experience was likely to be repeated in many other areas.

American industry was expected to produce 126 billion pounds of toxic wastes in 1981, enough to fill the mammoth New Orleans Superdome from floor to ceiling once every day. Traditionally, only 10 percent of this waste has been disposed of safely, the EPA says. The rest has been dumped into unsafe municipal landfills, open pits and lagoons or left in vacant lots by disreputable "midnight dumpers."

In recent years, these residues of the chemical revolution have begun oozing from under the nation's carpet. In 1978 in Love Canal, an area near Niagara Falls, New York, more than 200 families were evacuated after 82 chemicals seeped from an underground abandoned dump into basements and yards. President Carter declared the area an environmental disaster after residents complained of illnesses, miscarriages and birth defects.

Children were born with extra ears, fingers and toes and one child was born with two sets of teeth. One resident, Jim Clark, told a Senate subcommittee, "It got so bad that when someone had a kid, no one asked, 'Is it a boy or a girl?' but rather, 'Is it normal?' "

Some have called the hazardous waste problem "the sleeping giant of the decade." These are some incidents that received the most publicity in 1980:

- Officials cleaning up oil and chemicals spilling from an abandoned coal mine into Pennsylvania's Susquehanna River could not go into the mine because the chemicals formed hydrogen cyanide gas, the material used in gas chambers. As of September 1981, 100,000 gallons of the chemicals originally dumped into the shafts had been collected and disposed of by state officials. An estimated 100,000 gallons of remaining waste was believed by the EPA to be trapped inside the mountain where the coal mine was located. State and local officials estimated that an excess of $3 million had been spent to locate and identify the situation. Monitoring of the site was still going on.
- In Bullitt County, Ky., a 17-acre "Valley of the Drums" still contained 100,000 barrels of highly toxic chemicals. All EPA could do was stop the chemicals inside the rotting, rusting drums from leaking into a nearby stream. The agency was continuing to check the area in September 1981 for ground water contamination.
- The Velsicol Chemical Corp. dumped 300,000 drums of pesticide production waste in unlined trenches on a 242-acre site near Toone, Tenn. The water table became contaminated and residents brought a $2.5 billion class action law suit. EPA, state and Velsicol officials formed a task force to review conditions at the dumpsite. In September 1980, the task force capped the site. One year later, samples of chemicals from the site were distributed among the three groups for investigation. Monitoring of the site for signs of further ground water contamination was expected to continue for three years.
- In Elizabeth City, N.J., a fire broke out in April 1980 at a dump that had been used by the Chemical Control Corp. for highly explosive wastes. A major incident was averted when winds blew toxic clouds away from populated areas. The cost of the cleanup was estimated at $10 million to $15 million.

Danger Estimates Vary

The sheer quantity of garbage Americans produce is astonishing. Americans produced about 130 million metric tons of waste from residential, commercial and institutional sources in 1976. That figure was estimated to reach 180 million metric tons by 1985 with the average person contributing, by the 1976 figures, four pounds of refuse a day, or 1,300 pounds a year.

U.S. Surgeon General Julius Richmond stressed the problem to Congress in September 1980 when he said, "We believe that toxic chemicals are adding to the disease burden of the United States in a significant although as yet not precisely defined way."

In spite of the statements of Richmond and others, nobody really knew as the 1980s began how serious the nation's land pollution problem had become, and estimates varied widely.

The House Commerce Subcommittee on Oversight and Investigations in 1979 found 3,383 dumpsites. Some were beneath tennis courts, a yacht club, church parking lots, a cemetery, a raceway, botanical gardens, nurseries and an old silo. About 80 were private residences or farms, pastureland or gardens.

"Until recently, land was perceived to be an awesome sponge, a resilient reservoir which would readily absorb any chemical concoction that man could brew," wrote Rep. Albert Gore Jr., D-Tenn., in an Oversight Subcommittee report in 1980.

A private contractor hired by EPA estimated in 1979 that there were 32,000 to 50,000 disposal sites scattered throughout the country, and that 1,000 to 2,000 of these could be extremely dangerous. EPA suspected that 500 to 800 of those had been either abandoned or owned by operators who could not afford to clean them up.

An EPA hazardous waste task force compiled a list in 1980 of 4,598 dumpsites that needed to be investigated, a list that was growing by about 200 each month. Of those, about 8 percent were abandoned.

Another estimate came from the Chemical Manufacturers Association (CMA), which charged in 1980 that EPA's figures were "significantly overdrawn." A CMA survey showed, however, that there were 4,196 potentially hazardous dumpsites, only 174 of which were abandoned.

CMA estimated it would cost $247 million to $333 million to clean up the mess, compared to EPA's $22 billion to $44 billion. But both agreed that the cost would have been dramatically reduced if proper disposal methods had been used from the beginning.

Ironically, the land pollution problem of the 1980s developed partly because of the success of the air and water pollution programs of the 1970s.

Huge amounts of toxic materials removed from waterways and scrubbed from industrial smokestacks were solidified and dumped on land. Rain washed chemicals from dumpsites into nearby rivers and dangerous fumes escaped from incinerators to contaminate the air.

Danger to Water Supplies

Probably the most dangerous consequence of the improper dumping is contamination of underground water supplies. Half the nation depends on ground water for drinking. Once an underground reservoir is contaminated, it can take centuries for the danger to disappear.

Problems arise when landfills leak or bulldozers disrupt long-forgotten wastesites. One EPA study found that 90 percent of the landfills in the eastern half of the United States were leaking toxic substances into ground water.

For quite some time, it has been common practice for waste producers to collect chemical residues in containers and bury or dump them in empty fields, abandoned mines or rivers. Illegal dumping at night adds to the problem and even legal disposal by companies on their own property affords no safety unless pollutants are fixed firmly in place. Rainwater running through waste or chemicals from rusting drums can spread leachate as far as a mile and it may last for years.

Costs of Disposing of Hazardous Wastes, 1980

	Cost*
Land spreading	2-25
Chemical fixation	5-500
Surface impoundment	14-180
Secure chemical landfill	50-400
Incineration	75-2000
Physical, chemical or biological treatment	Varies

**Dollars per metric ton*

Source: U.S. Environmental Protection Agency

Chemical landfills never lie dormant. Water, when it penetrates buried wastes, removes dissoluble components, producing a polluted liquid leachate that flows out from the dump. Leachate can continue for more than 100 years and pick up dangerous material to spread around a large area. EPA's Office of Solid Waste in 1979 estimated that an average landfill site, about 17 acres in size, produces 4.6 million gallons of leachate a year after 10 inches of rainfall.

There are other ways improperly dumped wastes can threaten humans:

- Aging drums can explode, sending toxic fumes into the air. At least two persons have died from toxic fumes or explosions at landfulls and chemical lagoons.
- Fumes from buried drums can seep through the ground, killing grazing animals or causing illness and birth defects.
- Chemicals can seep into rivers and lakes, killing fish and wildlife.
- Chemicals can enter the food chain when wastes find their way into animal feed or onto pastureland.

Impact on Health

Hazardous wastes are defined by the EPA as wastes that are toxic, corrosive, ignitable or chemically reactive. They can include any by-product that poses a substantial present or potential threat to plants, animals and humans because it is harmful and nondegradiable. They can produce injury upon contact with the body or accumulation within the body and can enter through the mouth, nose or skin. They produce harmful effects upon the body's organs by stimulating or suppressing normal metabolic functions.

A chemical may have the effect of stopping proper oxidation of a cell, thereby halting adequate flow of energy to vital organs. It may combine chemically with tissues and cause them to grow abnormally or attach itself tightly to an enzyme, a complex protein that speeds chemical reactions throughout the body. When this attachment occurs, there is a severe lessening of energy production from food and a reduced capacity to renew worn-out tissue. When enough cells in organs such as the heart, liver or brain are harmed, serious debilitation and possibly death can result. Approximately 25 percent of industrial metals are toxic in high enough dosages.

Widespread Organic Wastes

Among the most hazardous substances are those that are carcinogenic (cancer-causing), teratogenic (a term used to mean causing defects in fetuses while in the womb) or mutagenic (causes mutations in genes).

Organic wastes make up 60 percent of hazardous waste emissions. Among these are plasticizers (a chemical added to rubbers and resins to give them flexibility), solvents and many other by-products of manufacturing.

The most potent organic chemicals are pesticides and defoliants. They are composed of the same elements, hydrogen and carbon, as human tissues. Because of this similarity to natural substances, many of them are biologically active. Many of these pesticides were created because they can combine with the outer fat of an insect and go on to destroy its nervous system. These chemicals are similar to those found in human beings and could react within the human system in much the same manner.

A report published by the U.S. surgeon general in 1979 said the National Cancer Institute listed at least 20 chemicals for which there is carefully researched evidence of human cancer causation. Among these were asbestos, benzene, vinyl chloride and arsenic. In addition, the institute listed over 2,300 specific chemicals as suspected carcinogens, including some insecticides, herbicides, asphalt fumes and wood dust.

The report also said that some of these chemicals produce mutations in the genetic material of cells that cause them to reproduce unchecked. The mutations also may stimulate the growth of tumor cells themselves, or they may somehow suppress innate systems that destroy tumor cells. In addition to cancer, environmental agents can cause other degenerative diseases such as arteriosclerosis, heart disease, hypertension, emphysema, chronic bronchitis, kidney disease, liver disease, diabetes and anemia.

Public pressure for better and earlier testing of chemicals for danger to human health and the environment contributed to passage of the 1976 Toxic Substances Control Act (TSCA). But there has been criticism that the law is being implemented too slowly. As of July 1980, according to the Council on Environmental Quality, only five classes of chemicals — PCBs (polychlorinated biphenyls), chlorofluorocarbons, phthalate esters, chlorinated benzenes and chloromethanes — had been subject to any regulatory action at all.

PCB Dangers

Some substances such as certain forms of PCBs are toxic even in concentrations of one part per billion. Dioxins are known to cause a variety of diseases in concentrations of parts per trillion.

PCBs (polychlorinated biphenyls) are a group of highly dangerous industrial chemicals long known as some of the most toxic substances created. PCBs are a synthetic organic chemical — they do not exist in any form in nature. PCBs, which have been in use since 1929, are used as insulating fluids in electrical equipment such as transformers used by utility companies. They also are employed in the production of adhesives, sealants, printing inks, coating, waxes and many other products.

Concerns about pollution from PCBs have been increasing since 1968, when some 1,000 Japanese citizens suffered health problems after ingesting PCB-contaminated rice oil. Japan halted production of the chemicals.

PCBs are long lived, resisting decomposition for many years. In many cases around the country PCB waste has been dumped illegally into the ground, into rivers and into quarries beside roads.

Common Hazardous Wastes

Chemical	Use	Manufacturing hazard
C - 56	Bug and insect killer	Acutely toxic, suspected carcinogen
Trichloroethylene (TCE)	Degreaser	Suspected carcinogen
Benzidene	Dye industry	Known human carcinogen
Curene 442	Plastics industry	Suspected carcinogen
Polychlorinated biphenyls (PCBs)	Insulaters, paints and electrical circuitry	Acutely toxic, suspected carcinogen
Benzene	Solvent	Suspected carcinogen
Tris	Fire retardant	Suspected carcinogen
DDT	Bug and insect killer	Acutely toxic
Vinyl chloride	Plastics industry	Known human carcinogen
Mercury	Multiple uses	Acutely toxic
Lead	Multiple uses	Acutely toxic, suspected carcinogen
Carbon tetrachloride	Solvent	Acutely toxic, suspected carcinogen
Polybrominated biphenyls (PBBs)	Fire retardant	Effects unknown

Source: Council on Environmental Quality

Cancer Incidence by Site and Sex†

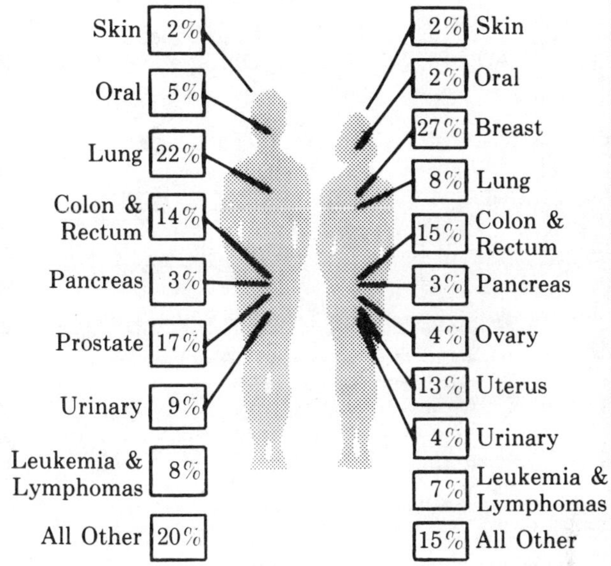

†Excluding non-melanoma skin cancer and carcinoma in situ.

Source: American Cancer Society

There is new evidence that PCBs, which have been shown to cause reproductive defects and death in fish, birds and mammals, are spreading up the food chain. Nearly one-third of 1,038 breast milk samples from nursing American women contained measurable amounts of PCBs, according to a survey conducted for EPA and released in 1978. Agency researchers theorized that most of the women were exposed to PCBs through their diet. PCBs have caused severe skin and eye irritations and have been linked to reproductive disorders, kidney damage and liver ailments in humans. Large doses have produced liver cancer in laboratory rats.

EPA estimated that 440 million pounds of PCBs were in landfills or dispersed throughout the environment in 1980. EPA regulations published under TSCA required that all PCB material be specially labeled and disposed of only at EPA-approved waste disposal sites — either chemical-waste landfills or high-temperature incinerators. Generally, solid materials — including power transformers, capacitors, contaminated soil, sludges and drain containers — must be disposed of at waste landfills. As of mid-1981, there were licensed incinerators for burning PCB waste in Deer Park, Texas, and El Dorado, Ark. Approved land disposal sites were located in Niagara Falls, N.Y., Model City, N.Y., Livingston, Ala., Williamsburg, Ohio, Casmalia, Calif., Beatty, Nev., Arlington, Ore., and Grand View, Idaho. Only two of those sites were approved for liquid waste disposal.

Other chemical substances such as dioxins created controversies throughout most of the 1970s. There were efforts to ban dioxins and rejoinders that not enough evidence existed about their potential effects on health. According to Dr. Irving Selikoff of the Mount Sinai School of Medicine, dioxins might interfere in the body's basic metabolic processes by stimulating abnormal enzyme production by the liver. Enzymes are essential to such body processes as producing hormones, converting food into energy and thinking.

Metabolic disorder is a relatively new concept whose effects may not be entirely understood. Accidental industrial exposure to dioxins have provided the only evidence to date on human health effects. Research on monkeys has shown that five parts of dioxin for every trillion of food could lead to cancer.

Carcinogens

Medical researchers still do not know what causes cell growth to continue unchecked and cause cancer. Such influences and substances as radiation, tobacco smoke, asbestos and vinyl chloride definitely have been proven to promote abnormal cell growth, but the exact reason why is still not clear. Cancer, unlike heart disease, the country's number one killer, is less dependent upon hereditary factors. Researchers believe that environmental factors, rather than genes, are likely to make one person more susceptible to cancer than another.

Carcinogens may take as long as 15 years to affect the body after exposure. For example, fatal cancer of the chest in men who handled asbestos in shipyards and elsewhere during World War II did not show up until 1960. Long time lags pose serious problems for scientists trying to link cancer to causes.

Some chemicals produce cancer directly by initiating the growth of malignant tumors. Even when such carcinogens do not trigger cancer, they may permanently alter cells, leaving them susceptible to other unhealthy elements. Tobacco smoke, for instance, can be both a direct carcinogen and also an agent for unleashing cancer-causing powers of other environmental influences. Noncarcinogenic poisons, on the other hand, usually stop damaging cells as soon as exposure is ended. If the poisoned person survives the exposure, healthy cells will replace the damaged cells.

Carcinogenic substances affect cells differently. Many scientists believe that they damage DNA and cause other cellular mutations that remain as cells replace themselves. The effect of contact with carcinogens can be cumulative, gradually increasing the chances that cancer will occur.

The dangers of drugs that may be carcinogenic are difficult to estimate because safe exposure levels are almost impossible to determine. A panel of U.S. cancer researchers in 1970 reported that no level of exposure to a chemical carcinogen should be considered insignificant. The panel went on to say that single carcinogens could not be evaluated out of context of total environmental exposure. Cumulative effects of a variety of carcinogenetic substances that a person may be exposed to at the same time must be taken into consideration. When the profits and jobs made available from the production of these chemicals are considered in decisions on whether to ban them or not, the task becomes even more complicated.

Agent Orange

Agent Orange was a chemical used by the U.S. Army in Vietnam to defoliate the dense jungles providing cover for enemy forces, and to destroy food crops. It was a combination of two herbicides — 2,4-D and 2,4,5-T that have been used domestically for about 30 years to control broad-leaf weeds.

Thousands of U.S. soldiers were exposed to Agent Orange in Vietnam, according to a General Accounting Office (GAO) study done at the request of Sen. Charles H. Percy, R-Ill. Many veterans later blamed exposure to Agent Orange for a variety of health disorders and sued the manufacturers of the substance for damages.

The veterans claimed the chemical caused cancer, liver damage, psychological and neurological symptoms such as depression, sleeplessness, tingling or loss of sensation in limbs, malfunctioning of the body's disease-fighting ("immune") system, miscarriages, stillbirths, and a broad range of birth defects in their children.

The component of Agent Orange that was suspected of causing diseases, TCDD, is a contaminant of 2,4,5-T — that is, a substance inadvertently created in varying amounts in the manufacturing process. TCDD is the "most toxic" of approximately 75 chemical compounds known as dioxins, according to Dr. Marion Moses of the Environmental Sciences Laboratory at Mount Sinai School of Medicine in New York.

"Very few toxic substances have been shown to affect such a wide range of [human] body systems, and nothing in the industrial environment approaches TCDD in how very little of it" can affect biological systems, he told a House Commerce Oversight and Investigations Subcommittee hearing in June 1979.

But the manufacturers insisted the herbicide was safe. Dow Chemical Co. said that in the 30-year history of producing it, there had been only one incident of illness among exposed workers — a 1963 outbreak of chloracne, a persistent and sometimes painful skin rash. That exposure resulted from an accident, not from normal manufacturing processes, and produced no "excess" illnesses or deaths, according to Dow attorney Don Freyer.

Dow and four other manufacturers that were fighting the veterans' class action lawsuit said the Veterans Administration (VA) should be responsible for any claims.

The only condition the VA recognized as Agent Orange-related was chloracne.

In May 1970 the Agriculture Department (USDA) moved to end the use of 2,4,5-T products on food crops and near homes, recreation sites and other areas. According to Steven D. Jellinek, who traced dioxin regulatory efforts for a House Commerce subcommittee in 1979, the USDA action was based on a National Institutes of Health study linking TCDD to stillbirths and malformations in laboratory animals. Jellinek subsequently directed the toxic substances program at the Environmental Protection Agency.

The Defense Department ended its Agent Orange spraying in Vietnam in 1970. Between 1965 and 1970 the department sprayed 10.7 million gallons of Agent Orange, at a rate of about three undiluted gallons per acre, concentrations much stronger than those used domestically.

Also in 1970, the Monsanto Co. ceased 2,4,5-T production, but "not at all" for health reasons, according to spokesman Dan R. Bishop. The subcontractor that fabricated the basic chemical was no longer able to supply it to Monsanto because of Defense Department priorities, and Monsanto's own plant at Nitro, W.Va., was "too old" to be put back into production, Bishop said at the time.

In 1972, the ban on 2,4,5-T products was successfully challenged by Dow in a court suit against the EPA, which had taken over most of the Agriculture Department's regulatory responsibilities for agricultural chemicals.

EPA resumed ban proceedings again the following year, but abandoned the process and turned to studies instead. While laboratory data showed that "even ... minute quantities of dioxin" could cause cancer, birth defects and other problems in animals, EPA needed a firm link — then lacking — between that animal evidence and human health risk.

A comprehensive 1974 National Academy of Sciences study of Agent Orange found no "definitive indication of direct damage by herbicides to human health," but suggested that was because there wasn't enough research on human exposure to show what the hazards might be. It urged further studies because stories of dioxin-related illness among Vietnamese were "so consistent that they could not be dismissed."

By 1977, Vietnam veterans were beginning to contact the VA about health problems they believed were caused by their exposure to the defoliant. The issue made headlines early in 1978 when a Chicago television station broadcast a program on the veterans' claims.

1979 Developments

In 1979 EPA suspended the use of 2,4,5-T on forests, rights of way and pastures on the basis of a study prompted by complaints from women in Alsea, Ore., that they suffered miscarriages shortly after the herbicide was sprayed near their homes.

Agent Orange victims formed an organization and launched a class action suit in New York against the five corporations that had supplied the federal government with the herbicide: Dow Chemical, Monsanto, Thompson-Hayward Chemical Co., Hercules Inc. and Diamond Shamrock Corp. On behalf of themselves and their children who had been born with birth defects, the veterans asked the court to order the companies to set up a fund to pay medical and disability expenses. More than 300 persons had become parties to the suit.

Two GAO reports, in April and November 1979, urged a long-term study of persons exposed to Agent Orange during military service. The second report also backed up veterans' claims that they had been sprayed directly or moved into areas immediately after spraying, contrary to Defense Department assertions that ground troops did not enter defoliated areas until many weeks after spraying.

Studies proliferated. The Air Force began developing a six-year study of 1,200 persons who participated in one of the major spraying missions ("Operation Ranch Hand"). Congress ordered the VA to undertake a study of Agent Orange victims. President Carter vetoed a companion bill calling for a study of civilian exposure to the substance, but established an Agent Orange task force to coordinate federal agency studies and directed the then Health, Education and Welfare (HEW) Department to study the problem. The VA ran a quick, small-scale study and found traces of dioxins in the body fat of both Vietnam veterans and a control group of individuals who had not been in Southeast Asia. It then made plans for the long-range study ordered by Congress. The VA and HEW established registries of persons exposed to the herbicides.

In December 1979 Congress approved by voice vote in both the House and Senate a bill to authorize studies on the effects of chemicals used in Agent Orange. A separate bill passed by Congress mandated two HEW studies relating to health effects of dioxin exposure:

•An epidemiological study of agricultural, Forest Service and chemical workers and other civilians who have come in contact with dioxins.

•A review of existing scientific studies of long-range health effects of Agent Orange by the Office of Technology Assessment (OTA) and coordination of the HHS work with any other agency studies of dioxins, including the VA's.

On June 2, 1981, over the Reagan administration's token opposition, the House passed four veterans' bills, including a measure to provide medical care to Vietnam veterans who were exposed to Agent Orange. The House action on the bill was the first time either house of Congress had approved legislation calling for treatment of Vietnam veterans suffering from exposure to Agent Orange. The bill would provide VA hospital care to Vietnam veterans if VA doctors determined that such care was necessary to treat a condition that "may be associated with exposure" to Agent Orange. The VA also would have to provide medical treatment if it was necessary to prevent hospitalization for such a condition.

The committee said that until scientists can determine the cause-and-effect relationship of the herbicide, the VA should do everything possible to provide care to exposed veterans. "When a doubt exists, the doubt should be resolved in favor of the veteran," the committee said in its report on the bill.

According to the VA, the bill would have the effect of extending hospital care to all Vietnam veterans for almost any medical or psychiatric condition. The agency said the costs of this provision could not be measured but would be "of considerable magnitude."

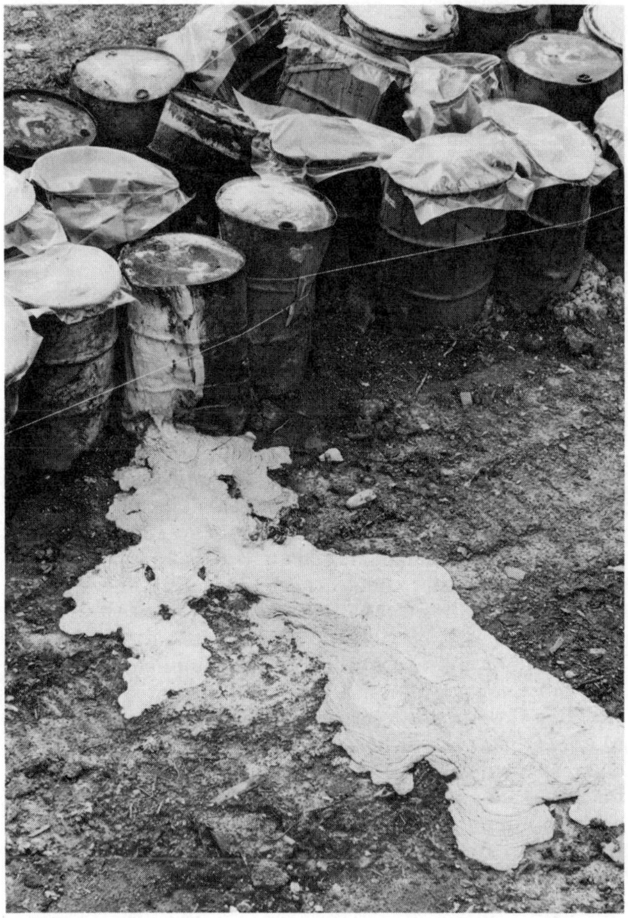

Hazardous Waste Accidents

The worst industrial accident in recent years involving toxic chemicals occurred in 1973 when a worker at the Michigan Chemical Co. near Lansing accidentally substituted polybrominated biphenyls (PBBs), a highly toxic fire-retardant, for magnesium oxide in feed prepared for the Michigan Farm Bureau. The mistake was not uncovered until after the feed was distributed to hundreds of Michigan dairy farms. Through the meat, milk and eggs of tens of thousands of farm animals, PBBs passed into the diets of an estimated 9 million Michigan residents. After the mistake was uncovered some 500 farms were quarantined and 23,000 cattle, 150,000 chickens and other farm animals slaughtered.

Health researchers conducted a study in November that compared 1,000 Michigan farm residents with a similar group of Wisconsin farm families. The study found that nearly one-third of the Michigan group suffered adverse health effects that could have been caused by PBBs. The researchers, headed by Dr. Irving Selikoff of the Mount Sinai School of Medicine, found that the Michigan group had an unusual number of medical problems, including memory loss, muscular weakness, sleep problems and abdominal pains. More studies are under way to determine the exact relationship between the PBBs and the health problems, including possible links to cancer.

In another incident, approximately 6,000 pounds of plastic and other wastes were buried between 1972 and 1979 in the Suller landfill near Gassville, Ark. In November 1979, the dump ignited and burned out of control for 12 days, producing a cloud of toxic hydrogen chloride. Dangerous levels of the gas were detectable more than two miles away, prompting the Arkansas governor to declare a state of emergency. When hydrogen chloride gas mixes with water it forms highly corrosive hydrochloric acid. Hydrogen chloride when inhaled in high concentrations can be fatal. In low concentrations, inhalation can produce irritation, burns, and ulceration of the skin, eyes and mucous membranes. It can cause reduced vision and blindness, laryngitis and bronchitis.

In 1979, in Rehoboth, Mass., 1,000 cubic yards of resins left over from a redistilling process were ordered removed from a dumpsite that the owner had placed within 10 feet of his own house. Assorted toxic wastes amounting to some 15,000 drums and 43 tanks were removed that same year in Lowell, Mass., where chemicals were leaking from drums within 200 yards of homes.

These examples are typical of developments in different locations throughout the United States. Vast stretches through much of the East, Louisiana, Texas, Washington, Oregon and California, according to the U.S. comptroller general in 1979, face the greatest potential for trouble. Farmlands have been used repeatedly as illegal dumpsites. In Persham, Minn., according to a report in *The New York Times,* 11 persons were poisoned by arsenic leaching from grasshopper bait. The victims worked for a building contractor who drilled a well close to where the bait had been buried by a farmer 30 years before. One of the workers lost the use of his legs for six months as a result.

New Jersey has been a favorite spot for midnight dumpers or "scavengers" paid to cart off wastes and dump them in swamps, rivers and streams to avoid paying disposal costs at a legitimate dumpsite. The most blatant offenders simply loosen tank-truck valves and get rid of contaminants along roadways in the middle of the night.

Disposal Technology

In 1980, the Council on Environmental Quality estimated that 56 tons of hazardous wastes would be generated nationwide in the next year and that approximately 60 percent of those wastes would be generated within 10 states: New Jersey, Illinois, Ohio, California, Pennsylvania, Texas, New York, Michigan, Tennessee and Indiana.

The most common method of disposing of solid wastes in this country is by landfill. Wastes are also scattered across the land in a process called land farming. In this process, wastes are incorporated into the soil, thus reducing their hazardous elements. Liquid wastes can be injected into deep wells that penetrate underground cavities where the wastes can be stored. This method is relatively low in cost, but unless injection wells are located in geologically stable areas, well below ground water supplies, there is an inherent danger of ground water contamination.

The Resource Conservation and Recovery Act already requires that landfills be secure, that operators show financial responsibility for up to $10 million per year in damages for any accidents and that landfills be monitored for 20 years to minimize the chance of hazardous wastes escaping into the environment. For a landfill to be listed as secure, it must have an impenetrable bottom to prevent chemicals from leaching into ground waters. It must also be capped to stop rain and surface water from leaching through wastes contained in the landfill.

Public opposition to siting and construction of landfills has become a problem in recent years. Most people feel that hazardous wastes should be properly disposed of, but not in their own backyards. States have taken over major responsibility for deciding where dumpsites are to be built and EPA has created a committee to assist states on the siting process.

Another method of waste disposal is to mix wastes with other chemicals to form a chemically stable substance that will not leach. These substances can then be disposed of in an unsecured landfill. Energy and materials can also be recovered from wastes that contain valuable materials. In fact, the extraction of these materials can often be accomplished with less energy depletion than the mining and processing of virgin materials. Only small percentages of wastes are suitable for recovery and new technologies must be developed to make the process a viable option for many waste producers. Recycling, according to the EPA, can reduce hazardous wastes by 20 percent.

Ways have already been developed to render wastes less hazardous or nonhazardous. For example, carbon or resin adsorption, distillation, centrifugation, flocculation, de-sedimentation, reverse osmosis and ultrafiltration are all processes that can transform waste into more desirable material. Biological processes include sludge treatment to destroy organic compounds, composting of organic-rich wastes and trickling filters to promote decomposition. Sound disposal of hazardous wastes is costly, but it is ultimately less costly than improper disposal.

Injection Wells

Well injection involves the emplacement of fluids into the ground through a bored, drilled, driven or dug well. Constructed like oil wells with steel and concrete casings to contain toxic and radioactive wastes, injection wells are a favorite disposal method for many industries. In 1981, as many as 400,000 wells were operating in the United States.

Defenders of the injection method of waste disposal say it is harmless and economically feasible. They claim it makes use of a virtually unlimited natural resource — isolated geological strata — that is cut off from the surface by layers of impermeable rock well below any level that could lead to pollution of ground water supplies. Deep-well injection is often less expensive than chemically neutralizing wastes or dumping them above ground.

Critics argue that drinking water could be contaminated by the process. According to the Environmental Protection Agency (EPA), injection practices can cause fluids to leak through faults or fissures in well casings. Wastes may also be forced upward by underground pressures into nearby wells.

In 1976 the EPA proposed Underground Injection Control (UIC) regulations as mandated by the Safe Drinking Water Act of 1974. After the oil well industry extensively criticized the proposed regulations, the EPA withdrew them until February 1979 when it issued a new set of guidelines. To implement the revised controls, EPA categorized well injection activities into the following five classes:

- *Class I* wells are used to inject industrial, nuclear and municipal wastes beneath the deepest geological layer containing underground drinking water supplies. Approximatley 400 of these wells were in use as of September 1981.

- *Class II* wells are used to deposit wastes generated by oil and gas production. They are the second most frequently used class of wells; 40,000 are currently in use.

- *Class III* wells are used at approximately 2,000 special-process mining sites across the country.

- *Class IV* wells are classified by the EPA as potentially the most dangerous type. They are used for disposal of hazardous wastes. Approximately 7,500 are in current use.

- *Class V* wells are all those not classified into categories I-IV. The largest number of wells currently in use, class V wells include recharge wells and air conditioning return flow wells.

New technologies currently under review often involve incineration. One method uses multiple hearth incinerators to repeatedly burn wastes until they are completely destroyed. The latest method — fluidized bed-burning — involves passing superheated wastes through a bed of sand that serves as a catalyst to speed combustion.

In February 1981 a new disposal method was announced at the University of California at Riverside that avoids incineration. The new process is based upon the discovery that a negatively charged form of oxygen called superoxide could break down many chlorinated compounds into harmless substances. Such a method could be used both by big industries and small companies that need to dispose of solvents. It does not, however, work in water and cannot be used to clean up already contaminated ground water.

High heat generated by cement-making kilns is another method under research that has the potential to eliminate both PCBs and dioxin contaminants. In 1981, a cement kiln in Puerto Rico was federally financed for $500,000 to conduct studies to determine the effectiveness of this method. The kiln at San Juan was used three days a week for 12 weeks and burned around 160,000 gallons of chemical wastes. For the test, no compounds had high percentages of chlorine (the higher the chlorine content, the hotter the burn must be).

A popular approach to burning toxic wastes in the past had been to use industrial incinerators that had been used as capacitators and transformers. Many of these incinerators are now banned in this country. The EPA has granted two permits for operation of incinerators, one in Deer Park, Texas, and the other in Eldorado, Ark. According to EPA, both facilities have been 99 percent effective in destroying PCBs but in the process have produced small amounts of a dioxin contaminant called TCDD. TCDD is regarded as a dangerous cancer-causing molecule and is one of the agents found in the defoliant Agent Orange. There are no known safe levels established for human exposure to the dioxin. In March 1980, a municipal waste-burning plant in Hempstead, L.I., was closed because of a dioxin problem and has not been reopened.

Scientists in recent years have shown renewed interest is waste burning at sea. *Vulcanus,* a vessel converted to a waste incinerator in 1972 is the best known example of sea incineration. The ship burned 10,400 metric tons of the defoliant Agent Orange in March 1977. *Vulcanus* was one of three incinerator ships operating in the world in 1981. The vessel has two ceramic-lined incinerators in the stern, a double hull and a double bottom and 15 tanks within the inner hull for carrying various chemical wastes. In an emergency the *Vulcanus* can dump her toxic burden into the sea.

LOVE CANAL: A TIME BOMB WENT OFF

Perhaps more than any other event in recent years, the Love Canal near New York's Niagara Falls represented, to environmentalists, the beginning of a new age of land pollution problems in this country. Environmentalists said the situation at Love Canal was so blatantly harmful to residents that it awakened the country to a new movement against improper disposal of hazardous wastes.

U.S. Sources of Hazardous Waste

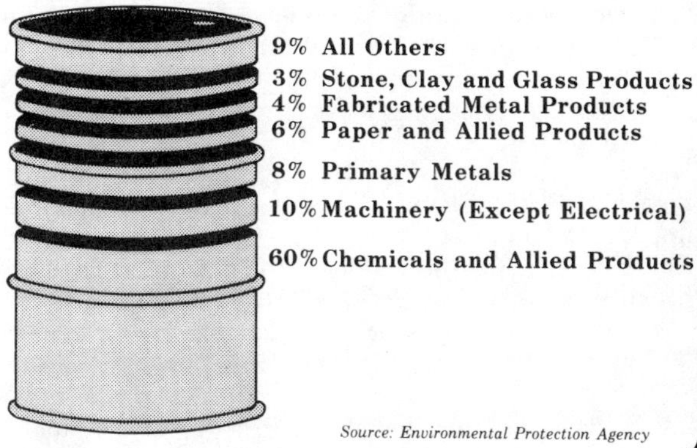

Source: Environmental Protection Agency

"We have learned that Love Canal was merely the first detonation of a string of chemical time bombs literally strewn across the nation," said Eckardt C. Beck, EPA's administrator for water and waste management at the time the dumpsite was first uncovered.

How It Developed

The Love Canal was originally built in the 19th century by William T. Love, an entrepreneur who wanted to construct an industrial city near the point where the canal would feed back into the Niagara River. State leaders, taken by the idea, allowed Love to use public property to divert large amounts of water from the nearby river to build the canal. Love's ambition exceeded his ability. The 20-yard wide canal was soon abandoned by Love and eventually purchased by the Hooker Chemical Co. In 1953, Hooker deeded the land to the Niagara Falls Board of Education for a token $1.

It has not been proven whether Hooker knew the extent to which the land was contaminated when the company transferred it to the school board. It was later learned, however, that Hooker Chemical dumped 21,800 tons of pesticides, cleaning solution and other toxic wastes into the canal between 1947 and 1952.

In 1953 the school board began to build a school and playground at the Love Canal's midsection. Construction workers hit a drainage trench filled with chemicals, but rather than halt work authorities decided to move the school 80 feet away. Families began to settle near the dump, knowing that the field close by was to be a park and recreation area for children.

According to the *Washington Star*, a March 21, 1968, Hooker document described samples of material taken from the canal site: "The sample was an oil-like residue that burned much like a 4th of July 'sparkler', " the memo said. At that time, Hooker employees found "traces above the surface of various toxic chemicals." Hooker gave no evidence of this.

While dumping from Hooker was still going on, children occasionally swam at the opposite end of the canal, sometimes arriving home with hard pimples on their bodies. Children who played in the area often came home with tears in their eyes.

By 1977, the Love Canal had been filled by years of heavy snowfall and rain that caused large quantities of the contents to overflow. Chemicals that had seeped into clay, silt and sandy loam appeared in nearby creeks.

Although residents were aware of the danger, most were financially unable to move away. The homes could not be sold, and residents' salaries were too low to finance two homes. Hooker Chemical Co. was also an economically important employer to the depressed area and a difficult establishment for the residents to confront. The company provided an estimated 3,000 blue-collar jobs to the general vicinity and was thinking of building a $17 million headquarters in downtown Niagara Falls.

City officials were aware of the chemicals and even knew they contained halogenated hydrocarbons including PCBs that were highly injurious to human health. High on the list of poisonous materials was hexachlorocyclopentadiene or C-56, which was produced from the manufacture of pesticides. The chemical, in certain doses, can cause damage to every organ in the body.

Early in 1978, EPA conducted tests in basements of homes near the canal to see if the chemicals had vaporized off the walls and were present in household air. Michael H. Brown, a reporter for *The Niagara Gazette,* at the time described the results of EPA's study in an article on Love Canal in the *Atlantic Monthly*. He reported that benzene, a known cause of cancer in humans, had been detected in the household air up and down the streets. A widely used solvent, benzene was known in chronic-exposure cases to cause headaches, fatigue, loss of weight, and dizziness.

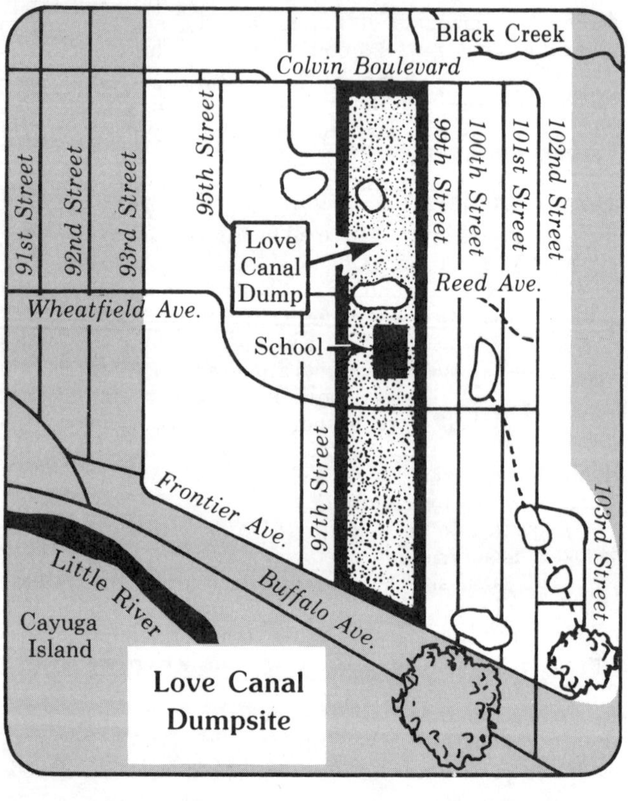

Love Canal Dumpsite

Brown went on to describe the residents' list of ailments after he conducted his own inspection of the area:

> Though unafflicted before they moved there, many people were now plagued with ear infections, nervous disorders, rashes and headaches. One young man, James Gizzarelli, said he had missed four months of work owing to breathing troubles. His wife was suffering epileptic-like seizures which her doctor was unable to explain. Meanwhile freshly applied paint was inexplicably peeling from the interior of their houses. Pets too were suffering, most seriously if they had been penned in the backyards nearest to the canal, constantly breathing air that smelled like mothballs and weed killer. They lost their fur, exhibited skin lesions, and while still quite young, developed internal tumors. A great many cases of cancer were reported among the women, along with deafness.

When the state finally conducted a health study at the dump in May 1978, the results were even more astonishing. Eighty or more compounds were found in the dump, 10 of which were potential carcinogens. Fourteen could damage the brain and central nervous system. EPA announced that tests had found four suspected carcinogens — benzene, chloroform, trichloroethylene and tetrachloroethylene — in air samples taken near the contaminated area. Two of them could cause narcotic or anesthetic consequences. Others were known to cause headaches, seizures, loss of hair, anemia or skin rashes. One federal report indicated that the odds of Love Canal residents contracting cancer were as high as one in 10.

National Attention

By this time the Love Canal story was attracting attention from the national media. President Carter had officially declared the Hooker dumpsite a national emergency. New York's Gov. Hugh L. Carey, D., went to the site and announced that the state, through its Urban Development Corp., would purchase, at fair market value, homes made uninhabitable by the chemicals.

The first evacuation was in August 1978, following accounts of a high incidence of birth defects and illness in the neighborhood. At that time, the state declared a health emergency and agreed to relocate and buy the homes of 239 first-ring and second-ring residents bordering the dumpsites. Most of those have since found new permanent housing.

One couple in the Love Canal area, Leonard and Phyllis Whitenight, had been unaware of any danger prior to the declaration of a health emergency by the state in August 1978. Leonard Whitenight, a printer by trade, held down three jobs at a time to meet the mortgage payments on their home. When the emergency was declared, the Whitenights were not particularly alarmed. They assumed the state would buy their home and they would look for another place to live. But the Whitenights were not one of the 239 families that were evacuated. They were assured, however, that they were in no danger by remaining.

Meanwhile, an environmental researcher, Dr. Beverly Paigen, at the Roswell Park Memorial Institute in Buffalo, began examining streams in the area around the Whitenights' home. The researcher theorized that water contaminated by toxic chemicals was being carried from the canal sight in underground streams. Miscarriages, birth defects and other ailments were prevalent in homes near these underground streams. Her epidemiological findings were confirmed by the first genetic tests on residents.

When the Whitenights first heard about Paigen's findings they recalled that 800 loads of fill had been dumped on their lot before they built their home and that the land on the street behind their home was often soggy and filled with puddles. Eventually traces of the poison dioxin, which is contained in Agent Orange, was found in a nearby creek where the Whitenight children had played.

The state set up a $5 million program to purchase homes in the area where the Whitenights lived. The Whitenights received $36,500 for their home. After this second evacuation, the federal government agreed in August 1979 to lend the state $15 million for the purchase of as many as 550 houses within a 30-square block area surrounding the 15-acre dumpsite. The state agreed to buy the houses at "fair market value" usually in the range of $30,000 to $35,000. The homeowners had three years from October 1979 to accept the offer.

Since Love Canal was first unearthed, Hooker Chemical has acknowledged burying up to 3,700 tons of trichlorophenol waste, which contains the chemical dioxin, at various other sites in Niagara County between 1947 and 1972. At last count, there was believed to be an estimated 141 pounds of dioxin in the canal site and as much as 2,000 pounds buried elsewhere in the county. Three ounces of dioxin are enough to kill more than a million people.

In April 1978, a House subcommittee released documents indicating that the Hooker Company had known as early as June 1958 that toxic chemical waste was seeping into the area. A company official testified that local residents had not been informed of the situation because the company feared a "substantial legal liability." In 1979, 15 dumps in Niagara County alone had been discovered to contain toxic chemicals.

The federal government filed suit against Hooker Chemical for $125 million in 1979, but suits by local citizens now total more than $3 billion. The government's suit charged that from 1942 to 1975, Hooker dumped 199,900 tons of chemical waste at four places: the Love Canal, Hyde Park, 102nd Street and a dump known as the "S" area. The EPA charged that the material was "migrating from the sites, contaminating the environment and endangering persons exposed to the chemicals."

Public sentiment had been aroused by Love Canal, putting Congress under increased pressure from constituents for a federal program to deal with toxic wastes. The end result was $1.6 billion legislation designed to protect the environment from disasters similar to the one at Love Canal.

FEDERAL ACTION TO COMBAT WASTES

The Resource Conservation and Recovery Act of 1976 dealt with land pollution for the first time and gave the Environmental Protection Agency the power to tell manufacturers how to deposit their waste materials.

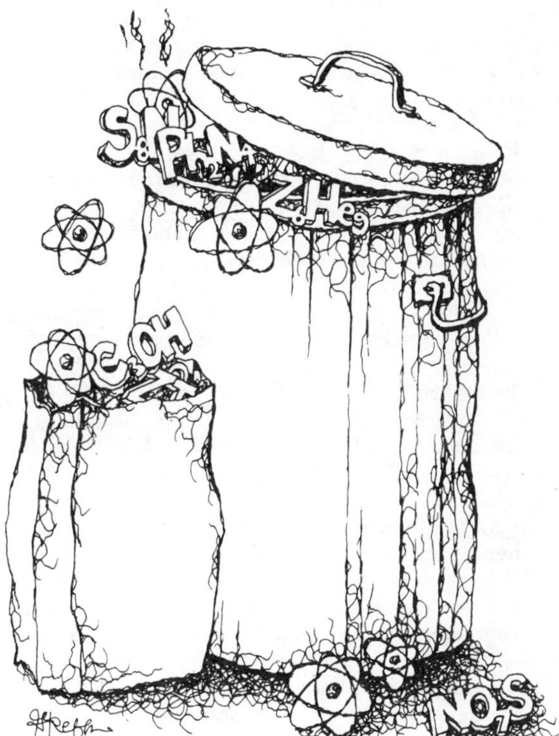

The Toxic Substances Control Act of 1976 (TSCA) expanded federal regulation of industrial and commercial chemicals and, for the first time, required pre-market testing for potentially dangerous chemicals. The bill directed the EPA to require that chemical manufacturers test products that pose a risk to human health or the environment. Companies planning to produce a new chemical or to market an existing substance for a new purpose would have to notify the agency 90 days in advance, giving the agency a chance to hold up marketing while more testing was done or even to ban a chemical in an extreme case.

The Resource Conservation and Recovery Act authorized a system to track hazardous wastes from their origin through all phases of treatment, storage and disposal. States were encouraged and given financial aid to oversee regulation of wastes. Permits from the EPA were required before wastes could be stored at facilities.

But implementation was slow. The EPA was still writing regulations for the law nearly three and a half years after President Ford signed the legislation. The law gave EPA 18 months to complete the task, until April 1978.

EPA missed the 1978 deadline and was sued by several environmental groups. But a federal court said the agency was doing the best it could and set a new deadline. EPA had told the court it was still processing the more than 1,000 comments from industry, states and environmental groups about the proposed regulations.

Congressional advocates of tough EPA action were not pleased. In a report issued March 18, 1980, the Senate Governmental Affairs Oversight Committee charged that EPA "has failed to make full use of its authority to identify and mitigate the hazards posed by the improper disposal of hazardous wastes. Enforcement actions taken by the agency to remedy inadequate disposal problems have been insufficient to date."

The report also reprimanded EPA for not recognizing sooner the seriousness of the hazardous waste problem and for not using all the funds Congress appropriated to carry out the law. EPA admitted what the subcommittee's year-long study found: that neither the agency nor Congress knew the enormity of the hazardous waste dumpsite problem when RCRA was drafted.

As a result of public and congressional pressure, the EPA finally adopted regulations under authority of the RCRA that became effective in November 1980. The regulations defined hazardous wastes and established a cradle-to-grave management system, including standards for transporters and permit requirements for owners and operators of facilities that treat, store or dispose of hazardous wastes.

The most important of the new regulations was the requirement that a manifest or inventory be kept on all waste. The regulations required a waste producer to keep track of hazardous wastes throughout the movement of the wastes from point of origination to point of disposal. Hence the name, "cradle-to-grave." First, a producer must check the EPA hazardous wastes list. If a waste is hazardous, it must be properly packaged and labeled and a manifest provided to the transporter. The transporter may deliver the waste only to an authorized disposal site.

The new plan also allowed states to operate a hazardous waste program in place of the national program if the state meets the standards. Failure to comply with the law was punishable by civil penalties and, in certain cases, by fines and imprisonment.

Also under the law every producer of hazardous waste in the country was required to register with the Environmental Protection Agency and every treatment center was required to obtain a permit. The law authorized EPA to investigate any dump and force the owner to clean it up if it posed an "imminent or substantial" danger to human health or the environment. It also provided the agency with authority to clean up the site when the operator could not. The requirements were the largest regulatory program ever launched by the EPA.

Douglas M. Costle, then EPA Administrator, said at the time the requirements were approved that the regulations will "turn up information and situations that will shock our nation. We will find waste sites that are currently unknown ... and gather hard data on a problem whose dimensions we can only guess."

The cost of abiding by the new regulations, according to Joan Berkowitz, vice-president of Arthur D. Little Inc., a research and consulting firm in Cambridge, Mass., would be about 10 times greater than using a municipal trash disposal. Industry officials, however, believed the large chemical-producing companies would comply with the regulations to avoid lawsuits. Individuals who knowingly violated the law and endangered human lives were subject to criminal penalties of up to $250,000 per violation and two-to-five years in prison.

The Justice Department's Land and Natural Resources Division stepped up its prosecution of waste violators. The division doubled its caseload between 1973 and 1979 to 28,000 incidents of litigation.

In December 1979, the Justice Department and the EPA filed the largest environmental protection action suit to date. The suits charged Hooker Chemical Company, its parent company Occidental Petroleum Corp. and Olin Corp. with violating federal pollution laws and endangering human health and the environment at Love Canal and three other sites in Niagara Falls, N.Y. The government sought $125 million — $68 million from Hooker, $50 million from Hooker and Olin and $7 million from Hooker for reimbursement of federal funds already spent to clean up the Love Canal area.

Public reaction to Love Canal brought congressional attention to the toxic waste disposal problem and added fuel to the movement to establish legislation to provide funds for disposal site cleanup and victim compensation.

SUPERFUND: PAYING FOR THE CLEANUP

Passed in the waning days of the 96th Congress in 1980, the Hazardous Substances and Hazardous Waste Response Liability and Compensation Act (commonly called the superfund law) established a $1.6 billion fund for cleanup of spills of hazardous substances and inactive hazardous waste disposal sites. The superfund bill was intended to finance cleanup of leaks into the environment of hazardous wastes when no responsible party could be identified or when the responsible party refused or was unable to pay. The bill gave the federal government the authority and money to act in emergencies to clean up chemical spills or dumps that threaten public health or the environment. The government could then sue those who caused the damages — if they could be found — to recoup the cleanup costs.

Part of the fund (87.5 percent) was to be financed by a tax on oil and specified chemicals; the remaining 12.5 percent was to come from regular appropriation of funds by Congress.

Liability Controversy

The chemical industry's major concern over the new legislation focused on the sticky question of legal liability. The Carter administration originally had wanted a "strict, joint and several liability" policy to be applied to chemical accidents. Strict liability would have made most parties involved in the disposal process — generators, disposers, haulers — open to damage suits regardless of negligence or compliance with contemporary waste disposal standards. Joint and several liability would have made any participant liable in an action, regardless of the extent of participation. Within Congress, supporters of a tough law backed a proposal that, in effect, would have established a new "toxic tort law" which departed from traditional theories of regulation and common law. Instead of being required to furnish direct proof that a substance caused injury, a plaintiff would merely have to provide evidence of statistical probability — that he was exposed to a known or suspected carcinogen and that he developed cancer.

These concepts of liability were not adopted. The final bill provided that those who own or operate waste disposal sites, produce wastes or transport them are liable for all cleanup costs and for up to $50 million for each incident of damage to government-owned natural resources. But injured persons would receive no compensation and had to seek redress through litigation in state courts, an expensive and time-consuming process that critics of the liability portions of the bill said effectively precluded many injured persons from being compensated. One version of the bill would have allowed victims direct access to federal courts to seek damages, but that was not in the final bill.

The final measure did not cover oil spills, as President Carter had proposed, and contained weaker liability provisions than the Justice Department had sought to impose on persons who leak or dump chemicals.

Chemical companies were to begin paying federal taxes in April 1981 on major chemical feedstocks and certain petroleum products. The law called for a national hazardous-substance response plan. The new plan was to establish priorities for correcting disposal site problems, and to assure that remedial actions were cost-effective.

The superfund law also called for the Public Health Service to establish an agency for toxic substance and disease registrations in cooperation with the states. The law specified penalties for various types of violations of waste disposal regulations: up to $10,000 or one year in jail for failure to notify the government of existence of a site; $10,000 a day for failure to prove financial responsibility; and punitive damages of up to three times the cost of a cleanup operation in some cases.

Costs of Legislation

The superfund was to finance the cleanup of from 100 to 300 abandoned dumpsites, "a fraction of the overall problem," according to Marc Tipermas, former chief of EPA's superfund office. As a result, he said, states would have to pick up a large share of the cost of cleaning up abandoned dumpsites. EPA officials were concerned that the $1.6 billion fund would not be large enough. States were expected to look to superfund money to help them finance their own cleanups. The bill also set up a $200 million liability fund to deal with costs that might arise from dumps permitted under the Resource Conservation and Recovery Act.

The EPA estimated that implementation of the bill would cost industry about a billion dollars a year, only about two-tenths of 1 percent of the companies' total sales and less than $2.50 for every person in the country. The agency estimated that the cost of compliance for industries would amount to less than 3 percent of the value industries add to final products before they are sold. Certain industries would have to pay more, including chlorine producers, manufacturers of chrome pigments and some producers of inorganic compounds. Producers of sodium dichromate, an inorganic substance used in the paint industry, in leather tanning and in electroplating faced costs amounting to 40 percent of the value they add to the materials they buy, according to EPA.

Future Controversies

Passage of the legislation did not mean the issue was settled. Advocates of a strong law were disappointed with many aspects of the bill that was finally approved, particularly the sections on liability of companies that dispose of hazardous wastes.

A major environment group, the Sierra Club, said it would lobby in later Congresses for more benefits for victims. The superfund itself called for a number of studies, including one dealing with the adequacy of existing common law to provide redress for people harmed by the release of hazardous substances. For most persons suffering losses, the primary avenue of redress is through claims against the polluter. This process is often a tough route to follow. The actual losses must be determined, the polluter identified and the relationship between the pollutant and damages proven. Delays during litigation are often long and can force settlements that may not be fair to victims. In addition, total damages may exceed the polluter's ability to pay.

The real cost of waste cleanup is another major issue that was expected to come before Congress in future years. There were indications that a lot more money will have to come from somewhere. One study done for EPA estimated that remedying problem sites similar to Love Canal could cost anywhere from $3.6 billion to $44 billion, depending upon whether wastes are actually removed or rendered harmless. The Council on Environmental Quality estimated the cost at between $28.4 billion and $55 billion.

As an example of the huge costs that may be lurking over the horizon, damage suits against the Velsicol Chemical Co. for contaminated wells near the company's 300-acre waste-disposal site in Hardeman County, Tenn., totaled about $2.5 billion.

During the superfund debates, a Chemical Manufacturers Association study suggested that the average cost of correcting each failing dumpsite would be $1 million. Yet the same study also concluded that costs of correcting conditions at Love Canal would be $23 million. The state of New York and city of Niagara as of June 1980 had already spent close to $36 million, with estimates on the total cost going as high as $300 million.

The 20th Century's Plague

The chemical industry has acknowledged that problems of safe waste disposal do exist, and that past practices have been deficient. But the industry also claims a "chemophobia" has overtaken the country that could lead to staggering costs for cleanup beyond efforts that are reasonably necessary for public health.

On the other side of the issue, advocates of stronger controls respond that chemical contamination is so serious that the issue cannot be avoided in an industrial society where people demand more potent medicines, more types of plastics and stronger pesticides. They argue that huge sums of money must be expended for cleanup and that strict laws must be passed to make companies producing hazardous wastes liable for financial damages if those wastes harm humans.

Health problems associated with chemical waste have increased since World War II. There remains much scientific controversy over the relationship between hazardous substances and human health, even when the substances are known to produce illness in test animals. In spite of this controversy, Congress has begun to accept the view that a relationship does exist and to deal with that link by passing such legislation as the Resource Conservation and Recovery Act of 1976 and the 1980 superfund law.

The problem is expected to worsen in years ahead as the amount of toxic waste increases. Waste sludges of nearly 8 million tons annually are being created at new wastewater treatment plants. New research efforts will be needed to learn how to properly dispose of these wastes and also to better understand the effects they have on human health.

There is considerable agreement that hazardous waste disposal is one of the most serious environmental problems faced by this country. There also is agreement that protecting human health and the environment from the effects of toxic chemicals is a complex undertaking. A vast number of chemicals touch the everyday lives of nearly all Americans. Only a small percentage of these chemicals pose threats to humans and the environment, but some can cause serious problems.

"It just boggles the mind to think how little is known," said Carrol Bastion, a toxic substances expert for the Council on Environmental Quality. "There will never be a way to reduce the hazards of toxic substances to zero even if we return to a much simpler society."

The Reagan administration's philosophy of reducing federal regulation of business and federal spending may shrink efforts aimed at cleaning hazardous wastes by reducing the EPA's role and giving states greater authority to identify and deal with contamination caused by dangerous dumpsites. Regardless of whether the administration succeeds or not in accomplishing this, the waste control program faces some lengthy delays. Before the funding controversy began, EPA officials said they expected to have emergency cleanup started at no fewer than 100 sites in 1981. By February 1981 the officials dropped that number to only a few dozen.

Some persons who have been involved in the problem think the only satisfactory answer is some significant changes in the lifestyles and habits of Americans and the industries they operate. But because dozens of chemicals suspected of being hazardous play a role in the way Americans live and work, changes will be extraordinarily difficult to accomplish. The most pessimistic observers believe that basic change will occur only after a major environmental or health disaster directly attributable to a widely used chemical.

4

Water: Is It Safe to Drink?

The problem of polluted drinking water is everywhere. It is not a matter, simply, of legislation, treatment reports and bureaucratic fumbling. It is a matter of life and health.

Carol Keough, *Water Fit to Drink*

History gives ample evidence of the penalties paid by past civilizations that failed, through ignorance or neglect, to provide for the safety of their water systems. The dangers of cholera and typhoid once transported through water supplies in the 19th century have been eliminated, but they have been replaced by an equally dangerous health hazard — carcinogens and viruses. Evidence supporting these threats is inconclusive, but research is beginning to provide alarming facts. The effluvia of an industrial society, especially its thousands of synthetic chemicals, toxic metals and pesticides, have led Americans to begin questioning the sources and quality of the water they drink.

Drinking water is usually considered the first priority in water management. Yet drinking water has received little attention on the national scene. And while there has been progress in the cleanup of rivers and lakes, largely due to the Clean Water Act of 1972, the nation has ignored the problem of ground water contamination from toxic chemicals — a problem that has reached significant proportions, in the opinion of many health experts.

Water and Health

Because unsafe drinking water is so hard to detect, most people drink contaminated water and don't know it.

Homeowners are reluctant to invest time and money in discovering the true quality of the water they drink. They assume state and local officials have tested water and upheld federal water quality regulations that may not even exist.

A report published by the Water Resources Research Institute in 1975, *The State of America's Drinking Water,* said that half of the water systems that serve fewer than 500 people did not meet minimum health standards, and nearly one quarter exceeded the mandatory limits for contamination.

The same report estimated that as many as 40 percent of the private systems, wells and cisterms, are even more contaminated than public systems. Among the many ingredients in drinking water are a number of chemicals that received attention as health hazards.

Nitrates, for example, are found naturally in vegetables, water and soil. When ingested into the body, they can be harmful, especially to infants. Nitrates are changed inside a baby's stomach into nitrites, which then change the hemoglobin so that it can no longer carry sufficient oxygen to the body's tissues. The tissues suffocate and the baby turns blue.

Another health problem related to nitrates found in drinking water is caused by the formation of powerful carcinogens called nitrosamines. Scientists are still uncertain how nitrosamines cause cancer. Apparently a chain reaction occurs within the body that changes nitrates into the cancer-causing substance. According to scientists, any nitrate a person eats or drinks can be changed into a nitrosamine.

Large amounts of nitrates come from saliva and from vegetables. About 90 percent of the nitrates humans consume come from our food, and about 9 percent from cured meats. Less than 1 percent comes from drinking water.

Nitrates in water come from septic systems, animal feed lots, industrial waste waters, sanitary landfills and garbage dumps. Technical problems in the operation of wastewater treatment plants have made the removal of nitrates from waste water difficult. Only one plant, in Nassau County, New York, had managed to remove nitrates with any success by the end of the 1970s.

Asbestos also has been showing up in water tests and, unlike nitrites, is a proven deadly contaminant in relatively small doses. Studies at the Mayo Clinic in Rochester, Minn., have shown that inhaled or swallowed asbestos fibers can travel once they get inside the body and cause gastrointestinal cancers.

The single most frequent source of asbestos in drinking water is the cement used to make large water mains. An estimated 200,000 miles of this pipe are in use in the United States. According to EPA, the pipes are beginning to disintegrate and release asbestos fibers into the water.

The EPA can regulate asbestos levels in drinking water under the federal Clean Water Act, but few towns or cities can afford to replace entire water supply systems. The EPA also has difficulty definitely proving that asbestos in water causes cancer.

Lead is perhaps the most dangerous mineral found in drinking water. Researchers have found that the connec-

Annual Production of Synthetic Organic Chemicals, 1920-78

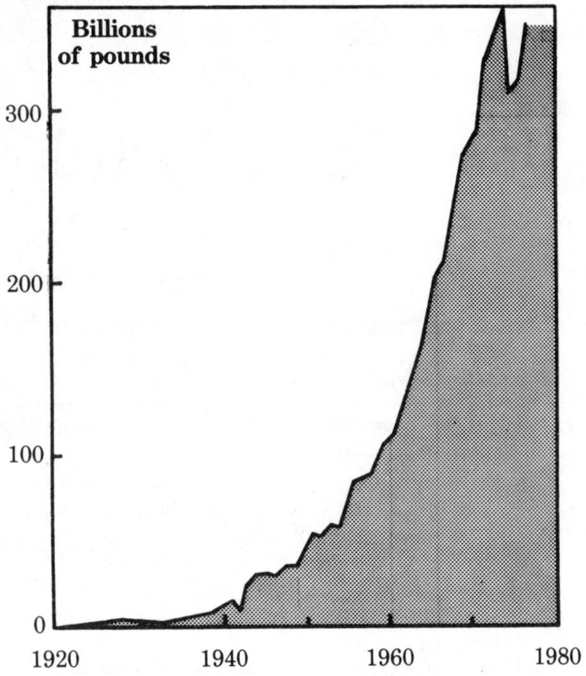

Source: Council on Environmental Quality

tion between lead intake and mental retardation is much stronger than previously assumed. They also have recently discovered that high blood pressure and the body's ability to fight off infections can be affected by high levels of lead in the bloodstream.

In addition to hazards such as nitrites, asbestos and lead, the use of chlorine to disinfect water may have adverse health effects. The federal government's Council on Environmental Quality (CEQ) issued a report in December 1980 that strengthened previous studies that have linked rectal, colon and bladder cancer to chlorine use. Chlorine combines with natural organic matter in water to produce chemicals — trihalogenated methanes — that have been shown to cause cancer at high doses in laboratory animals.

"While these studies are preliminary and subject to a number of limitations, they do provide significant evidence of increased cancer risks from drinking chlorinated water, which should be of concern," said CEQ member Dr. Robert Harris, in releasing the report.

On the positive side, good water should contain certain trace minerals that are essential to normal body functioning, such as iron, zinc, copper, manganese, chromium, cobalt, molybdenum, iodine and selenium. Other minerals such as lead, cadmium, mercury and arsenic can be harmful.

Mining and municipal solid waste landfills are two prominent contributors to harmful trace minerals in water systems. Steel plants, iron foundries or zinc mines, for example, may be served by water supplies contaminated with copper, zinc or aluminum which, in higher than average doses, could be harmful to human health.

Solid waste landfills — which include food waste, yard waste, glass, metals, pesticide containers, batteries, tin cans, and dead animals — can contaminate surrounding water supplies, especially when rainfall causes contaminates to sink into the ground water.

With cancer rates rising yearly, the presence of possible carcinogens and other harmful substances in water is worrying public officials in all parts of the nation. They fear that contaminated ground water could affect generations to come.

Water Quality and Quantity

Water experts warn that unless Congress and the states improve the way they manage the nation's water supply the United States will face a water crisis in the 1980s that will equal or surpass the energy crisis of the 1970s. The problem will not be an actual national shortage of water. Rather, the experts predict, the crisis will be caused by pollution, waste and dramatic increases in demand in water-short areas such as the West. These problems are created or exacerbated by poor management by government agencies at all levels, the experts say.

"The water crisis is not going to be a crisis in terms of a physical shortage, but will be caused by institutional problems that prevent us from using and managing the water efficiently," said Warren Viessman Jr., a senior engineering and public works specialist for the Congressional Research Service.

Water experts who criticize government mismanagement always point to one overriding problem: water agencies have not acknowledged the interdependence between water quantity and quality in a region or river basin, even though they are intimately related. One example, cited by Larry Silverman, legislative director of the Clean Water Action Project, a Washington-based environmental lobby, is in New Orleans, where chemical contamination of the city's drinking water is caused by pollutants dumped into the Mississippi River upstream.

"Water is a renewable resource, but it is being engineered in such a way that it is being made into a finite resource," said Silverman. Congress enacted major laws dealing with quantity or quality but never merged the two into a single statute. As a result, the nation's water is managed by a mélange of agencies, departments, laws and programs with overlapping and sometimes conflicting missions. Water supply and pollution control projects, for example, are planned, financed and constructed by separate agencies. Just how many federal programs deal with water supply and pollution is unknown.

A 1974 survey by the federal Water Resources Council (WRC) identified 25 federal waste programs that were spending $7.4 billion approved by Congress in 70 separate funding accounts. The programs were administered under more than 200 federal rules, regulations, orders and laws dealing with chemical wastes threatening water supplies, strip mining runoff and conservation of the nation's soil and water resources. The Clean Water Action Project has identified 35 federal programs dealing with water supply and pollution, and an Environmental Protection Agency (EPA) study found 39 federal water conservation agencies. The WRC's 1974 study has never been updated to determine how much the nation spends annually on water programs. This information is not known even by the Office of Management and Budget, the federal government's central budgeting office.

Another major factor nudging Congress to act is that water problems now are so widespread that nearly every congressional district has a problem — leaky municipal water mains, disappearing or contaminated ground water, lakes destroyed by acid rain or increasing flood damages.

In addition, the drought in February and March 1981 — which resulted in below normal river flows in 46 states — has increased Congress' awareness that many local water problems result from lack of coordination in federal water programs. A House water resources panel that held hearings on the drought in March 1981 was besieged by pleas from local officials for better federal coordination of water supply and pollution control agencies.

Four government policies said to exacerbate water problems were highlighted during those hearings:

- Lack of coordination between federal and state programs dealing with water quality and quantity.
- The failure of water agencies to recognize the interdependence between ground water and surface water.
- Government policies that discourage conservation.
- The proliferation of cost-sharing arrangements for federal grants which have led cities to solve their least pressing water problems first.

Past studies also indicate that the focus of attention on long-range abatement of the nation's lake, stream, river and coastal water pollution has inadvertently distracted attention from a more immediate part of the pollution problem — safeguarding ground water from chemical contamination. Ground and surface water, although interrelated, have not been given equal pollution control treatment over the past decade.

GROUND WATER: NEW POLLUTION THREATS

According to the Council on Environmental Quality, ground water is subsurface water that occurs in the soil beneath a water table (the level below which the ground is saturated) or in underground cavities called aquifers. An aquifer has walls of porous rock or sand. The term comes from two Latin words — aqua, water, and ferre, to bring. An aquifer can cover a few square yards or several thousand square feet. At the bottom of an aquifer is a layer of bedrock that makes the formation fairly watertight. When a well is dug, it taps water contained in an aquifer.

Ground water, found in soil and aquifers, and surface water, found in rivers, lakes and streams are intimately connected. One cannot be used without affecting the other. Ground water replenishes 30 percent of surface water by percolating up to the surface in springs. Thus it improves water quality by keeping the streams moving and diluting pollutants.

Water exists in the ground in many locations other than aquifers. There are two separate layers of water in the ground, separated from each other by the water table. The upper portion of the soil holds some water, where it is available to plant life. Immediately beneath that layer is the zone of water saturation in which water saturates all the pore spaces between soil particles. The line between the two layers is called the water table.

When water is pumped to the surface, as in a well, the water table around the site drops correspondingly. Nearby water in an aquifer is then pulled into an adjacent area.

Shallow ground water, found between soil particles, is usually of high quality because soil typically removes most of the contaminants before the water reaches an aquifer. Cleansing by filtration through the soil occurs as the water moves vertically and horizontally. With time, ground water tends toward chemical equilibrium with the minerals that it contacts, thereby increasing its mineral content.

Although soil filtration cleanses most pollutants from percolating water, ground water is still vulnerable to contamination. Plants and microorganisms, for example, do not break down most chlorinated hydrocarbons, a class of nonbiodegradable synthetic organic compounds that can be harmful to health. The long-range effects of groundwater pollution are more serious than surface water pollution because it takes many years to flush waste out of an aquifer. Most people who have bad wells simply choose to abandon them rather than try to cleanse them.

Because ground water moves slowly, a slug of contaminant moving with the ground water will flow and disperse into a plume, the dimensions of which are controlled by the structure of the aquifer. Because of the slow rate of travel and the vagaries of flow and dispersion, ground water may be heavily contaminated in one place, but remain pristine only a few hundred feet away. Size of the openings influences how fast water can flow through an aquifer.

Adding to the difficulty of detecting contaminated aquifers is the cost of testing and monitoring underground

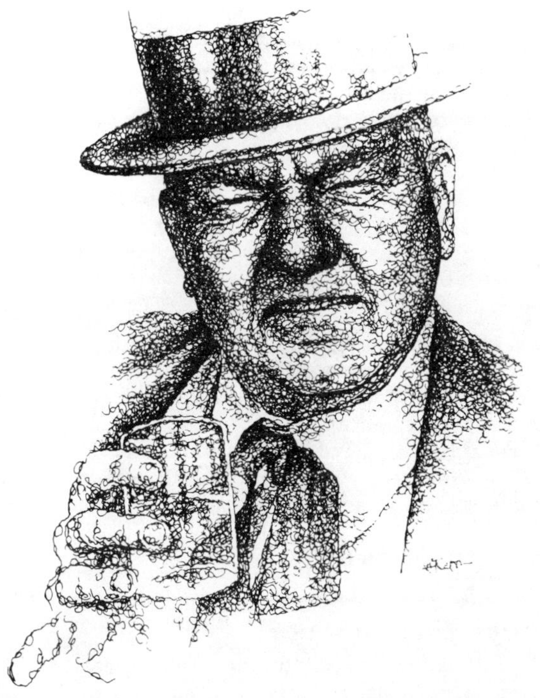

History of Water Management

Management problems in water programs and the lack of coordination among federal water agencies have been studied since 1908.

At that time, the Inland Waterways Commission in the administration of Theodore Roosevelt recommended coordinating all federal agencies involved in building waterways. A National Waterways Commission was authorized by Congress to coordinate the various water-related departments, but its members never were appointed, and in 1920 the authorization was repealed.

Since then there have been dozens of studies, commissions and reports calling for a unified national water policy. None prompted congressional action because states feared federal encroachment upon their water rights, and Congress resisted turning over water planning to the executive branch.

Then in 1961 the Senate Select Committee on Water Resources made five broad recommendations calling for:

- Comprehensive management plans for all the nation's river basins.
- Increased state involvement in water planning.
- Periodic assessment of regional water supplies.
- More federal water research.
- More federal emphasis on conservation.

Although the committee made no legislative proposals, most of its suggestions later were incorporated into two laws — The Water Resources Research Act of 1964 and the Water Resources Planning act of 1965.

The laws were touted as the long-sought answer to the coordination problem. Sponsors said they would put an end to the fragmented, project-oriented approach to water planning.

In signing the 1965 act, President Lyndon B. Johnson said, "The day is past when the nation can afford to listen to, or laugh smugly with, those who have gone about slandering our water resources projects as pork barrel and boondoggle."

But the acts failed to achieve that goal. The nation's water program still is criticized frequently by environmentalists as being riddled with economically unjustifiable projects built at the behest of politically powerful constituents or members of Congress.

The 1964 law set up an Office of Water Research and Technology, which provided grants to universities to develop better water conservation methods.

The 1965 act established the Water Resources Council (WRC), designed to be the focal point for national water planning. It was to encourage conservation and coordinate water quantity and quality programs. The law also established six river basin commissions to manage rivers on a regional basis.

But the council and the river basin commissions have been ineffective largely because neither has authority to enforce planning efforts. The WRC has been unable to coordinate quantity and quality programs, mostly because it cannot control the two most powerful water agencies — the Army Corps of Engineers and the Environmental Protection Agency. In addition, the council is chaired by the secretary of the interior, whose agency concentrates on Western water issues. That has led states and other federal agencies to distrust the council's objectivity.

President Carter tried unsuccessfully to establish a national water policy and to strengthen the WRC. The plan sparked a bitter confrontation between Carter and Congress, which refused to relinquish water policy making to the executive branch.

As a result of the standoff between Carter and Congress, no water project authorization bill was enacted during his administration.

---

wells. When ground water occurs in varying layers, several separate testing wells must be dug in order to test one aquifer. Further assessment of the quality of the water requires sophisticated and expensive equipment.

According to Robert H. Harris, a member of the Council on Environmental Quality in 1980, the volume of ground water under the United States is estimated to be about 50 times the volume of annual surface water flow. About 45 percent of this amount can be recovered.

Pollution from Sewage

Contamination of ground water from human activities may come from surface garbage disposal sites, landfills, agriculture, land disposal of waste waters, septic tanks, mining, petroleum and natural gas production, underground injection wells and other sources. In most cases, the source of contamination is from leachate from septic tanks or cesspools. Each year, according to Carol Keough in *Water Fit to Drink,* 1,700 billion gallons of waste liquids from toilets are placed in the ground, most of which are liquid wastes from domestic septic systems. Other wastes are found on the land, in landfills or in dumps.

In 1980, approximately 19.5 million housing units in the United States used onsite disposal systems. Some operated well, others did not. These systems discharge an estimated 1 trillion gallons of waste onto the ground each year. Septic tanks and cesspools rank highest in total volume of waste water discharged directly to ground water and are the most frequently reported sources of fecal, toxic and other contamination. Septic tank discharges often contaminate private wells.

In most areas, homeowners can buy septic tank cleaning fluids which usually contain trichloroethylene (TCE), benzene, or methylene chloride. A gallon or less of the fluid, when flushed down a toilet, dissolves the sludge in a septic tank so that it flows into the solid adsorption field. This practice causes two types of severe ground water contamination. The sludge itself is a contaminant, but more important, TCE is a known animal carcinogen. TCE and other chlorinated organic solvents spread with the ground water. An estimated 400,000 gallons of these septic tank cleaners were used by homeowners in 1979 on Long Island alone.

In most towns, domestic wastes are treated by municipal sewage plants that may dispose of domestic wastes in deep injection wells or shallow wells. The use of deep injection wells (wells drilled deep into the ground where waste is then disposed of in underground cavities) results in fewer cases of ground water contamination.

Most U.S. water supply systems filter water through beds of sand. This traps particles in the water, but organic compounds, including pesticides, are not in particle form and can get through. However, if the water is passed through a bed of activated carbon granules, a far more effective purification system is produced. Many organic compounds are "adsorbed" onto the surface of the carbon and held there. Activated carbon purification is in widespread use in U.S. food and beverage plants and in drinking-water plants in other countries, but it is rare in U.S. drinking systems.

Organic compounds in raw water supplies have long been a problem for designers of community water systems. In early summer and fall, vast collections of algae and other organisms bloom in lakes and reservoirs and then die, giving foul tastes and odors to the water. A test of the organic compounds that make the stench has been developed. Water samples are run through a test device containing activated carbon; organic compounds adhere to the carbon and are then extracted by means of chloroform and weighted. This test, however, is seldom run, although it is recommended in current drinking-water standards.

Contamination of drinking supplies can be attributed to pipes through which the water passes, cross connections between water lines and sewage lines or other possible sources of contamination. Finally, water can become contaminated after it leaves a treatment plant if the pressure in the distribution system falls too low. In that event, backflow may occur, returning polluted water to the system for redistribution.

Chemical Pollution

An estimated 500 to 1,000 new chemicals are being introduced by the nation's chemical industry each year, adding to the more than 100,000 chemical compounds that already exist. Industrial waste, generated by the manufacture of these synthetic compounds, is considered the major contributor of harmful substances to our drinking water. A 1980 EPA report found that one or more hazardous organic or inorganic substances had contaminated the ground water at 50 industrial waste disposal sites. Contaminants found in the ground water were selenium, arsenic, chromium, lead, cyanide, copper, nickel and barium. Organic contaminants include polychlorinated biphenyls, chlorinated phenols, benzene and other solvents.

When synthetic organic compounds such as these get into food and drinking water they can cause serious health problems. At high concentrations, many synthetic organic compounds can cause nausea, dizziness, tumors and blindness — problems that have not normally been associated with drinking water. At lower concentrations, humans may develop skin eruptions or nervous system impairment.

Other sources of contaminants are pesticides and soil sterilants that combine with normal runoff water generated by rains or snows or domestic wastes. Chlorine, when used to disinfect water, interacts with normal humic acid produced as organic matter decomposes. The combination forms chloro-organics, some of which are known carcinogens.

Perhaps the most difficult pollutants to control are those that come from non-point sources. A contaminant that can be traced to a specific source, such as a pipe discharging chemicals from a factory, is a point source. A non-point source is one in which the main source of the pollutant cannot be easily identified. In such a case, the source is diffuse, such as a pesticide that runs off a field and drains into a stream or well.

Injection wells also cause contamination because wastes are pumped thousands of feet beneath the ground's surface. Leakage from these wells is common. Deep well injection of liquid wastes has become a common practice over the last two decades, especially for the chemical, petrochemical and pharmaceutical industries. *(See box p. 34)*

Examples of Contamination Sites

Several instances of underground water contamination have occurred within the last three years in New England. In May 1978, four wells in Bedford, Mass., which provide 80 percent of the town's drinking water, were found to be contaminated with toxic chemicals. The contamination was discovered by accident when a resident engineer was testing the water for a paper he was writing.

Bedford was forced to restrict water use and ban new water connections. The town also bought water from four neighboring towns, until one of them closed two of its main wells because of trichloraethyline contamination. As a result of the contamination, state and federal officials conducted studies of an unexpected pattern of cancer deaths among women in the town of Bedford to see if it were due to statistical chance or some community-wide environmental cause. Analysis of Bedford death certificates from 1969 through 1978 by the state's Department of Public Health revealed a jump in cancer deaths among women, but not men, during the second four years following discovery of the water contamination.

In Gray, Maine, 16 private drinking wells were closed in 1977 after it was discovered that they were contaminated with toxic organic chemicals. All were located near an industrial waste handling facility built in 1972 to process waste oil. From 1972 to 1977, the facility was used as a transfer station. Materials were mixed, stored in tanks, and shipped to refiners. Approximately 100,000-200,000 gallons were processed annually at the Gray site.

Wastes spilled at the processing facility leached into the ground water. Offensive odors were reported in drinking water from nearby wells. The well water discolored laundry. Although samples were tested at the state laboratory, the contaminants were not identified. The residents then turned to alternate sources of water eventually extending the town pipeline.

In August 1979, a visiting cancer expert found children playing in and around drums and oily spills within the fenced off site where the gate of the transfer station facility had been left open. In a letter sent to a state health official, a cancer expert wrote that "in Gray homes of the 16 in which people had consumed water from wells now closed, seven reported skin rashes, five reported eye irritations, one reported a miscarriage, four mentioned urinary tract problems, seven mentioned central nervous or peripheral nervous system problems, eight reported gastrointestinal problems, and three reported respiratory problems."

Long Island has had a particularly tough time with contaminated water supplies. A two-year study of water pollution on Long Island concluded in August 1980 that toxic industrial wastes were gradually contaminating even the purest supplies of drinking water there and that federal and state regulatory programs have failed to stop the pollution.

In response to this, a 250-page study was written by the New York Public Interest Research Group that reviewed 1,453 federal and state discharge permits and found that none contained stringent controls on waterborne waste disposal by 100 Long Island companies. The report also said that 66 companies on Long Island avoided direct federal and state regulations by discharging nearly 10 million gallons of contaminated waste water into 11 municipal sewage systems each day.

As a result, according to the report, Long Island's cancer mortality rate was in the top 10 percent of the nation, adding that "high cancer mortality may be directly linked to toxic pollutants consumed in water or absorbed via other routes of exposure." Some of the more hazardous chemicals identified in the study were benzene, toluene, trichloroethylene and perchlorethylene, all manmade compounds that are part of industrial processes. "The entire underground water reserve will eventually become contaminated and unfit as a source of public water supply," said the report, unless new and costly purification programs are instituted.

Further complicating the ground water issue is the fact that underground aquifers often lie beneath several states. Depletion or pollution of an aquifer in one state can cause problems in another state.

For instance, the Ogalalla Aquifer underneath the High Plains stretches from South Dakota to Texas. The aquifer levels are dropping because landowners in some states are taking out water faster than it is being replenished.

Other examples abound of problems created because ground water and surface water are not jointly managed.

- The $1.7 billion Tennessee-Tombigbee Waterway being built in Tennessee, Mississippi and Alabama, will de-

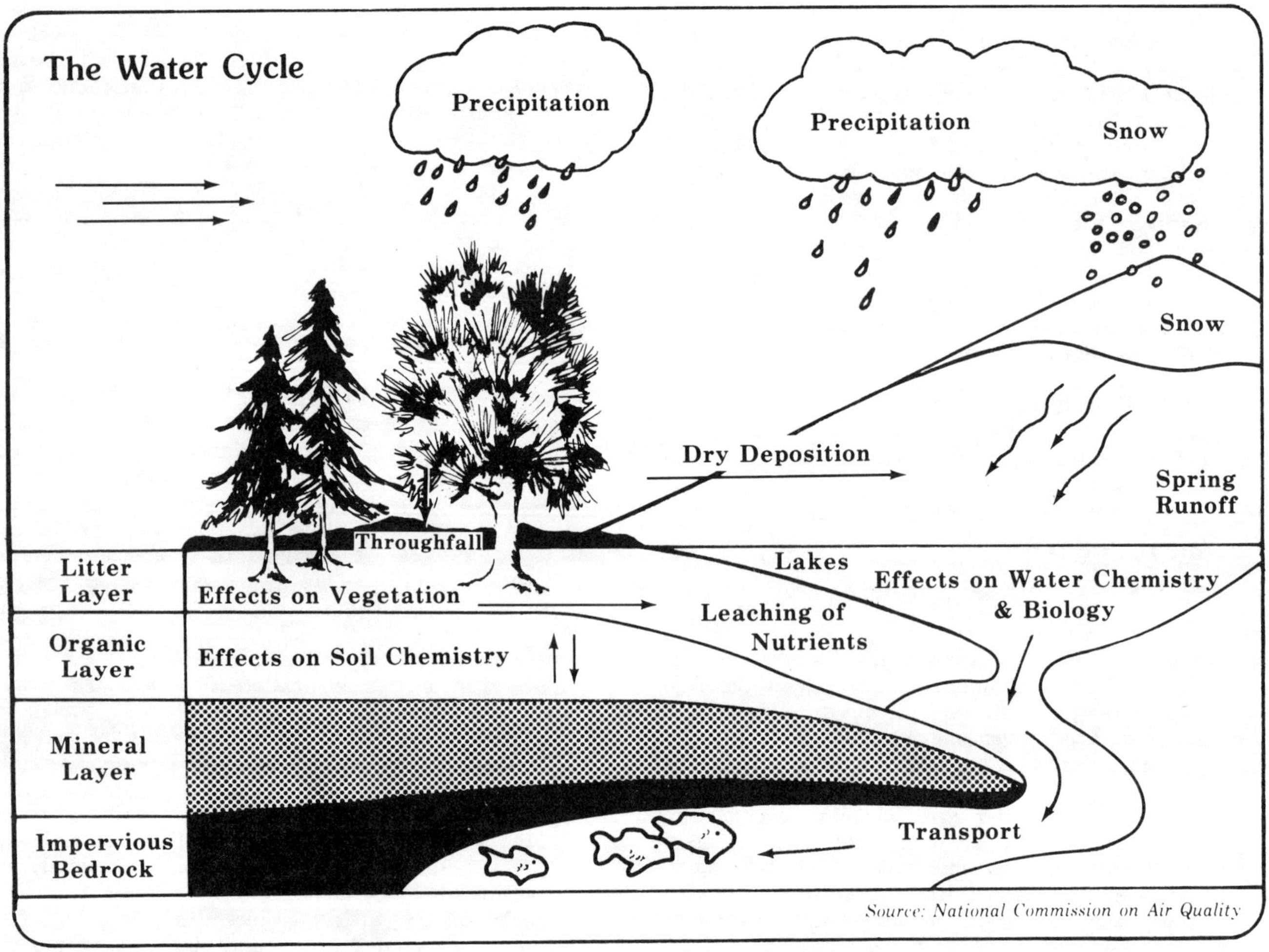

Source: National Commission on Air Quality

plete water tables nearby. Rep. Jamie L. Whitten, D-Miss., asked Congress in the spring of 1981 to compensate landowners for their lost water supplies.

- In Monmouth, N.J., officials wanted to build a dam in 1981 on the Manasquan River to provide water for coastal residents because their ground water was threatened by sea water seeping in. But upstream from the proposed reservoir was a chemical dump, leaking into the ground water that replenishes the river that would feed into the reservoir.
- To prevent flooding, millions of dollars in the 1930s and 1940s were spent to drain low-lying areas around south Florida's Lake Okeechobee. The water was pumped to the ocean, away from the wetlands that had helped recharge the ground water underneath. That ground water provides drinking water for coastal cities farther south, but as of early 1981 salt water was seeping into it from the ocean.

Pre-1980 Legislation

Congress has passed four laws that deal in part with ground water, but it has not coordinated those laws with state statutes. The four laws are the Federal Water Pollution Control Act, the Safe Drinking Water Act, the Resource Conservation and Recovery Act and the Surface Mining Control and Reclamation Act.

The Federal Water Pollution Control Act of 1970 replaced pollution laws going back to 1899 and greatly expanded sewage treatment grants.

The principal federal law on water pollution is the Federal Water Pollution Control Act Amendments of 1972, one of the most comprehensive and expensive environmental pieces of legislation in the nation's history. This law initiated a major change in the basic approach to water-pollution control in the United States by limiting effluent discharges and setting water-quality standards. It set a national goal of eliminating all pollutant discharges into U.S. waters by 1985 and an interim goal of making the waters safe for fish, shellfish, wildlife and people by July 1, 1983. To that end, it required all U.S. industries, by July 1, 1977, to use the "best practicable control technology currently available" for treatment of any discharges. By July 1, 1983, industries will have to use the "best available technology economically achievable."

Limits are based on categories and classes of industries, and are aimed at complete elimination of discharges if technologically and economically possible. Industries may seek relief from the requirements based on alleged lack of economic capability. The law authorized more than $24.6 billion to be spent in cleaning up the nation's waters, including $18 billion in federal construction grants to the states for building waste-water treatment plants. These are allotted on the basis of need, as determined by the Environmental Protection Agency. The federal government pays 75 percent of the costs and state and local governments provide the remaining 25 percent. Finally, a pollutant-discharge-permit program was established under strict guidelines administered by the agency.

The Safe Drinking Water Act of 1974 directed the EPA to establish national standards setting maximum allowable levels for certain chemical and bacteriological pollutants in some 240,000 water systems (those serving more than 25 customers). Previous federal drinking water programs were limited primarily to prevention of the spread of communicable diseases through drinking water involved in interstate commerce. The act was amended in 1977.

Suggested Distances Between Contamination Source and Well Site

Source of Contamination	Distance*
Waste disposal lagoons	300
Cesspools	150
Livestock and poultry yards	100
Privies, manure piles	100
Silo pits, seepage pits	150
Milkhouse drain outlets	100
Septic tanks and disposal fields	100
Gravity sewer or drain not pressure tight	50
Pressure-tight gravity sewer or drain	25

*in feet

Source: Water Fit to Drink

The Resource Conservation and Recovery Act of 1976 established a federal permit program to regulate hazardous wastes and required states receiving federal grants to ban all open dumping within five years of enactment. Finally, the Surface Mining and Reclamation Act of 1977 stated that mining operations could not interrupt, discontinue or permanently damage the quality or quantity of underground or surface water.

Renewed Concern in 1980

Most states do not recognize the hydrological connection between ground and surface water, and many states have no policies for water management. They often allow landowners to pump ground water without regard to the effect it has on nearby water supplies.

In response to growing alarm over the contamination problem, Toby Moffett, D-Conn., chairman of the House Government Operations Subcommittee on Environment, Energy and Natural Resources, held a two-day hearing in July 1980 to study the problems of ground water contamination.

Moffett, in his opening statement, stressed the urgency of the ground water pollution problem. "The hard lesson we must learn," said Moffett, "is that our Earth is not a bottomless sponge which will soak up poisons and somehow miraculously make them go away or become safe to consume. Now, not later, is the time to reverse this unseen and insidious trend toward the destruction of our precious ground water resources. We must develop a national policy on ground water."

During the hearings, Robert Harris of the Council on Environmental Quality testified that contamination of ground water was a largely irreversible process, very expensive to detect and impossible to predict.

"The discoveries of contamination of ground water by toxic, synthetic organic chemicals are particularly disturbing," Harris said. "The levels of contamination are in many cases far higher — orders of magnitude higher — than

Sources of Ground Water Contamination

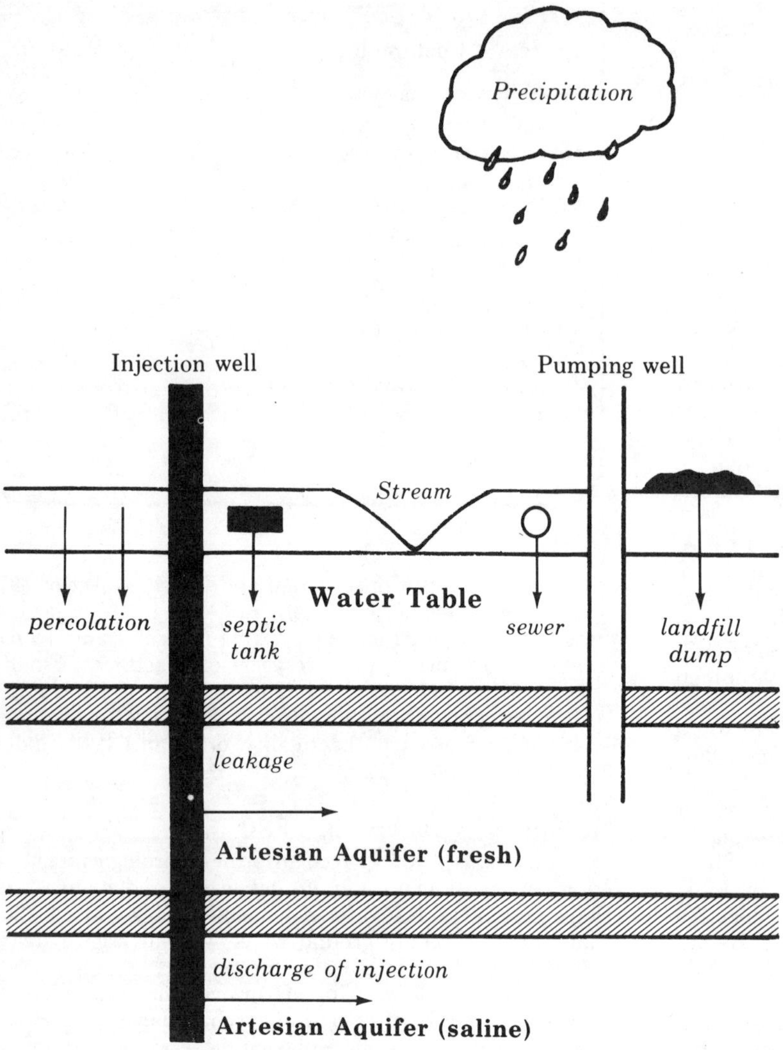

Source: Council on Environmental Quality

Contamination of ground water from human activities may come from a multitude of sources. Major contamination sources include injection and pumping wells, septic tanks, sewers, contaminated streams and landfill dumps.

those found in raw or finished drinking waters from the most contaminated surface supplies, such as the Ohio and Mississippi Rivers."

Other witnesses noted the tendency for chemicals previously dumped in rivers and lakes before passage of the Safe Drinking Water Act to show up in water supplies obtained from underground sources.

"....[C]ontaminants that we began observing in surface waters in 1973 and 1974 that led to the passage of the Safe Drinking Water Act, are now showing up in alarmingly high concentrations in much of the nation's drinking water supplies obtained from underground sources," Harris said.

Harris went on to outline the vastness of the nation's ground water sources. According to his testimony, 50 times as much water is present as ground water in this country than flows in all our rivers and streams over a year.

EPA Activity

As a result of the hearings, EPA proposed a strategy in the fall of 1980 for ground water protection that got mixed reviews from industrial leaders. EPA proposed setting up a three-tiered classification system for the protection of the nation's ground water based on use and protection of natural resources. The first category was to protect aquifers that are important sources of drinking water, the second category covered aquifers that could supply drinking water, and the third category limited degradation such as that normally associated with energy development, industrial activities and waste disposal.

"Our notion ... is that in the future the classification system will serve as the mechanism by which public debate is fostered on any major development with ground water and public policy implications," the EPA's deputy assistant administrator for drinking water, Victor Kimm, said at a hearing in 1980.

Thus, while the EPA has stated that a non-degradation goal is "impossible," a primary concern in the strategy will be to set up priority areas for protection. In addition, while the Chemical Manufacturers Association told the EPA it preferred that the goal of the strategy be to provide a technique for the efficient management of water, the EPA responded that the general thrust would be health and environmental concerns. Industrial leaders worried that the classification system would prove difficult to implement because of its land use control implications.

SURFACE WATER: KEEPING PROBLEM AT BAY

Surface water, as the term suggests, is water found on the surface of the earth. It is supplied by rain and includes puddles, rivers, creeks, lakes or streams. About half the country's population gets its drinking supply from surface water.

The Council on Environmental Quality reported in 1980 that the quality of the nation's surface water had changed little over the previous five years. This suggested the nation had stemmed pollution in rivers and lakes, but only to maintain the status quo of five years earlier. Evidence showed that pollution from toxic wastes remained widespread.

Approximately half of the pollutants received by rivers and lakes come from storm sewers, municipal sewage treatment plants and industries. The rest comes from untreated and uncontrolled runoff from parking lots, lawns, agricultural areas and construction sites. In some rivers and lakes of already dubious quality, this additional pollution is often just enough to make the water unacceptable.

Problems in the management of urban runoff have begun to appear. For example, according to CEQ, of the 6,623 municipal sewage treatment projects begun since 1972, only 1,552 were in operation as of December 1979. These facts suggested that the full effect of pollution control efforts would not be seen for several more years.

Nevertheless, some local areas have dealt successfully with surface water pollution problems:

- The Pemigewasset River, which runs through a well-known recreation area in New Hampshire, was so polluted by the mid-1960s that few fish survived in it and tourists spurned it. With the pollution control efforts of both industry and municipalities, 55 miles of the river are now suitable for fishing and swimming.
- In 1971, the Hackensack River in New Jersey was officially declared "virtually dead." The river was full of garbage and rusting cars, and many of the fish, shellfish and crustaceans that had thrived in it for years had disappeared. After an intensive five-year cleanup effort, the Hackensack Meadowlands Development Commission reported in 1976 that the river was coming back to life.

Rivers

Water quality degradation from toxic substances has continued to threaten the purity of the country's rivers. Since 1976, the James, Hudson, Shenandoah, Susquehanna, the Delaware, the Housatonic, the Coosa, the Shiawassee, the Mobile, the Tombigbee, and the Holston Rivers have been affected by toxic pollutants.

The 1978 State Water Quality reports to Congress, submitted under the Clean Water Act Amendments of 1977, revealed that 35 of the 37 states reporting had a problem with pollution by toxic substances. According to these reports, the most widely reported toxic substances contaminating rivers were heavy metal residues released by industries. Pollution by pesticides ranked as second to metals in the same category. Pollution from cyanides, phenols, polychlorinated biphenyls and other industrial chemicals also was reported by more than one-half of the reporting states. Polychlorinated biphenyls (PCBs) were reported as a problem in eight states; as a result, fishing was restricted in parts of the Hudson and Housatonic Rivers, and fish consumption bans or warnings were issued in Connecticut, New York, Michigan and other states.

Heavy metals include lead, cadmium and mercury. Because their concentrations are frequently below the detection limits of measuring equipment, data are often reported simply as "less than" a given value. Industrial wastes with dangerous lead contents have been dumped into rivers and lakes. Even at low levels, lead in the blood stream can poison the body's ability to fight off infections and other harmful substances. Many experiments with animals have shown that small doses of lead that produce no obvious signs of poisoning can severely hamper the body's ability to fight off bacterial and viral infections or survive the poisons bacteria produce.

Waste produced from electroplating, photography, insecticide and mining industries contain traces of cadmium, another highly toxic metal. Cadmium accumulates in the body and after 10 to 20 years of stockpiling can lead to health problems including high blood pressure, kidney disease, and emphysema. Mercury is also a deadly metal when ingested. It is used in some paints and other industrial products, causing an upswing in mercury contamination in recent years. Mercury affects the nervous system and kidneys where it can cause grave damage. Often mercury enters humans through the food chain from fish.

Pollution of rivers and streams by pesticides is also a serious problem. More than one-half of the states reporting in the 1978 state quality reports listed problems with pesticide pollution. The South Central states are most affected by pesticide pollution, but there is some evidence of improvements following certain restrictions on pesticide use. In Arkansas, for example, concentrations of DDT in river and streams have gradually decreased.

Lakes

According to the Council on Environmental Quality's 1980 report to Congress, 99 percent of the population lives within 50 miles of a publicly owned fresh water lake and at least one-third lives within five miles of a lake. Conservative estimates list more than 10,000 of these lakes as in need of pollution reduction or restoration.

EPA first acted to help clean up and protect publicly owned lakes by establishing the Clean Lakes Program in 1975. The program funded state and local demonstration

Pesticide-Related Water Pollution, 1978

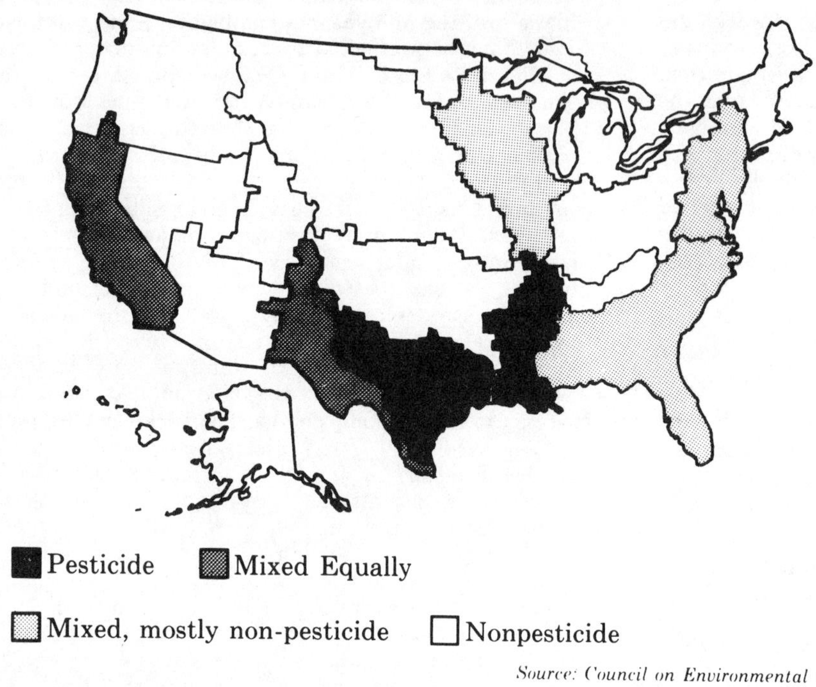

Pollution of rivers and streams by pesticides is a serious problem. The most prominent area of pesticide-related water pollution is in the South Central states.

projects to restore publicly owned fresh water lakes. In 1979, EPA made the program part of the state water quality planning and management effort of the state-EPA agreement process.

Perhaps the most widespread pollution problem connected with lakes is a process called eutrophication. Eutrophication begins with the increased production of plants within the lake. When they die, they settle to the bottom and decay. In the process, they use up dissolved oxygen in the water and gradually fill the lake. When pollutants are discharged into the lake, they provide excessive nutrients that accelerate this process. The algae grow and bloom, becoming so dense that they block sunlight from deeper parts of the lake or river. Fish and invertebrates can no longer live in such a place. When a lake or river eutrophies it is said to be dying.

Waste Management

The Senate began in spring 1981 to overhaul the multibillion-dollar sewage treatment plant construction program, the nation's second largest civilian public works program.

Second only to the federal highway system in cost, the Environmental Protection Agency's massive program to clean up the nation's waters has cost the taxpayers $33 billion since its inception in 1972 and at current spending rates could eventually cost $120 billion. EPA is authorized under the Clean Water Act to spend $5 billion a year through 1982 for construction grants to municipalities. From these funds, EPA makes grants for 75 to 85 percent of eligible costs of designing and constructing municipal wastewater treatment and collection facilities. Other monies have been appropriated for areawide planning grants and for state planning.

Yet the program has been criticized by nearly everyone involved in it: the states that receive the 75 percent federal construction grants, the engineers who build the plants, the General Accounting Office (GAO), congressional investigators and EPA.

Critics say the program has been too rigid, is riddled with fraud and costly bureaucratic delays, has produced huge "white elephant" plants that often do not work and has been a major catalyst for urban sprawl. Nobody really knows how much the program has improved the nation's waters, and many pollution control officials fear urban and agricultural runoff, which is largely unregulated, is negating many of the cleanup efforts.

The ambitious program to build thousands of sewage treatment plants was launched in 1972 with enactment of the Federal Water Pollution Control Act. The act was amended in 1977 when Congress passed the Clean Water Act.

The 1972 act, which replaced water pollution control laws dating back to 1899, set two goals: fishable and swimmable waters by 1983 and elimination of all polluted discharges into navigable waters by 1985.

It required industries to install certain equipment by July 1, 1977, and more stringent technology by July 1, 1983. Cities were to provide "secondary treatment" — removing 85 percent of pollutants — by July 1, 1977, and to use the "best practicable" technology by mid-1983. EPA was to define each of the technologies.

One persistent complaint about the 1972 law was that it required high-technology equipment nationwide — in order to achieve zero discharges by 1985 — regardless of how clean or dirty the water was where the treated water was being dumped.

Recognizing the need for more flexibility, Congress in 1977 allowed for "innovative and alternative" technologies — such as using treated sewage water for irrigation or recycling it for other uses.

The 1977 amendments, which authorized $5 billion a year through fiscal 1982, also gave industry until 1984 to clean up toxic and conventional pollutants, and until 1987 to clean up other pollutants. Cities won an additional six years, until 1983, to clean up their discharges if they had not received promised federal funds, as did industries tying into those plants.

In 1980 the act was amended again to repeal a requirement that industries discharging wastes into city-owned plants pay some of the cost of building those plants and to allow states to assume more than their normal 25 percent share.

Since 1972, $38.98 billion has been authorized and $33.3 billion appropriated for construction grants. Of the 13,000 grants awarded to date, about 3,200 plants are now operating.

The GAO, in 18 studies of the construction grants program in the years between 1978 and 1981 found that:

- Secondary treatment is often unnecessary and could be replaced by cheaper alternative technologies.
- Expensive advanced treatment facilities, which remove all pollutants from wastewater, often do not improve water quality but can cost five times more than secondary plants.
- Non-point sources of pollution such as agricultural and urban runoff may prevent many areas from meeting the 1983 cleanup deadline, yet they have received only 1 percent of the total water pollution control funds.
- Up to 87 percent of the treatment plants surveyed violated their discharge permits at least once a year, and 31 percent were in "serious" violation. The failures were caused by design and equipment deficiencies, overloads from storms and leaks, toxic effluents from industries, and lack of operator training.
- "Staggering" operation and maintenance costs, which could reach $30 billion by 1990, create a heavy financial burden on low-income families in small communities.
- Enforcement by EPA and the states varies from none to minimal, and virtually no one is held legally responsible for the failure of treatment plants.

"Billions of taxpayer dollars have been invested in these treatment plants, and much of it appears to have literally gone down the drain," said Rep. Elliott H. Levitas, D-Ga., chairman of the House Public Works Committee's Investigations and Oversight Subcommittee.

Escalating costs are a major problem. Initial estimates were that the program would require a total investment of $63 billion in 1972 dollars. But because of inflation, bureaucratic delays and population growth, EPA estimated that by the year 2000 it will cost $120 billion to reach the cleanup goals, with the federal share approaching $90 billion.

"It is apparent that the federal government cannot bear the financial burden of meeting all municipal wastewater treatment system eligibilities, including future growth and needs," John Hernandez, then deputy EPA administrator, told the Senate Environment Committee's Environmental Pollution Subcommittee in June 1981.

Hernandez said the administration is trying to streamline the program to speed up construction schedules. One effort is to "fast track" high priority plants: those that would result in the greatest improvement in water quality per dollar spent. The goal is to have 80 percent of those plants under design within 24 months of receipt of a grant application.

CHANGING POLICY: NEW VIEWS IN CONGRESS

There were strong indications in early 1981 that Congress — pressured by governors and state water officials — would be ready to rewrite federal water policy by 1982.

"You have a great amount of interest, and the problems are so pronounced that the opportunity for revising water policy is very real," said Don H. Clausen, R-Calif., ranking minority member of the House Public Works Committee.

Clausen was backed by Robert A. Roe, D-N.J., who became the new chairman of the House Public Works Subcommittee on Water Resources in 1981.

"We see the scattered jurisdiction throughout Congress and the executive branch as the crucial problem," Roe said. "We're spending tens of billions of dollars on programs that are countervening somebody else's effort."

As of 1981, no new federal water supply projects had been authorized in four years because of a water policy stalemate between the Carter administration and Congress. Members were eager to break that logjam because it has meant a loss of federal dollars for their states. However, federal government budget constraints will force a careful examination of how and where those dollars will be spent.

Congressional Water Jurisdiction

Here is a list of the congressional committees with jurisdiction over water issues. The number of subcommittees each panel has assigned to deal with water is in parentheses.

House Committees	Senate Committees
Agriculture (3)	Agriculture (3)
Appropriations (6)	Appropriations (6)
Banking (1)	Banking (2)
Budget	Budget
Energy and Commerce (4)	Commerce (1)
Government Operations (1)	Energy (2)
Interior (4)	Environment and Public Works (4)
Merchant Marine and Fisheries (4)	Finance
Public Works (3)	Governmental Affairs (2)
Science and Technology (2)	Small Business (1)
Small Business (1)	
Ways and Means	

In addition, several of the powerful, longtime chairmen of key water committees — men who favored the traditional approach to water policy — retired or were defeated for re-election in 1980. They were replaced by reform-minded members.

President Reagan on taking office in 1981 sent to Congress numerous changes in former President Carter's federal budget for fiscal 1982 beginning Oct. 1, 1981. Among the changes were several major revisions in water programs. The president wanted to abolish the federal Water Resources Council (WRC), which was designed to coordinate federal water programs; reform the Clean Water Act's sewer construction grants program; eliminate the coastal zone management program and increase inland waterway user fees.

Other water measures before Congress in mid-1981, separate from Reagan's budget, that could spark a water policy debate included a Senate bill to establish block grants for water project construction and a House measure to charge Western farmers more for their federally subsidized irrigation water.

Kepone Pollution

In July 1975, illness struck seven workers employed at Life Science Products in Hopewell, Va., a company that manufactured Kepone, a highly toxic insecticide, for Allied Chemical Co. It was found that the workers' trembling and shaking were a result of their exposure to the chemical.

The problem of Kepone poisoning extended far beyond Hopewell. Both Life Science and Allied, which developed Kepone and produced it from 1966 until Life Science took over in 1973, had discharged Kepone into the James River which empties into the Chesapeake Bay.

As a result of the Kepone discharge, the Life Science plant was closed, Kepone production was halted in Virginia, the state's then-Gov. Mills E. Godwin ordered a ban on fishing in the James River, the federal government prohibited the manufacture of all pesticides containing Kepone, and Congress and the state legislature began lengthy hearings on tightening environmental regulations. Life Science, Allied and the city of Hopewell were brought to court and charged with hundreds of violations of federal and state water pollution laws. They have been convicted on some of the charges. Some were dismissed or dropped while others were pursued.

Kepone poisoning was not limited to the air, water and soil around Hopewell nor even to the James River. Traces were found in the lower Chesapeake Bay and the Atlantic Ocean. Kepone causes neurological disorders and there is fear it may be harmful to the liver, spleen, brain and male fertility. It is also suspected of causing cancer.

Split Jurisdictions

One obstacle to the merger of water quantity and quality programs was the fragmented congressional jurisdiction over the two problems.

Twelve House panels and 29 of their subcommittees, and 10 Senate committees and 21 subcommittees had responsibilities for water in the 97th Congress that began in 1981. Most of them dealt with either supply or quality, and those with jurisdiction over both usually assigned them to separate subcommittees.

In addition to fostering inconsistencies among federal water agencies, the split jurisdictions had resulted in the same dichotomy of purpose in state agencies that administer grants handed out by the federal agencies.

Federal water supply money usually is channeled through four agencies: the Interior Department's Bureau of Reclamation, the U.S. Army Corps of Engineers, the Tennessee Valley Authority and the Soil Conservation Service in the Department of Agriculture. They handle dams, irrigation, flood control, navigation and hydroelectric power.

But their missions often conflict with the goals of agencies that control water pollution or protect wetland wildlife habitats, such as the EPA and the U.S. Fish and Wildlife Service.

State-Federal Coordination

In addition, federally funded water pollution programs often are not coordinated with local water supply problems. For example:

- Sewage lines often were constructed on rivers near drinking water intake lines built by cities.
- In the 1970s, EPA encouraged construction of massive regional sewage treatment plants that used large amounts of water. Cities drew their water from rivers and lakes, sent it to homes and then sent the sewage to treatment plants, usually located downstream. The plants then dumped the treated sewage — which is more than 90 percent pure water — into a river or the ocean. The treated water was rarely recycled into upstream lakes from which the original water had come. Water supply shortages in upstream cities resulted.
- EPA rules governing the temperature and content of discharges into rivers has meant that it often is cheaper for companies to divert their discharges into off-stream lagoons or storage tanks than to treat them and return them to the rivers. The result: less water flowing downstream, which creates more pollution because there is less water to dilute pollutants.
- The $1.7 billion Central Arizona Project, which will divert fresh water from the Colorado River to Phoenix and Tucson, is expected to cause salinity problems downstream. As a result, the government is building a $350 million desalting plant in Yuma, Ariz.

Another government policy that has added to water management problems is the large number of cost-sharing schemes offered by agencies distributing state and local grants. There are at least 160 different types of arrangements in which states pay back or share costs with the federal government.

The proliferation has encouraged states to "shop around" for the federal programs that require the least amount of local matching funds. Consequently, instead of

Lake Water Impairment, 1978

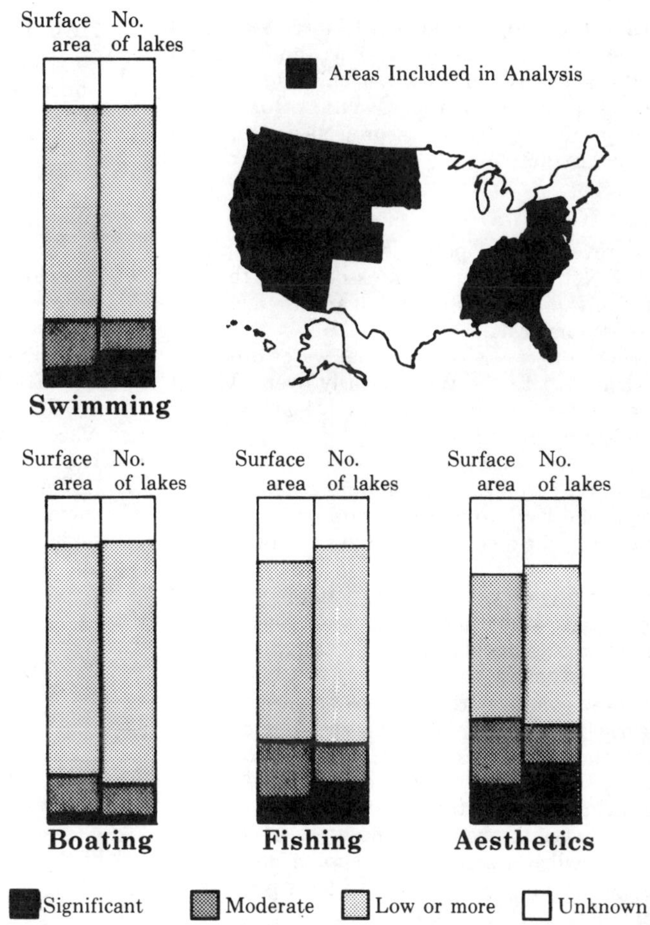

Source: Council on Environmental Quality

The level of pollution of lake water is determined largely by the quality of feeder streams and disposal of nearby wastes, land use practices, soil erosion and runoff of fertilizers and pesticides from farmlands and gardens. Airborne pollutants can also affect lake water quality.

solving their most urgent water needs, cities have solved those problems for which the federal government was most willing to provide help.

Rethinking in Congress

The drought, the continuing congressional logjam holding up new projects and a growing realization that the current method of approving water projects is not meeting certain needs have been factors pushing Congress toward action.

For example, it takes an average of 26 years to get a flood control project under way after it has been authorized. There is a $33 billion backlog of authorized but unfunded Corps of Engineers projects, according to the Senate Environment Subcommittee on Water Resources.

In addition, there is growing sentiment that the traditional "backscratching" method of doling out federal water dollars needs to be replaced.

Federal dams, navigation projects, levees and harbors have been the product of mutual accommodation among members of Congress. Water projects have been viewed as a way to aid districts and states, even if the expenditures did not always make good economic sense or damaged the environment. Water projects also are visible evidence to the voters back home that a representative or senator is doing his job.

Consequently, members seldom question projects in colleagues' districts.

Sen. Pete V. Domenici, R-N.M., a critic of federal water policy, has charged that it consists of "a willy-nilly listening to a few congressional witnesses on their pet projects."

Sen. Alan K. Simpson, R-Wyo., in 1979 characterized Congress' water project authorization process as "the most classic exercise extant of how to pour [federal money] down the rathole." Simpson vowed to help revamp the process, although he admitted the job would be "rougher than a stucco bathtub."

Budget pressures may force Congress to seek cheaper alternatives to traditional projects, and new members who campaigned on anti-spending platforms will be sensitive to charges of wasteful spending if they vote for economically unjustifiable projects. Environmentalists trying to reform water policy hope to recruit some of those members for the battle.

"Pressures of the budget are going to force a rational evaluation of water project authorizations, and rational evaluation is the antithesis of pork barrel," said Edward Osann, executive director of the Coalition for Water Project Review, a group that fights projects it considers environmentally destructive.

Pressure for Reform

Pressure to revamp water policy is coming from groups as diverse as the National Governors' Association, the National Academy of Public Administration and the National Society of Professional Engineers.

Also spurring Congress is the fact that water problems no longer are confined to the West. Nearly every district has experienced water shortages, pollution, leaking water mains or diminishing ground water.

Rising health issues, such as increased evidence of carcinogens in water supplies and contamination of previously pristine ground water sources are adding to the pressure on Congress to take a closer look at water control and regulation.

However, breaking down the institutional barriers and untangling the congressional jurisdictions will not be easy or popular. Members' parochialism has fostered the fragmentation, and it is deeply entrenched.

"Each of these overlapping programs has its own constituency, its own unique legislative history and congressional supporters, its own collection of regulations and customs, and its own set of priorities," said Larry Silverman of Clean Water Action in 1981.

Silverman believes the budget committees in Congress are the ones that will oversee the overlapping programs.

"The Budget Committee is in an excellent position to scrutinize all of the many federal water programs," Silverman told the House Budget Committee in early 1981. "Your budget cutting activities should cover the whole waterfront."

New Leadership

Advocates of water policy reform pointed to the changes in the leadership on the major committees controlling water that occurred at the beginning of 1981 when the 97th Congress convened. Most of the former chairmen, who supported the current approach to water projects, left at the end of 1980.

On the House Public Works Committee, former chairman Harold T. Johnson, D-Calif. (1959-81), former Water Resources Subcommittee Chairman Ray Roberts, D-Texas (1962-81), and former ranking minority member William H. Harsha, R-Ohio (1961-81), left Congress through retirement or election defeat.

In the 97th Congress, the new chairman of the Public Works Committee and the Water Resources subcommittee were New Jersey Democrats James J. Howard and Robert A. Roe, respectively. Because New Jersey has some of the nation's worst water supply and pollution problems, Howard and Roe were expected to be particularly sensitive to the need for revisions in water policy philosophy.

On the Senate Environment and Public Works Committee, former Water Resources Subcommittee Chairman Mike Gravel, D-Alaska (1969-81), was defeated in 1980. He strongly resisted efforts by panel members Pete V. Domenici, R-N.M. and Daniel Patrick Moynihan, D-N.Y., to change water projects' funding methods.

House, Senate

Roe in 1981 held hearings on the drought and questioned witnesses extensively on what should be done to better coordinate federal programs dealing with water quantity and quality.

Roe said his panel would try to draft legislation that deals with the conflicts between federal water quality and quantity problems. "We need to recognize that they are one and the same," he said.

Roe's subcommittee had jurisdiction over both water supply and pollution laws, including the omnibus water projects' authorization bill and the sewage treatment construction grants program, that were scheduled for review in the 97th Congress.

In the Senate, James Abdnor, R-S.D., took Gravel's place as head of the Environment Subcommittee on Water Resources. Although he supported traditional project funding methods as a House member (1972-81), Abdnor was thought to favor reform initiatives because limited federal budget resources was expected to make the financing of any undertakings more difficult.

Projected Water Consumption

(Percentage of total fresh water consumption. Bracketed figures are millions of gallons of water per day.)

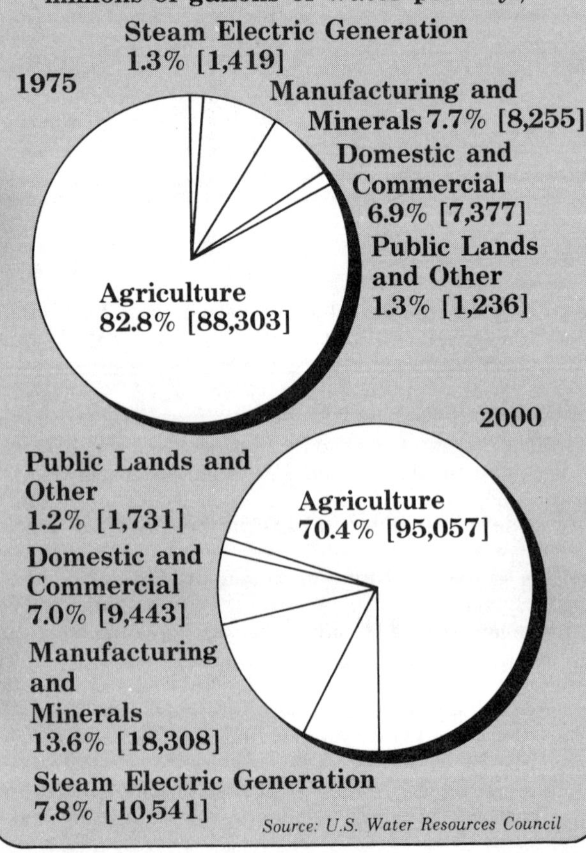

Source: U.S. Water Resources Council

A key player in the Senate debate was Domenici, who was a member of both Abdnor's panel and the Energy Committee. The latter committee authorizes Western reclamation projects. He also became the new chairman of the Budget Committee in 1981.

In March 1981, Domenici reintroduced with Moynihan a water policy reform package, first introduced in 1979, that would provide block grants to states based on population and size and let the states decide which projects should be built. States would be required to pay 25 percent of construction costs, with the federal government paying the rest.

Except for large interstate projects, such as navigational improvements, Congress would no longer be involved in project authorizations. That plan was criticized by some water officials because it would not improve coordination between federal water supply and pollution agencies. It dealt only with supply projects such as dams, not with funding for sewage treatment plants. Another criticism was that it would provide money to states based on their size, not their need.

Administration Review

However, much of what Congress does in 1982 or later was expected to depend on Reagan administration proposals. Through mid-1981, officials still refused comment on their plans, primarily because most officials who would help formulate policy still had not been confirmed.

Reagan proposed no new water projects in his fiscal 1982 budget revisions, cut out three Army Corps dams and refused to fund the sewer construction grants program until Congress revised it.

Interior Secretary James G. Watt said the administration hoped to propose new construction in fiscal 1983 and asked Western governors to help him set priorities. Watt indicated he might favor block grants for water projects and more state cost-sharing.

Because the current sewage treatment plant construction program is so expensive and troubled, President Reagan told Congress in March 1981 that he did not want to spend additional funds on sewage construction grants until the program was overhauled. He asked Congress to rescind or cancel $1.7 billion in fiscal 1981 grant funds that had already been approved, and said if Congress made the program more cost-effective he would seek $2.4 billion in fiscal 1982 grants. Congress in 1981 approved the rescission.

Reagan also wanted to reduce the federal government's future obligation from a projected $90 billion to $23 billion. He proposed eliminating federal funding for most projects serving rural areas and those providing for future growth. Instead, he said the money should be targeted to plants in large cities. His plan shifted federal sewer spending from rural and high-growth areas in the South and West to older cities in the Northeast and was expected to produce tough battles between representatives from those regions.

EPA Budget '82

Significant to continued upgrading of water quality will be the distribution of funds planned under "superfund" legislation passed by Congress in 1980. The superfund was financed over a period of five years by a combination of federal appropriations and taxes levied against chemical manufacturers. The fund was created to pay for cleaning up leaks into the environment of hazardous wastes when no responsible party could be identified or when the responsible party refuses to do so. In addition to the 1982 budget request of 503 personnel and a total of $200 million to support the program in its first year, EPA also requested a 1981 supplemental appropriation of $68 million for initial implementation.

On the other hand, President Reagan proposed reducing funds for EPA from approximately $1.43 billion and 10,621 workyears in 1981 to $1.39 billion and 10,387 workyears. These cuts were expected to affect EPA's grant program for sewage treatment construction. About $1.7 billion of 1981 and earlier year construction funds already appropriated were to be cancelled. Although the new construction grants budget for fiscal 1982 called for $2.4 billion, this was only for projects designed to improve significantly the quality of water in the near future.

The 1982 budget also eliminated both area-wide water planning grants funding, for a $34 million savings, and Clean Lakes, Solid Waste and Resource Recovery grants, for a $23 million decrease. The reductions reflected the fact that regulations and planning called for in the 1977 Clean Water Act amendments were to be largely completed in 1981. As a result, the program's principal focus was directed at carrying out existing requirements.

However, some of EPA's water cleanup efforts were to gain funds under the proposed budget. The ocean disposal program was to increase by $3.1 million to study the environmental effects of additional ocean dumping sites and EPA's enforcement of controls on toxic industrial discharges would be increased by $2.4 million.

Summary

Since 1974, there have been more than a dozen epidemiologic studies conducted on the health effects of contaminants generated by toxic wastes. Read together, these studies suggest an increased cancer risk associated with drinking water that has been contaminated by hazardous chemicals. Efforts to control the influx of these materials into rivers and lakes began in 1972 under the Clean Water Act, but the law did not cover ground water contamination. It is the ground water problem — in alarming contrast to the contamination of rivers and lakes — that will become the crucial issue of the next decade. The level of contaminants in our ground water, according to Robert Harris of the Council on Environmental Quality, sometimes is 1,000 times the concentration of the same contaminants that were in drinking water supplies when the Safe Drinking Water Act was debated in 1974. As of 1981, there were no federal health standards for most of these contaminants.

State and local governments, as well as Congress, are beginning to recognize the problem as a national one that can no longer be ignored. The effort begun with the Clean Water Act of 1972 to clean up surface water will most likely be expanded to include underground sources that produce at least 50 percent of the water humans consume. But the Reagan administration, as part of its overall goal to reduce the cost and size of government, was expected to slash funding for wastewater treatment. New funds generated under 1980 superfund legislation should aid water cleanup by controlling the proliferation of toxic dumpsites; however, the size of expenditures under this program was in controversy in late 1981. Stricter regulations proposed by the EPA under the Resource Control and Recovery Act could put a tighter cap on toxic chemicals leaking into vital water sources.

5

Nuclear Power and Radiation

When the character that actor Jack Lemmon portrayed in the movie *The China Syndrome* was shot trying to prevent a nuclear core meltdown, he became a hero to a vocal group of viewers who in the late 1970s embraced the anti-nuclear movement with born-again zeal. The subsequent accident at the Three Mile Island nuclear power plant near Harrisburg, Pa., lent an eerie authenticity to the movie and focused even more attention on what had been a largely grass-roots movement.

In fact, the Hollywood treatment of a nuclear accident as seen in *The China Syndrome* was a simplistic view of the issue. The nuclear debate cannot be so easily separated into a good guys versus bad guys plot; the scales swing back and forth when the dangers from radiation are weighed against the benefits of relatively cheap energy production.

A staff report to the Nuclear Regulatory Commission following the Three Mile Island accident said some radioactivity was released into the atmosphere at the site but posed only "minimal risks" to the people who lived nearby. However, the report noted that emissions of some radioactive gases were 11 times above recommended levels.

As a result of the accident, the safety practices of nuclear plant operators were called into question. The Kemeny report, an independent study commissioned after the Three Mile Island accident to examine the state of the nuclear industry, severely reprimanded the Nuclear Regulatory Commission for relying too heavily on licensing and paying insufficient attention to ensuring the safety of plants once they were in operation.

The issue is emotional partly because many people have only a sketchy knowledge of how a nuclear reactor actually works. What really causes a meltdown? Can a plant blow up? A survey conducted by the Council on Environmental Quality in 1980 showed that 52 percent of those polled did not know whether a nuclear power plant could explode into a Hiroshima-like mushroom cloud (the answer is no). Twenty-seven percent did not know that nuclear plants had to be built near water that is needed in the plant's extensive cooling system.

As more people begin to suspect that they have contracted cancer or other debilitating illnesses from radiation exposure, claims for compensation are piling up with the government and in the courts.

Although experts differ, it appears that radiation at low levels of exposure is more dangerous than generally appreciated. In any case, it will be years before science will be able to produce any definitive results on the effects of radiation on human health. At stake in the growing controversy over low-level radiation are not only widespread medical practices but also certain military policies and, above all else, the future of the nuclear power industry.

How to dispose of nuclear wastes has become a politically explosive issue in recent years. Many experts see waste disposal as the most serious obstacle to further nuclear power development. States are refusing to permit disposal sites within their boundaries or even movement of wastes across state lines. As of mid-1981, all three plants originally built to reprocess high-level nuclear waste in this country had been closed.

The prognosis for the nuclear industry in the 1980s looks uncertain. Reeling from the accident at Three Mile Island and the embarrassing light it shed on the Nuclear Regulatory Commission's performance, the industry in 1981 was struggling to stand on its own feet again. Many critics argued that nuclear power simply had become too expensive to survive. For example, the cost of constructing two nuclear plants and three companion reactors in Hanford, Wash., grew from an estimated $6.5 billion at conception to $23.8 billion by 1981, a nearly 300 percent increase.

Increasing costs, consumer energy needs and continued governmental support will play a large part in the success of the industry in the future. The Kemeny Commission said the future of nuclear power was undoubtedly a political question. "The ultimate resolution of the question," its report said, "involves the kind of economic, environmental and foreign policy considerations that can only be evaluated through the political process."

NUCLEAR SAFETY: EXPECTATIONS GONE AWRY

In 1954, when Congress was considering whether to allow private industry to develop electricity from the still government-controlled nuclear fission process, advocates of public power argued for a federal nuclear electricity program. With a massive government investment, they said, the cheap power could be made available even more quickly across the nation — and at lower cost — than if done by private industry. Their chief argument was that the government, at great expense, had developed the nuclear power program, and the public should benefit from that use of tax funds. By letting private industry take over, they contended, the companies would get the major benefit of billions of dollars in public funds spent for present and future research and development.

The public power supporters lost the 1954 fight. Private industry was given responsibility for marketing nuclear power, and, in fact, the Atomic Energy Commission (later the Nuclear Regulatory Commission) was even prohibited from operating commercial nuclear power plants. But the AEC's development and promotion of nuclear power continued, along with regulation. As the commission cajoled the infant industry along, it was more as a booster than a watchdog.

By the mid-1970s, though, the situation was changing. The government continued to spend money on nuclear research and regulation, as predicted in the 1954 debate, but the earlier promotion of nuclear energy was tempered by concern about safety of reactors and disposal of wastes.

Congress in 1974 abolished the Atomic Energy Commission, giving its regulatory functions to a new Nuclear Regulatory Commission, and its research and development operations to the Energy Research and Development Administration, which was later incorporated into the Energy Department.

Perhaps more significant for the new nuclear industry, though, was the financial bind faced by many utilities as electricity demand grew slowly after the Arab oil embargo launched a period of rapidly rising fuel costs. Utilities' solution was to cancel orders for nuclear reactors and put on hold planning for new ones. Another blow to the industry was President Carter's opposition to completion of a breeder reactor demonstration project in Tennessee. The breeder technology, which generates its own fuel, had been considered by the industry as the key to its future, with the demonstration project seen as crucial and timely.

Nevertheless, the federal government was still favorably disposed to nuclear power as a necessary energy source. The Carter administration decided to help by speeding the federal reactor licensing process, which industry had blamed for part of the 12-year lag between planning and operation of a reactor. In early 1979, the industry, which was by then living on back orders, was hoping for a boost from the licensing reform legislation. But in March 1979 came the accident at the Three Mile Island plant in Pennsylvania, the worst mishap in the history of commercial nuclear power. By 1980, more than 140 of the 170 new units once anticipated before the end of the century had been deferred or canceled. Reactor manufacturers later privately predicted that no new orders were likely until the late 1980s.

To the existing financial difficulties were added new public worries about safety and the prospect of expensive modification of existing plants with new safety features. Although a group of senators interested in giving the industry a boost won Senate passage of a nuclear waste disposal bill in July 1980, that chamber and the House could not resolve differences in their respective versions of the bill and the legislation died. The outlook for the nuclear industry was bleaker than ever.

Congress indicated its continuing support for nuclear power after the Three Mile Island accident, but many questions — both practical and philosophical — still faced the legislators in the 1980s. Congress had not given clear directions to the executive branch in years about issues such as disposal of radioactive wastes, the extent to which costly safety features should be required, changes in licensing procedures, standards for radiation exposure and allocation of the costs of accidents and of decommissioning plants. Proponents of nuclear power still sought a hearty endorsement from Congress, while opponents looked for a vote halting expansion until controversies such as waste disposal had been resolved.

The majority of Congress apparently fell in neither camp as 1981 began. Most representatives and senators didn't want to abandon nuclear power, but did want operation of reactors and disposal of waste to be as safe as possible. Exactly what that meant, they weren't sure.

The Industry Is Launched

Controlled nuclear fission was first demonstrated in 1942 by Enrico Fermi, who was conducting experiments at the University of Chicago. But it was 1951 before electricity was generated from nuclear power, even on an experimental basis. The research was funded by the Atomic Energy Commission.

When Fermi was doing his research, responsibility for atom splitting still rested with the Army Corps of Engineers' Manhattan Project, which secretly developed the atomic bomb. Congress in 1946 shifted that responsibility to a new five-member civilian organization, the Atomic Energy Commission, which was directed to encourage development of atomic energy. To help oversee the new agency, Congress took the unprecedented step of providing in the law for a special joint legislative committee. The Joint Committee on Atomic Energy became one of the most powerful congressional panels ever to exist, but was disbanded in 1977 when Congress decided it had outlived its usefulness.

The same year the AEC lab first generated nuclear electricity, the commission set up an industrial participation program under which private companies could help develop electricity from atomic power, with the idea of eventually marketing it commercially. In 1953, Congress provided funding for a demonstration power plant, and the contract was awarded to Westinghouse, for the reactor, and to the Duquesne Light Company, for operation and construction of the plant. The facility was located near Shippingport, Pa., and went into operation in 1957.

Private Companies Involved

The AEC could contract with utilities and power companies for development of nuclear power plants, but the 1946 law had made nuclear materials a government monopoly. Legally, only the government could own and operate the plants. As commercial production and sale of nuclear electricity appeared more feasible, President Eisenhower and Republicans in Congress sought to revise the 1946 law. Private industry involvement was opposed by Democrats who thought the government should retain some responsibility for commercial power development, but Republicans won and the Atomic Energy Act of 1954 launched a new industry.

Under that law, the AEC would give a utility a permit to construct and then a license to operate a nuclear power plant. The AEC was to retain control of the nuclear fuel by leasing it to utilities and then taking it back. In 1964, however, Congress changed this procedure, authorizing sale to private industry of uranium enriched at government plants. The government still had responsibility for disposing of the wastes left after the fuel had been used. In addition, after no one assumed responsibility, Congress in 1978 provided federal funds for the clean up of radioactive uranium "mill tailings" at abandoned mills and dumps.

In order to compete with coal fired power plants, designers originally drew up plans for extremely large plants that could produce power cheaply. These large reactors would be difficult to control, but the AEC accepted the risk. Safety was considered by plant designers but it was seldom the dominant factor, according to Daniel Ford of the Union for Concerned Scientists.

Liability Insurance Law

Another obstacle to private development of nuclear electricity was removed in 1957 when Congress adopted an amendment to the 1954 law limiting industry liability to $560 million in case of a nuclear accident. The risk of a catastrophic accident had scared away private insurers. Under the 1957 law — the Price-Anderson Act — if private insurance that was available could not cover utilities for the $560 million, the government would make up the difference. Congress renewed the law in 1965 for 10 years, and again in 1975, extending the liability limit to reactors for which licenses had been granted as of Aug. 1, 1987.

While the AEC continued to prod along the infant nuclear industry, the commissioners did show concern for public safety. In 1961, the AEC issued guidelines that required siting of reactors away from densely populated areas. However, within six years the siting rules had been relaxed as the AEC had decided that safety features built into the reactor design were adequate protection.

Industry Increases Efforts

The first nuclear reactor that produced electricity actually marketed by a utility was the Shippingport plant in Pennsylvania. But the first utility-owned reactor was the Dresden plant in Morris, Ill., owned by Commonwealth Edison Co. It began commercial operation in 1960. Two other plants of that era were the Yankee Nuclear Power Station in Massachusetts and New York Consolidated Edison's Indian Point plant.

In the late 1960s, the reactor manufacturers began to offer special contracts to utilities that required the reactor builders to absorb any cost overruns or cost increases resulting from inflation. They wanted business, and they got it. The four reactor vendors were Westinghouse Electric Corp., General Electric Company, Babcock & Wilcox Company and Combustion Engineering Inc.

State public utility commissions had responsibility for deciding whether a power plant, including a nuclear one, was necessary. If such a finding of need were made, then the commission issued a certificate of public convenience and necessity, which guaranteed the utility that it could charge ratepayers for construction and operating costs once the plant had gone into service. The AEC got involved usually only after this step.

The environmental movement prompted a major change in this procedure. A lawsuit was filed by opponents of the Calvert Cliffs plant, which the Baltimore Gas and Electric Company wanted to build on the Chesapeake Bay.

Status of Nuclear Power Plants

	1977	1978	1979	1980
Licensed to operate	65	70	70	68[2]
Licensed for testing[1]	—	—	—	1
Construction permits issued	78	88	91	85
Construction permits requested	59	37	25	11
Total	202	195	186	165

Figures are as of Sept. 30 of each year.

[1] After the March 1979 accident at Three Mile Island in Pennsylvania, licensing procedures were revised, adding another stage of review by the Nuclear Regulatory Commission after the testing period and prior to granting a commercial operating license.

[2] Does not include three plants shut down indefinitely: Three Mile Island in Pennsylvania; Humboldt Bay in California; and Dresden 1, in Illinois.

Source: Nuclear Regulatory Commission

Based on the National Environmental Policy Act (NEPA), the local environmentalists charged that the AEC, in issuing the plant permit and license, had not adequately considered the environmental impacts. In 1971, the federal circuit court in the District of Columbia ruled that the AEC had failed to comply with NEPA in this and other decisions. In the future, the court said, the AEC would have to ask four key questions: was there a need for power from the plant; was the site suitable; was nuclear energy satisfactory as a source for the plant; and were any additional safety precautions needed.

Issues in the Early 1970s

Environmentalists and consumer advocates, such as Ralph Nader, kept raising questions about nuclear safety. At the same time, government officials continued to issue scenarios for the future that called for increasing reliance on nuclear power. Most were more realistic than a 1962 AEC report that said nuclear reactors would provide half of all electricity in the year 2000, but the role for nuclear power was expected to be significant by 1985. This optimism about nuclear growth was clouded, though, by increasing concern about nuclear safety.

Rasmussen Report

By 1973 and 1974, when the Joint Committee on Atomic Energy held hearings on nuclear safety, AEC officials contended that reactors were safe and that a special study they had commissioned would prove their point. The study, being directed by Norman C. Rasmussen of the Massachusetts Institute of Technology, piqued the interest of Congress. Those concerned about safety managed to add a special provision to a five-year extension of the Price-Anderson Act that they approved in 1975. If warranted by the Rasmussen report, the new provision said, Congress could repeal the extension of the liability limit. However, President Ford did not like that restriction and vetoed the bill.

In late 1975, the Rasmussen report was completed. Called the "Reactor Safety Study (WASH-1400)," the report said an accident causing loss of reactor coolant, melting of the core and breach of the containment was likely to occur only once in 10 million years of reactor operation or, as the report declared, was as probable as a single meteorite striking an individual on earth. The Rasmussen report also concluded that damages in the worst possible nuclear accident could run as high as $14 billion. The probability of this worst accident, however, was only about one in one billion.

In the wake of the Arab oil embargo, the hopes of nuclear supporters soared. At first it seemed the new awareness of oil scarcity might be a boon to the still new nuclear industry. In 1975, there were 56 reactors in operation and more than 150 were in various stages of development. But the surge of orders placed in the late 1960s and early 1970s had already started to dwindle. The embargo and resulting recession ended up curbing demand for electricity, the only outlet for nuclear energy. At the same time, higher bills for fuel forced utilities to scramble to stay out of the red financially. The result was a hold on plans for new power plants, including new nuclear reactors, which had turned out to be far more costly to build than the initial rosy predictions by reactor makers interested in drumming up business.

By early 1978, utilities had cancelled more than 30 earlier decisions to build reactors and deferred construction of dozens more. The slowdown gradually began to show up in government estimates of future nuclear power generation.

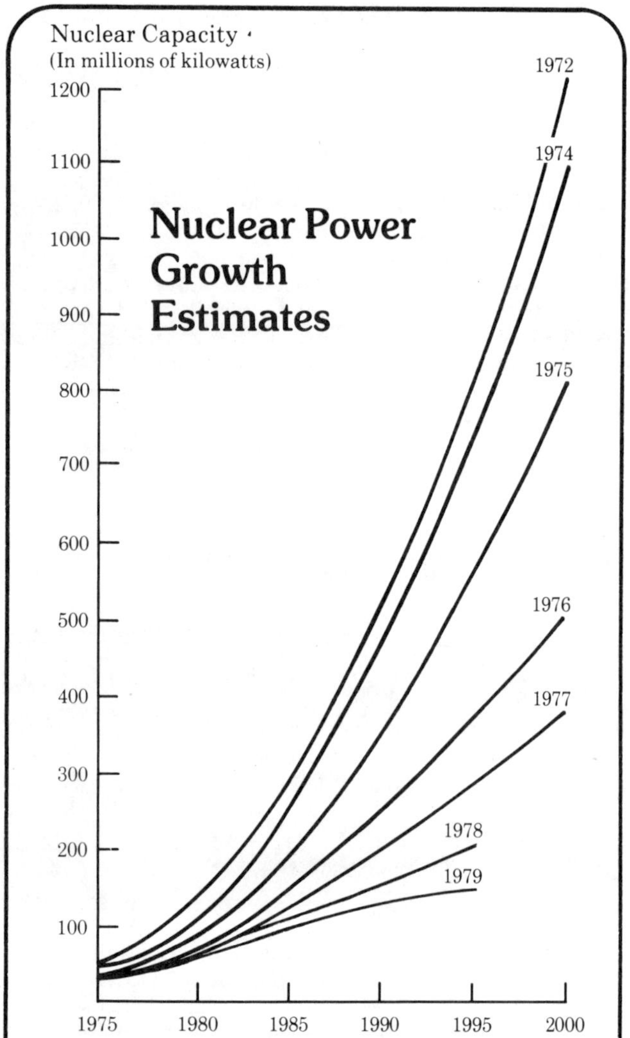

Source: Department of Energy

Industry Doubts Spread

By 1977, even the industry's leaders were conceding the future was cloudy. Craig Hosmer, president of the American Nuclear Energy Council, wrote in an October 1977 letter to a senior White House aide that unless new reactor orders came soon, "the U.S. nuclear industry will move quietly to extinction." Hosmer, a member of the House from 1953 to 1975, had once been ranking Republican on the Joint Committee on Atomic Energy.

Nuclear opponents shared that view in comments made in 1978. "The nuclear industry is dead in the water because they can't finance it — and we don't need it," said Mark Reis, Washington representative for Friends of the Earth, an environmental organization.

"It's like an endangered species," suggested Anthony Z. Roisman, an attorney with the Natural Resources Defense Council in Washington. "When it gets below a certain level, it cannot reproduce." Roisman cautioned that his group was not flatly against nuclear power. "Our position on nuclear power is that it is a last resort technology — which will not be needed," he said.

The already troubled nuclear industry was particularly frustrated by the Carter administration. The 1977 decision to cancel the plutonium-powered breeder reactor project at Clinch River, Tenn., and the ban on reprocessing of spent fuel to create plutonium had been blows to the industry, even though Congress kept pushing the breeder project.

The year 1979 turned out to be a very bad year for nuclear power.

In January, the NRC repudiated sections of the 1975 Rasmussen report. The commission had asked for a new safety study by a panel of scientists, known as the Risk Assessment Review Group, or the Lewis Panel, after its head, University of California physicist Harold Lewis. The Lewis report said the methodology used by Rasmussen was legitimate, but that the 1975 report was "inscrutable" to peer review.

Later that month, the Union of Concerned Scientists, the most respected of the groups critical of nuclear regulation, called on the government to shut down 16 U.S. reactors because of safety problems.

On March 13, the Nuclear Regulatory Commission ordered the temporary shutdown of five nuclear plants after it determined that a computer model used to establish their ability to resist earthquakes had been faulty. The same day a special 14-agency governmental review unit raised questions about the scientific and technical feasibility of safely disposing of radioactive wastes created by commercial reactors. The report called into question a matter the industry had long argued it would have no problem resolving.

Then came Three Mile Island.

Nuclear Reactor Operation

In a controlled nuclear reaction, uranium nuclei are split apart and heat is released. This heat can convert water into steam to power a turbine which generates electricity. At the center of the system is a reactor vessel that is connected to one of the most elaborate plumbing systems ever devised. There are several types of commercial power reactors. Some use ordinary water to cool their fuel, some use gas, such as carbon dioxide, and some use liquid metal.

There were in 1981 43 pressurized water reactors licensed to operate in the United States, and 64 more were operating around the world. In this type of reactor, the water is kept under extremely high pressure so that it can absorb heat from the reactor but not turn to steam. In order to do this, the water must be kept moving through the reactor to prevent it from overheating. The water that goes through the reactor is known as the primary cooling water and the water supplied by the main feedwater pumps is the secondary cooling water. The heated water from the reactor does not mix with water that goes to the steam generators by the feedwater pumps. Instead, it flows through thousands of small tubes inside each steam generator. Like a conventional radiator, heated water from the reactor, moving through tiny steam-generator tubes, heats the colder secondary cooling water surrounding the tubes. The reactor-cooling system is designed so that the heat added to the primary cooling water is transferred to the secondary cooling water.

The water in the second cooling system boils and turns into steam. This steam is piped into a turbine where it expands and spins large turbine blades. The shaft of the turbine is connected to a generator that produces electric current. If the delicate equilibrium between output of heat by the reactor and uptake of heat by steam generators is upset, the uranium fuel has the potential to overheat, perhaps uncontrollably.

As the reactor operates, the fissioning of uranium nuclei causes radioactive waste to accumulate. These wastes give off radiation that generates a significant amount of heat. Water must, therefore, be continually pumped through the system, even when the reactors are shut down. Inadequate core cooling can give rise to what is popularly known as a meltdown accident. If the cooling system fails, the nuclear core would turn into a mass of molten radioactive metal and melt to the bottom of the reactor, where it would penetrate the floor of the containment building in which it is housed. The containment building is not designed to stop the fuel from flowing down into the ground. This sequence of events has been called the China Syndrome — a fictionalized reference to the general direction in which the molten core would be traveling. The formation of hydrogen and carbon-dioxide gases, explosive reactions between molten metal and residual water in the building and other phenomena could damage the containment building and allow radioactive elements to escape into the surrounding area.

What Happened at Three Mile Island Plant

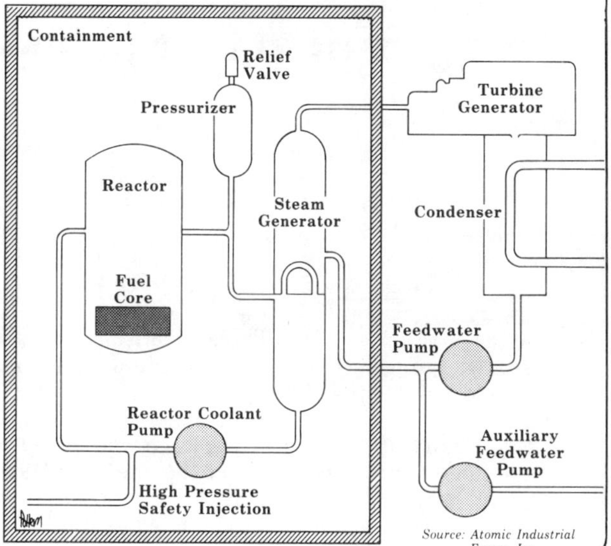

Source: Atomic Industrial Forum, Inc.

Three Mile Island Accident

The problem at the reactor near Harrisburg, Pa., began at 4 a.m. on March 28, 1979, with a breakdown of water pumps that were part of the cooling system that kept water flowing over the fuel rods.

Several different mechanical problems contributed to the failure of the TMI cooling system, including poor overall plant design, but key factors were: the shutdown of two auxiliary cooling pumps for maintenance two weeks before the accident; the failure of relief valves to close properly, which allowed too much water to drain from the cooling system; and a stuck pressure indicator, which gave operators in the control room erroneous information.

According to an article in the April 6, 1981, *New Yorker* by Daniel Ford of the Union of Concerned Scientists, the accident involved what is known as a common-mode failure — a single event or condition that can cause simultaneous multiple malfunctions and create a widespread failure in the plant's safety system.

According to Ford, a NRC official had written a series of reports prior to the Three Mile Island accident outlining the "disastrous effect" that common mode failures could have on the safety of nuclear reactors. The official involved had urged that the problem be corrected while the Three Mile Island plant was being constructed. The NRC ignored the report.

Equally important, other investigators said later, were the actions of reactor operators who turned off the emergency and primary cooling systems, thus unintentionally thwarting the built-in "defense-in-depth" against a failure of the cooling system. Their training had not prepared them for the series of events that took place at TMI. In addition, the utility, General Public Utilities Corp., its subsidiary that operated TMI, Metropolitan Edison and the reactor manufacturer, Babcock & Wilcox, were faulted for safety procedures and equipment. The Nuclear Regulatory Commission was criticized for its overall regulation of nuclear safety.

Who Will Pay for Three Mile Island?

As the second anniversary of the accident at Three Mile Island arrived in 1981, members of Pennsylvania's House delegation were preparing to seek a congressional "bailout" for the beleaguered plant's owner.

One proposal would in effect force U.S. electric utility customers to pay the multimillion-dollar cost of cleaning up after the Three Mile Island accident. However, some members said the federal government should pay for the cleanup.

Like Pennsylvania's politicians, utilities and the nuclear industry were widely split on who should pay for the cleanup. The owner of the damaged nuclear plant, General Public Utilities Corp. (GPU), said the problem was a national one, and hired a former member of Congress to try to work out a solution.

By early 1981, inspection teams, wearing special protective suits, had entered the reactor building six times since the accident. During the entry in February 1981, they positioned television cameras near the reactor to monitor it.

As of spring 1981, about 700,000 gallons of radioactive water remained in the reactor building, and more was accumulating daily. The water eventually would have to be pumped out, cleaned and shipped to a disposal site. The reactor building, highly radioactive, would have to be scrubbed, and the damaged reactor core removed.

GPU and the rest of the nuclear industry would like this cleanup finished as quickly as possible, but it was expected to take several years beyond 1981. A spokesman said the industry considers the problem "like a wart that must be removed" so that nuclear power can progress.

Pennsylvania officials were even more anxious. They pointed to the health and safety dangers to the immediate area, arguing that the reactor building was not built to store highly radioactive liquid waste.

Because the cleanup was to take longer than originally expected, costs also rose — to at least $1 billion. Bernard Cherry, GPU vice president for planning, said the company could not afford $700 million above the insurance payment. Until it could determine where the rest of the money was to come from, GPU slowed cleanup work to the minimum pace it said was necessary to maintain health and safety. At that rate, Cherry said, the insurance money would last about two more years.

In the summer of 1980, after GPU asked for federal help, the Pennsylvania House delegation formed a task force to consider the role of the federal government at Three Mile Island. The task force was headed by Rep. Allen E. Ertel, D-Pa., in whose district the plant was located.

The task force drew up a bill to establish a national, quasi-public insurance corporation to provide additional property insurance to nuclear utilities. The bill included a retroactive provision authorizing the funding of three-quarters of Three Mile Island cleanup costs not covered by existing insurance. Half of this payment would be repaid by GPU.

The corporation would be funded by charging annual premiums to utilities that have nuclear power plants. Utilities that refused to pay would not be allowed to operate nuclear reactors.

The utilities in turn would pass their multimillion-dollar premium costs on to their customers. The effect would be that the users of nuclear-generated electricity nationwide would pay for cleaning up Three Mile Island. The bill also would provide nuclear utilities with additional property insurance, which the 1979 accident showed was needed.

In a letter to President Reagan asking for help, Rep. Bill Goodling, R-Pa., a member of the task force, said the potential risk at Three Mile Island was 100,000 times greater than the hazard from the Mount St. Helens volcano in Washington state, "and is equally unpredictable. Unless the cleanup takes place promptly, the growing fear of people in that area will be exacerbated tremendously. We cannot wait for the legislative process to work. We do not have that kind of time."

Environmental groups opposed the task force bill. They said that by spreading the risk, the insurance scheme would decrease the incentive to operate safely.

Howard Symons of Congress Watch, a Ralph Nader organization, called the bill a "bailout" that used the problem of Three Mile Island to solve some of the nuclear industry's larger financial problems. He said Congress should vote directly on whether to have federal funds pay for the cleanup of TMI.

These findings were made in an October 1979 report by a presidential commission on the accident, headed by John G. Kemeny, president of Dartmouth College. In addition, most findings were supported by a study done for the NRC by Washington lawyer Mitchell Rogovin, as well as by a special Senate investigation by the Environment and Public Works Subcommittee on Nuclear Regulation.

Several weeks passed before the reactor cooled to an acceptable level. Cleanup of the contaminated reactor containment had been completed at the end of 1980. Unresolved by 1981 was who would pay for the $900 million-plus cleanup operation.

At the height of the crisis, officials had considered evacuating thousands of residents from the area because of the chance that the plant's nuclear fuel could overheat and "melt down," releasing dangerous radiation.

Pennsylvania Gov. Richard L. Thornburgh, R, March 30, 1979, asked young children and pregnant women living within five miles of the plant to leave because of leaking radiation. They were joined by hundreds, possibly thousands, of others. Thousands more stayed home from work April 2, and most area schools closed.

Conflicting information from state, federal and utility company officials about the accident and potential hazards caused additional confusion, particularly in the first two days after the incident. Plans to handle such an emergency were being written on the spot because, apparently, no evacuation plans had been ready prior to the accident.

Graphic Images Remain

The week's events left the public with a series of graphic images: top level government officials debating evacuation of a half million people; the voluntary evacuation of children and pregnant women; the federal government's deep involvement in the operation of the local utility; Pennsylvania's capital at Harrisburg temporarily reduced to a veritable ghost town as residents stayed inside; the Pentagon flying in tons of lead bricks to assist a team of government officials in bringing the overheated reactor under control, and the federal government flying in hundreds of thousands of bottles of potassium iodide to counteract absorption of radioactive iodine 131 in the event of a catastrophe. It was a week of news reports of industry spokesmen minimizing the safety risks of the accident, of contradictions by government officials taking a more cautious approach and of sharp challenges to both by nuclear experts and anti-nuclear groups.

Cautiously assessing the accident during its early stages, President Carter said the events "will make all of us reassess our present safety regulations ... and probably lead inexorably toward even more stringent safety design mechanisms and standards."

Pennsylvania Sen. Richard Schweiker, R, said the accident showed that "we have seriously underestimated both the safety problems associated with nuclear power generation and our ability to cope with a nuclear emergency."

A grimmer view came from Rep. Morris K. Udall, D-Ariz., who chaired the House Interior Committee which handled most nuclear regulatory legislation. He declared, "The aura of confidence in nuclear energy has been shattered."

Industry officials reacted defensively, repeatedly referring to statements by Department of Energy Secretary James Schlesinger that "we will have to have nuclear power" to meet energy needs.

Charles F. Luce, chairman of Consolidated Edison of New York, predicted: "When the need is looked at with the alternatives, nuclear will remain an important part of our future."

"You can look at the situation in two ways," said an official with Westinghouse Electric Corp. who asked not to be identified. "From a technical viewpoint Three Mile Island is no problem. It sounds bad but there was no major accident.... From the political point of view it's next to a disaster. And public perception determines the political view.... It looks like this incident will have a profound effect on the industry."

Two years after the accident, the Unit 2 in the plant at Three Mile Island remained shut down. The plant's containment building and auxiliary tanks were flooded with more than a million gallons of radioactive water. The cost of the clean-up was estimated at a billion dollars.

Reports showed that the types of human error involved in the accident were not uncommon. Government records indicated that as many as 18 percent of all serious nuclear plant malfunctions reported to the NRC in 1978 were a result of human error.

NRC Response to Accident

The Nuclear Regulatory Commission's practice, according to Peter Bradford, one of the agency's five commissioners, "was never designed to be an effective regulatory system" but "was constructed for the stamping out of nuclear power plant construction permits or operating licenses at the assembly-line rate of one or two per week for every week in the years from 1975-2000."

In the wake of the accident, President Carter appointed a commission to study government and industry safety practices regarding nuclear energy.

The 12-member panel, headed by Dartmouth College President John Kemeny, found that the underlying problem at Three Mile Island stemmed not from deficient equipment, but rather from compounded human failures. Kemeny commission members concluded that the NRC relied too heavily on licensing, and paid insufficient attention to ensuring the safety of plants once they were in operation.

In the months after the March accident, industry officials did not even mention licensing reform. The public mood was for more, not less, regulation of nuclear power.

Utilities stepped up their advertising campaign in support of nuclear power. "The safety system worked," was a headline in a full-page ad in *The New York Times,* bought by a group called America's Electric Energy Companies.

"One thing is certain," the advertisement continued. "What happened at Three Mile Island does *not* justify a halt to nuclear power development...."

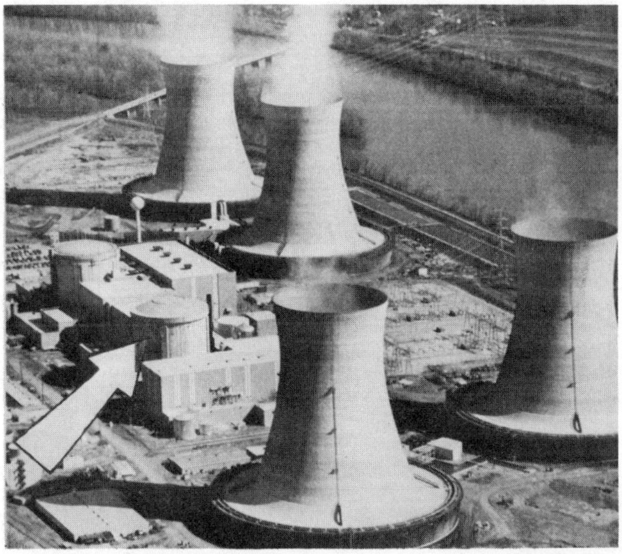

Arrow shows reactor number two at the Three Mile Island power plant near Harrisburg, Pa.

The importance of public opinion to the future of nuclear power had led to a warning from the Kemeny Commission. "We are convinced that, unless portions of the industry and its regulatory agency undergo fundamental changes, they will over time totally destroy public confidence and, hence, they will be responsible for the elimination of nuclear power as a viable source of energy," the panel said.

Nuclear Industry Takes Action

The utilities that used nuclear power, along with other nuclear-related companies, took several steps they hoped would improve nuclear safety and public opinion.

They set up an Institute of Nuclear Power Operations in Atlanta that provided an in-house training program for plant operators, used auditors to monitor reactor operations and distributed information about potential problems. Its initial annual budget was to be between $11 million and $12 million.

"Altogether it will be a kind of watchdog," said Carl Goldstein of the Atomic Industrial Forum, an international association of companies involved with nuclear power. The institute would "prod a utility into action" if a deficiency were found, he said.

The utilities also set up a mutual insurance program to help cover the costs of buying more expensive substitute electricity in the event of an accident or shutdown.

One sanction the institute would have against plants that did not meet safety requirements would be to keep them out of the insurance program, Goldstein said.

Still another industry program developed in response to the Three Mile Island accident was the Nuclear Safety Analysis Center, which was to be part of the Edison Electric Institute. The center was to concentrate on technical analysis and long-term research on reactor safety and operations.

The question of a moratorium had been ducked by the Kemeny Commission. The 12 members failed to agree on whether the growth of nuclear power should be halted until the changes it recommended had been made. Although eight commission members wanted a pause in construction, they could not agree on what events would lift a moratorium.

In the midst of congressional debate on the issue, the NRC made a decision on its own. The commission Nov. 5, 1979, announced that it would continue to hold off for an indefinite period on the issuance of operating licenses and construction permits for new plants. The NRC had decided just after the March accident to delay licensing for a few months in order to concentrate on the TMI accident. The NRC action continued what was essentially a *de facto* moratorium.

"Our first and most important responsibility is to apply those remedies and lessons [from Three Mile Island and the Kemeny report] to the operating plants," said NRC Chairman Joseph Hendrie at a Nov. 5, 1979, congressional hearing. "We have a pause in licensing. I've been trying to stay away from the word 'moratorium.' "

The delay in licensing immediately affected four newly constructed plants that were ready or almost ready to start up. The plants were Salem 2 in New Jersey, North Anna 2 in Virginia, Diablo Canyon in California and Sequoyah 1 in Tennessee.

The "pause" in licensing ended in August 1980 when the first post-TMI license was issued to the North Anna 2 unit, a Virginia Electric and Power Co. plant. The NRC moratorium was months longer than that sought by congressional proponents of the moratorium amendments.

Greater reliance on coal has also added to the lessening demand for nuclear power. Proponents of nuclear power argue that the trend toward coal makes the public more vulnerable to strikes in the coal fields and causes air and water pollution. Opponents respond that pollution control equipment now makes coal-fired plants cleaner than most existing oil-fired plants. They also argue that coal-fired plants do not carry the risks of transporting nuclear fuel, the possibility of a meltdown or the risks associated with radioactive waste that are connected with nuclear reactors.

The NRC and other federal officials have been hampered because major policy and philosophical questions about nuclear power have not been addressed by Congress in years. For example, NRC officials have received little guidance on how to balance possible risks to the public against the costs to utilities of making safety improvements. Congress had never expanded on the few words in the 1954 Atomic Energy Act that said there should be "adequate assurance of no undue risk" from nuclear power.

"Congress needs to say either we want it [nuclear power] under the following conditions or we don't want it," said one NRC official. "Lacking those kinds of decisions, we're all in a quandary — and nuclear power is slowly going down the tubes."

Although most legislators generally agree that safety must be improved, they are less united on just how to accomplish that. And safety questions tend to breed other, politically loaded questions.

- If evacuation plans are required but are not feasible for a reactor near a major city, does that mean the plant should be shut down?
- If better designed control rooms could prevent accidents, does that mean existing plants should be modified, at great expense?
- If safety must be improved, does that mean no additional reactors should be built until the new safety rules are completed?

Carter Response

In his first response to the Kemeny Commission report, in December 1979, which was also his first detailed statement on nuclear power since the accident, President Carter urged a resumption of plant licensing by the NRC as soon as possible, but no later than six months. Safety was important, "my top priority," Carter said, but he added: "We cannot shut the door on nuclear power for the United States."

Nuclear power was "critical if we are to free our country from its overdependence on unstable sources of high-priced foreign oil," Carter said. "We do not have the luxury of abandoning nuclear power or imposing a lengthy moratorium on its further use.

"As I have said before, in this country nuclear power is an energy source of last resort," Carter said. "By this I mean that as we reach our goals on conservation, on the direct use of coal, on development of solar power and synthetic fuels and enhanced production of American oil and natural gas, as we reach those goals, then we can minimize our reliance on nuclear power."

Congressional Reaction

In Congress, the initial reaction to the Three Mile Island accident was a spate of hearings and investigations, led primarily by the House Interior and Senate Environment and Public Works committees, which had jurisdiction over the NRC and nuclear regulation. Rep. Udall chaired Interior, as well as its energy subcommittee. Sen. Gary Hart, D-Colo., chaired the Nuclear Regulation Subcommittee in the Senate. Both men had in the past criticized the nuclear industry and the NRC, and both favored pushing for additional federal controls. They were countered by nuclear power advocates who downplayed the accident. For example, Rep. Mike McCormack, D-Wash., said the Three Mile Island incident was not unexpected by nuclear experts. He then cited the lack of injury as a demonstration of the safety of nuclear energy. "Nuclear power is still hundreds of times safer than coal," said McCormack, referring to the deaths of coal miners.

When faced with divergent views and complicated and controversial questions, Congress often will require years and sometimes decades to act on major issues. The delay is lengthened when the signals from the public are mixed, as they have been on nuclear power. As Udall put it, "People tell you they are willing to have nuclear power, and then they say, 'But don't put it in my neighborhood.' "

The compromises needed to pass legislation were not forthcoming in the months after the TMI accident. Improved emergency preparedness and stiffer fines for violators of NRC rules were the most Congress could agree on. A bold Senate plan in 1980 to shut down reactors in states without approved evacuation plans was watered down, so that in an uncooperative state a utility could submit a plan of its own to the NRC, thus reducing the chance of reactor shutdowns.

During 1979 action on the same bill, a move by nuclear critics to pass a six-month moratorium on NRC issuance of new construction permits, failed badly. The Senate vote, in July, was 35-57; the House vote, in November, was 135-254. Supporters of the moratorium argued that safety problems should be resolved before the industry expanded. Opponents said a moratorium would kill the nuclear industry.

Reagan Position

President Reagan campaigned on a strongly pro-nuclear position and had said that Three Mile Island must be cleaned up. But as of late 1981 his administration had not formally taken a position on the issue of who should pay.

Energy Secretary James B. Edwards, an outspoken nuclear supporter, told the Senate Energy Committee in February 1981 that he hoped to use research money to help clean up TMI. "They need help and the nuclear industry is in trouble," he said. He added that the federal government would not pay the whole bill.

Edwards had established an Energy Department task force to consider what to do about Three Mile Island. Some observors considered it unlikely that Edwards would be able to pry much cleanup money loose from David A. Stockman, Office of Management and Budget director, who generally had opposed industry subsidies.

The federal government had spent about $12 million on the Three Mile Island cleanup since the 1979 accident occurred. President Carter had budgeted another $10 million for fiscal 1982. Pennsylvania House members had asked Reagan to increase that amount dramatically.

The Nuclear Safety Oversight Committee, established by Carter after the 1979 accident, told Reagan in February 1981 that not enough progress was being made toward cleaning up TMI. The committee suggested that the federal government pay half of the uninsured cleanup costs and provide the remainder with a federal loan.

"The precise division of federal assistance between direct support and loan is of secondary importance compared to the compelling need to provide financing for an expedited cleanup," the committee said.

RADIATION: HOW HARMFUL IS IT?

The kind of radiation of concern in the debate over health hazards connected with the nuclear industry is called "ionizing radiation," that is, electrically charged radiation which ruptures the chemical bonds that join atoms together in molecules. Ionizing radiation which passes through biological tissue can prevent a cell from dividing, or it can damage the genetic material contained in the cell's nucleus, causing it to divide abnormally. Harmful effects can be somatic, which shows up in damage to the individual organism, or genetic, mutations which show up only in future generations.

There are five kinds of ionizing radiation of biological significance: alpha particles, beta particles, gamma rays, neutrons, and X-rays. Although primarily artificial in the human environment, X-rays also enter the atmosphere as part of cosmic radiation. The other forms of radiation are

Nuclear Terminology

Scientists use the following units to measure levels of radiation that "ionize" or cause changes in human cells.

Roentgen: A measure of the quantity of radiation in the air.

Rad (radiation absorbed dose): A measure of the amount of ionizing radiation absorbed by a human cell.

Rem (Roentgen equivalent man): A measure of the biological effects of the energy produced by radiation. One rem is equal to one rad. High levels of radiation are considered to be doses above 50 rems.

Millirem: One rem equals 1,000 millirems. Current standards set maximum safety levels for workers exposed to radioactive materials at five rems a year and levels for the general population at 500 millirems a year or .5 rems.

Person-rem or Man-rem: A measurement of doses received by entire populations. It is calculated by multiplying the number of people exposed by the dose.

Compensation Sought for Radiation . . .

"During the time the radiation was out, we worked and we played in it, but we thought it would be okay because we believed it was safe like we were told. . . ."

—Agatha Barnum to Sen. Jake Garn, R-Utah, at St. George, Utah, April 20, 1979

Between 1945 and 1963, the year of the nuclear test ban treaty, the United States exploded some 235 nuclear devices in atmospheric tests in the Pacific and in Nevada.

The trials at the Nevada test site began in 1951, and radioactive fallout was thought to have drifted into that state, neighboring portions of Utah and Arizona, and perhaps farther. The major population groups who were exposed to fallout and who were seeking compensation from the government were civilians who lived in the path of the drift, and civilian and military personnel — as many as 250,000 soldiers, according to one estimate — who took part in the tests.

"Many units were marched or helicoptered to ground zero soon after the explosion. . . . At one test, six volunteers stood at ground zero under an airburst some 20,000 feet above them," Sen. Alan Cranston, D-Calif., told a 1979 Senate hearing.

Evidence on the health effects of relatively small doses of radiation is confusing and not well developed; most of the data linking radiation with human illness come from studies of the massive "doses" at Nagasaki and Hiroshima. Scientists have not developed a definitive method for relating the size of a low-level dose to its impact, if any, on human health.

At the time of the atmospheric weapons tests, most researchers thought low doses were safe. However, later studies suggested that the risk at low levels is in fact 10 or 20 times greater than was believed.

The major sources of low-level exposure were "background" radiation, from cosmic rays and naturally radioactive substances in the environment, and medical exposures such as X-rays. The next largest source was radioactive fallout. Other sources were nuclear energy and consumer products, according to the task force.

Tests Safe, AEC Said

The Atomic Energy Commission (AEC), which was abolished and had its functions split up in 1974, was responsible both for conducting the nuclear tests and monitoring their health effects.

AEC's public position during the 1950s was that the tests were safe. Utah Gov. Scott M. Matheson, D, remembers that "on occasion, residents were advised to remain indoors for an hour or two" during tests, but "the AEC [radio] announcements were quick to remind listeners that 'there was no danger'."

Those public announcements masked internal warnings, which the AEC disregarded and sought to discredit as "Communist inspired" scare stories, according to evidence produced at joint Senate-House committee hearings in April 1979. The warnings were that actual doses were significantly higher than "safe" levels and that they could cause human illness.

emitted by radioactive substances such as radium, uranium and thorium.

The absorption of radiation by other substances is measured in rads, a precise physical quantity defined as the amount of radiation that will cause one kilogram (2.2 pounds) of material to absorb 0.01 joules of energy. Different kinds of radiation do different amounts of damage to living tissue at any given level of exposure; exposure to one rad of beta radiation, in other words, is not precisely as harmful as exposure to one rad of alpha radiation. The rad therefore is adjusted by a measure of biological effectiveness called the "quality factor"; the factor is one for beta and gamma radiation, and roughly 10 to 20 for neutrons and alpha particles. Multiplication of the dose absorbed by the quality factor yields the "dose equivalent," expressed in rems, the standard measure of biological impact. Since the rem is a large quantity, human exposure to radiation generally is expressed in millirems. One millirem is one-thousandth of a rem.

However, even millirems provide only the crudest estimate of how radiation affects tissue. Rapidly dividing cells, such as are found in the human fetus, are exceptionally vulnerable. Radiation is more harmful to women than to men, and some age groups are unusually susceptible to certain kinds of cancer. Young children, for example, are especially vulnerable to leukemia. Certain radioactive elements, moreover, tend to concentrate in specific parts of the body, where they can emit harmful radiation over a longer period of time. Strontium-90 migrates to the bones; plütonium concentrates in the liver and in the bones, and secondarily in human gonads. Many radioactive substances enter the food chain on which both animals and humans depend.

Radiation Sources

Most radiation to which humans are exposed comes from natural sources. Cosmic rays account for about one-third of the natural background radiation on average — more in high altitudes and less closer to sea-level — and terrestrial sources for close to one-half. A building material

... Damage from U.S. Nuclear Tests

One dramatic early warning came in 1953, when about 17,000 sheep that had been grazing in the path of test fallout died. Exposed sheep herds also showed large numbers of stillbirths and birth defects. Radiation dose levels for those herds were "almost 1,000 times the permissible count for human beings," and public health officials in internal AEC memos questioned what the implications might be for human health.

But the AEC ruled out paying damages for the dead sheep, because, as an AEC official told sheepherders at the time, "If we paid for them, every woman that got pregnant and every woman that didn't would sue us."

Another witness at the hearing, Dr. Harold A. Knapp, testified that his 1962-63 study concluded that the AEC had grossly "miscalculated" — by a factor of 1,000 — radiation doses to infants' and children's thyroids from drinking contaminated cow's milk. Reconstructing the sequence from old memoranda, Knapp found that the AEC refused to lower acceptable exposure levels because a change could create public doubts about the earlier standard, and because of the "world situation." In 1965, Public Health Service officer Edward S. Weiss suggested a link between increased leukemia in southern Utah and the tests, but the report remained an internal, unpublished document until 1979, according to Sen. Orrin G. Hatch, R-Utah.

Over the years, at least 15 congressional panels have concerned themselves with radiation. Department of Health and Human Services studies of exposed children who were victims of leukemia, bone cancer, thyroid abnormalities and congenital defects were begun, but dropped in 1971. The visibility of the issue in 1979 and 1980 stemmed from 1978 radiation hearings by the House Commerce Health Subcommittee headed by Rep. Paul G. Rogers, D-Fla. Rogers' hearings, pressures from Utah Gov. Matheson for disclosure of accurate exposure data and two new studies prompted another round of congressional hearings in 1979.

A 1977 study by HEW's Center for Disease Control found double the expected rate of leukemia among participants in a 1957 nuclear test that was code-named "Smoky."

In 1977-78, Dr. Joseph Lyon of the University of Utah again looked at childhood leukemia rates, and discovered that children born during the test years in areas downwind from the test sites had twice as much incidence of leukemia as children born both before and after the tests. The significance of this finding has been questioned by Dr. Marvin Schneiderman of the National Cancer Institute. He said other types of cancer in that group decreased during the years leukemia was on the increase.

A Feb. 21, 1980, report in *The Washington Post* raised the possibility that the 1979 Three Mile Island nuclear accident may have produced a new group of "victims."

After the accident an unusually large number of children were born with serious thyroid defects in the three Pennsylvania counties near the nuclear plant, according to the story, which also included official denials that the amount of radiation released could have caused the problems.

such as granite contains small amounts of radioactive materials and emits appreciable amounts of radiation.

Among the sources of radiation not ordinarily found in nature, X-rays account for overwhelmingly the largest portion of average human exposure, while radionuclides used in medical diagnosis and therapy make a small but noticeable contribution. A typical chest X-ray series can expose the patient to roughly 250 millirems — more than the total radiation dose a U.S. resident ordinarily receives in a year. In 1978, about 162 million diagnostic X-rays were administered for medical purposes and 86 million for dental purposes; radionuclides were administered in close to 8 million cases.

Many leading health physicists believe that current levels of exposure to X-rays are unwarranted by any standard and could be sharply reduced without detriment to medical practices. It has been argued that the dose delivered by medical diagnostic X-rays could be reduced by 90 percent, while at the same time increasing the quality and amount of diagnostic information available.

Under new guidelines, issued at the recommendation of a special task force headed by the Environmental Protection Agency, dental X-rays are not to be given as part of a routine screening test in government hospitals. While still further restrictions may follow, X-rays will continue to be used, but more sparingly. They provide medical information that cannot otherwise be obtained.

The situation is quite different with the other main artificial sources of radiation: nuclear weapons testing and the nuclear power industry. Concern about nuclear fallout was the single most important factor leading to the 1963 treaty banning atmospheric testing of atomic devices. That concern also helped persuade France to stop its atmospheric testing in the mid-1970s. By 1981, only China continued to conduct atmospheric tests.

The nuclear power industry could be profoundly affected by the controversy. Nuclear power in the early 1980s accounted for less than one millirem of the average American's annual exposure to radiation. The level of exposure would rise with expansion of nuclear power.

From X-Rays to Hiroshima

When radiation first was discovered, the excitement of uncovering a heretofore unknown world far outweighed any thought of detrimental biological effects. Wilhelm Conrad Roentgen's discovery of X-rays in 1895 and Henry Becquerel's finding in 1896 that uranium spontaneously emits radiation ushered in one of the great eras of science.

Scientists were quick to learn that radiation in large doses could cause skin lesions, and some early experimentalists burned themselves intentionally with radioactive substances in order to study the biological effects firsthand. But the most detrimental effects appeared only in time when the early experimenters fell prey to cancer. Marie Curie, who with her husband discovered the element radium, was but one of many such victims.

The atomic bombing of Hiroshima and Nagasaki at the end of World War II for the first time exposed large populations to the lingering effects of radiation. Of some 350,000 people in Hiroshima at the time of the blast, 140,000 had died by the end of 1945, according to the best available estimates; in Nagasaki roughly 74,000 out of 280,000 died. The survivors provided the raw material for the first large-scale study of the biological effects of exposure to varying levels of radiation.

Results of Hiroshima-Nagasaki research, as summarized by the Natural Science Group — a body organized by the Geneva-based International Peace Bureau to appraise the Japanese studies — were in some ways predictable and in some ways surprising. The incidence of leukemia among survivors increased rapidly for a decade, peaking at a level 30 times the normal Japanese rate. Thyroid, breast and lung cancers appeared at significantly higher-than-normal rates among those exposed to initial radiation in both cities. Malignant tumors — salivary gland tumors, gastric carcinoma, bone tumors, prostate cancer and malignant lymphona, etc. — appeared at an abnormally high rate after an average latency period of about 20 years.

However, death rates from non-malignant causes have been lower than average among survivors. While children exposed in the womb suffered an increase in birth defects, they have not proved to be more susceptible to leukemia than other Japanese children. Most startling of all, even though it has been established since 1927 that radiation causes genetic mutations, no significant genetic effects have been found in the survivor population.

People who entered the cities after the atomic explosions may provide a better basis for calculating health hazards from low-level radiation. Studies of some 40,000 Japanese who went to look for friends and relatives suggest a high incidence of radiation-related cancer, according to a recent report from Dr. Alice Stewart, a leading British radiologist. Norman Solomon, a free-lance writer, has reported that U.S. soldiers who performed clean-up duties in the two cities show "many confirmed cases of leukemia, other unusual blood diseases, and bone marrow cancers." Survivor studies have been criticized on the grounds that much of the information collected is not open to public scrutiny. The Casualty Commission classified all of its data, and during the years immediately after World War II, U.S. occupation forces in Japan "censored all articles about the A-bombs."

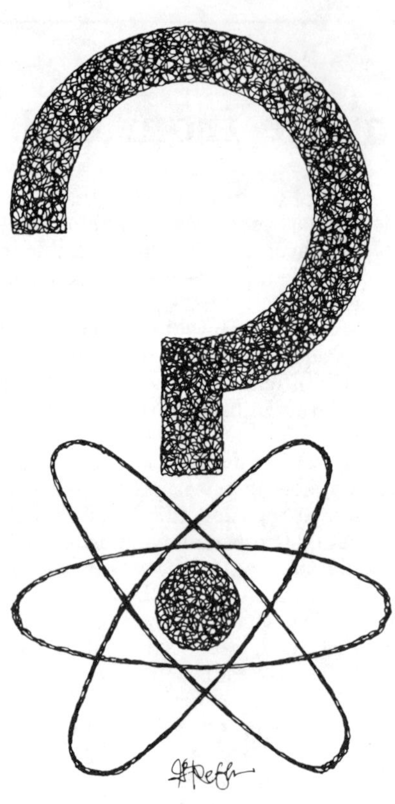

Scientific Basis for Controversy

The controversy over low-level radiation revolves around the relationship of biological effects to radiation doses at low ranges of exposure.

Under the "threshold" hypothesis, the potential danger of radiation drops sharply at low levels of exposure. It is assumed that human cells generally must incur radiation damage more than one time before serious biological effects show up, and that in most cases cell damage is repaired before the critical threshold is reached. The "threshold" theorists frequently argue that humans have built up an immunity to radiation at levels found in nature and small additional amounts make little difference.

Other persons contend that radiation is harmful at any level. Proponents of what probably is the most widely accepted hypothesis, the "linear" theory, believe that biological effects are directly proportional to doses at all levels of exposure.

Some scientists take an even more cautious view of radiation dangers, and argue that more biological effects may occur per unit of radiation dose at low levels of exposure than at high levels. At high levels, according to this reasoning, many cells are killed outright and no further damage occurs.

Experts disagree about which of the three theories is correct not only for radiation in general but also for each kind of radiation. Some experts think, for example, that the relationship between dose and effect is super-linear for high radiation (alpha particles and neutrons), while the threshold theory correctly describes low radiation such as X-rays and gamma rays.

Because radioactive substance came into widespread use only a generation ago, and because the latency period for more cancers is quite long, there are few groups of people suitable for study. Moreover, the few groups that have made studies frequently turn up unexpected and seemingly bizarre results — such as the lack of genetic effects in the Hiroshima-Nagasaki studies — which cast doubt on the methodology used or the suitability of the people selected.

The quest for reform of government research into radiation reflects a hope that it may still be possible to resolve the key issues by scientific means, a hope that may be in vain.

In any case, years will pass before science can produce definitive radiation research. Meantime policy decisions on nuclear energy, nuclear war strategy and medical practices face public officials.

Even if the risks associated with low-level radiation were precisely known, the policy decisions now facing the United States would involve painful choices. Some people invariably must bear a disproportionate amount of the risk that use of radiation entails, and somehow it must be determined how much risk certain social benefits are worth. There seems to be no way of making such determinations without ultimately putting a price on human life, and yet a cold calculation of this kind necessarily violates strong sentiments about the sanctity of life.

NUCLEAR WASTE: CENTRAL SAFETY ISSUE

Although radioactive wastes are generated at each stage of the nuclear fuel cycle, the most dangerous wastes are created in the operation of the reactors. Various decay products of nuclear fission build up in the fuel as the reaction proceeds and soon begin to interfere with fission activity. Because of this, and because the uranium fuel is gradually being consumed, about a third of the fuel in a reactor must be removed each year and replaced by new fuel. The spent fuel can be processed to recover usable

The Nuclear Fuel Cycle

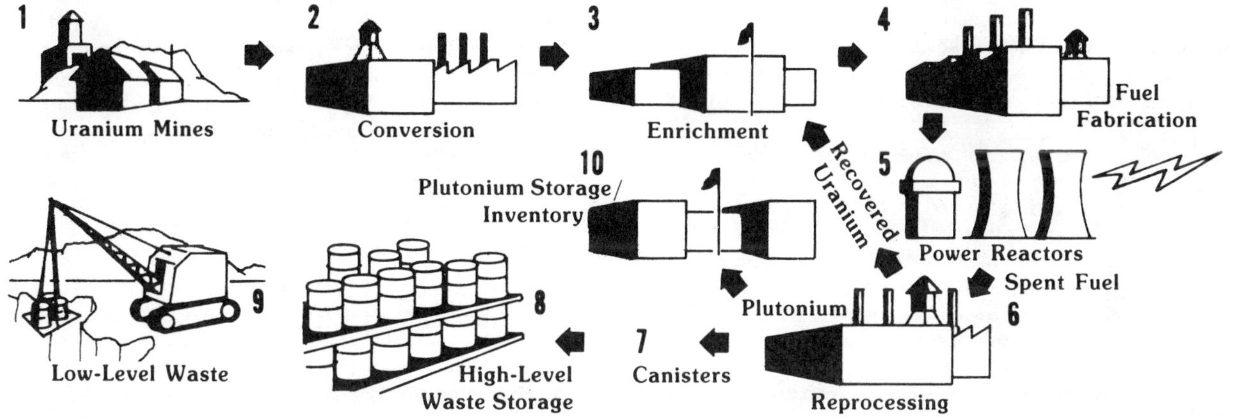

1. Mining and milling of ore to obtain raw uranium, called yellowcake, generates large quantities of low-level wastes called uranium tailings.
2. Removal of the impurities from the yellowcake and conversion.
3. Enrichment of the uranium from step 2 to a level suitable for power reactor fuel.
4. Conversion of the uranium from step 3 to leave a powder, which is fabricated into fuel elements for the power reactor.
5. Insertion of the fuel elements into the power reactor; operation of the reactor to produce electricity; removal of the spent or partially consumed fuel from the reactor; and storage of the highly radioactive spent fuel rods in cooling tanks at power plant.
6. Reprocessing of the spent fuel to separate unconsumed fuel from the radioactive wastes for future recycle.
7. Solidification of high-level liquid wastes left over after reprocessing to reduce the risks of accidential release and allow for permanent disposal.
8. Storage of high-level radioactive wastes for indefinite periods of time.
9. Burial of contaminated equipment, clothing and other low-level wastes.
10. Plutonium storage; recycling of recovered uranium.

SOURCE: Office of Technology Assessment

uranium and plutonium, but a lethal residue of liquid waste remains. The total amount of atomic waste produced by commercial nuclear power plants as of July 1981 was 4,880 cubic meters.

High-level radioactive wastes are classified as either fission products or fission byproducts. Although they have different properties and life spans, all must be isolated from the human environment for hundreds of years. In general, fission products have shorter toxic lives than fission byproducts. The most troublesome fission products, strontium-90 and cesium-137, have half-lives of about 30 years — which means that they remain dangerous for 600 to 1,000 years. (A half-life is the time required for half of the atoms of a radioactive substance to disintegrate.) The fission byproduct, plutonium-239, has a half-life of over 24,000 years, which means that it must be isolated from the biosphere for nearly 500,000 years. And because current reprocessing techniques do not physically separate the fission products from the fission byproducts, all high-level nuclear wastes must be contained for nearly half a million years.

Primary sources of radioactive waste are nuclear reactors used to produce electric power, drive nuclear submarines or produce plutonium for nuclear explosives. A number of byproducts from nuclear reactors are used in medicine, industry and research. Wastes produced by these byproducts are usually only slightly radioactive.

Another source of radioactive waste is the mining and milling of uranium. When uranium is separated from its ore in the milling process, the tailings from the milling retain radium and radon and are, thus, sources of radioactivity.

The mill tailing problem arose in August 1980 when 100 Navajo families filed a suit for damage over a large spill of radioactive waste that occurred in July 1979. The lawsuit filed by the Navajo people's legal service was entered in two tribal courts in New Mexico and Arizona against the United Nuclear Corp., which operated a uranium mill at Church Rock, New Mexico.

In 1979, a dam at the company's mill tailing pond broke and spilled 100 million gallons of low-level radioactive waste into the bed of the Rio Puerco. A resulting flash flood ran 90 miles downstream and finally ended about 45 miles from Arizona. At the time, Navajos living near the flood area were told not to let their livestock drink or graze near the riverbed.

Because of the low levels of radiation emanating from uranium tailings, a number of tailing piles for mills operating for the weapons program in the 1950s and 1960s were abandoned with little precaution to prevent their exposing the surrounding environment to radioactivity.

Sheldon Novick, in his book *The Careless Atom* (1969), wrote, "In other forms of air and water pollution, we have to reach the point of real disaster before beginning to think of control. This must not be allowed to happen with radioactive wastes — once entered on their winding course through the environment, radioactive isotopes are out of reach of man's control. The damage, once done, is irremediable."

Despite the dangers posed by the accumulation of large quantities of highly radioactive materials, waste management has had a relatively low priority in nuclear development. Many technical people familiar with the subject regard waste disposal as a difficult but soluble problem, and not a major obstacle to widespread adoption of nuclear power.

Nuclear Waste: Storage Pools Are Filling

Commercial nuclear reactors are fueled with enriched uranium which is contained in long metal rods. The nuclear reaction creates relatively short-lived fission products and what are called "transuranics."

The fission products, such as strontium-90 and cesium-137, are radioactive and hazardous for 300 to 600 years. The transuranics, such as plutonium-239, are even more radioactively dangerous and remain so for a much longer period — at least 245,000 years.

When commercial nuclear power was first promoted by the federal government, it was assumed that spent fuel from reactors would be reprocessed, an additional step that separates the fission products from the transuranics. The fission products would be stored and the transuranics used again as fuel. The spent fuel would again be reprocessed, and the cycle would continue.

Reprocessing never became a commercial success, however, and subsequently was banned by President Carter. He argued that the plutonium produced in reprocessing could eventually lead to the proliferation of nuclear weapons. (The Energy Department reprocesses spent fuel from military reactors to make atomic weapons for the Defense Department.)

How Reprocessing Works

Periodically, a portion of the fuel core of a nuclear reactor must be replaced with fresh uranium fuel. The spent fuel is stored in pools of water at the reactor site. The water cools the fuel and serves as a barrier preventing the escape of radioactivity.

Utility engineers have come up with several different methods for increasing the capacity of storage pools. They can stack the rods differently, for example, or add other materials that prevent interaction among the radioactive matter in the rods.

According to Owen Gormley, acting director of the Energy Department's fuel storage division in 1980, most plants were built on the assumption that they would store spent fuel for a year or so, then ship it to a reprocessing plant. Their storage pools are filling up.

Some utilities have put in more efficient racks, enabling them to store more fuel in the pools, but there is a limit to that. The Energy Department in 1980 said 27 nuclear plants would require away-from-reactor storage by 1985.

Critics suggest the department may be overestimating the need, as it has in the past. In 1979, for example, it said 1,180 tons of spent fuel would have to be stored away from reactors by 1985; in 1980 that estimate was reduced to 755 tons.

Making Up for the Past

Between 1946 and 1970, the United States dumped 62,000 steel drums containing low-level nuclear wastes into the Atlantic and Pacific oceans at various places. This practice was gradually discontinued and supplanted by land burial. In 1981, however, some states were becoming reluctant to accept any more radioactive wastes for land burial. This has prompted the federal government to investigate other options, including a return to ocean dumping. As a first step the Environmental Protection Agency initiated field studies to determine what had happened to low-level wastes dumped into oceans in past years.

The findings were not encouraging. Scientists in the mid-1970s found traces of radioactive cesium leaking from containers at a site 120 miles east of Ocean City, Md. They also found traces of plutonium in ocean sediment off the coast of San Francisco.

Between 1975 and 1980, the government grappled with several different plans for effective waste storage. In 1976, the Energy Research and Development Administration (ERDA) issued a five-volume report analyzing various technical alternatives for handling and storing commercial radioactive wastes. At that time, the processes included: 1) solidify liquid high-level wastes into glass, ceramics or calcine powder; 2) encapsulate them in cement, concrete or a glass medium, and 3) bury them in stable geologic formations, such as salt beds.

Salt beds are considered the most likely repositories because the presence of the bed indicates that no water has penetrated the area for a long time; otherwise the salt would have dissolved.

A water-tight cavity is important because flowing water can carry particles of waste from burial sites into the environment. In addition, salt beds are geologically stable; they are not likely to be affected by earthquakes. Finally, salt can mend itself when it is fractured. Consequently, a disposal site in salt would be protected against geologic stress which might cause fissures in other formations.

In 1966, salt mines in central Kansas were studied as possible burial grounds for nuclear waste. In 1970, the then Atomic Energy Commission selected an abandoned salt mine near Lyons, Kansas, as a demonstration facility for waste emplacement. Residents and local officials, unwilling to have dangerous materials stored near their homes, forced the AEC to abandon the facility. Residents also feared that numerous drill holes and shafts would make the depository unstable.

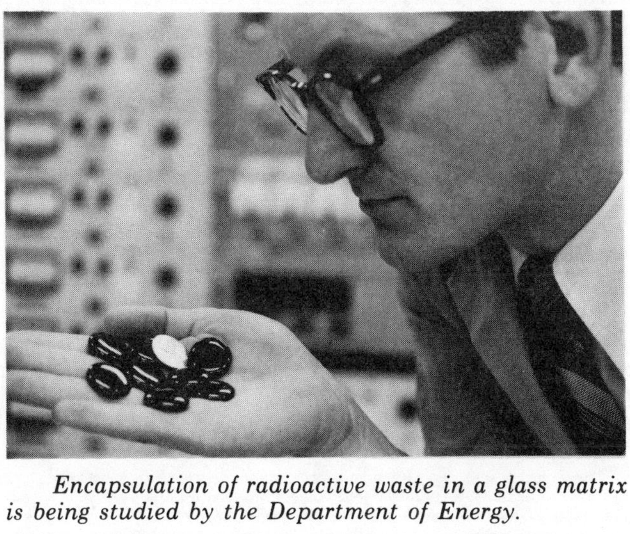

Encapsulation of radioactive waste in a glass matrix is being studied by the Department of Energy.

The bedded salt concept is still looked upon as the most satisfactory. Other options include: disposal in other geological formations, such as granite and domed salt; transportation to outer space; disposal under the ocean floor; or transmutation of long-lived radioactive elements into less troublesome forms.

The Department of Energy also is investigating the possibility of creating a very deep underground cavity — possibly with an atomic explosion — and injecting liquid nuclear wastes into it. The theory is that the hot wastes would melt the surrounding underground rocks, which would resolidify so tightly they would contain wastes.

Another possibility involves a process called transmutation; in which long-lived radioactive wastes are bombarded with neutrons inside a reactor to burn off more of the fissionable material, thus shortening their hazardous life. However, the engineering problems are enormous and some radioactive waste products, such as cesium-137 and strontium-90 cannot easily be changed by this bombardment process.

Future of Plutonium Processing

Spent nuclear fuel rods are intensely radioactive and generate tremendous amounts of heat. After removal from the reactor, they are temporarily stored in a large concrete chamber, open at the top and filled with about 40 feet of water. They are positioned in a rigid storage rock at the bottom of the chamber to allow the water to circulate continuously and prevent a chain reaction.

Most people assume that the only way to handle nuclear wastes is to store them safely until they lose their radioactivity. But some scientists say there could be alternatives to storage.

Dixy Lee Ray, former chairman of the Atomic Energy Commission and a strong advocate of nuclear power, has said, "It has happened before, that today's garbage turns out to be tomorrow's useful product, and this can happen with radioactive wastes too, at least to some extent." She noted that various radioisotopes already were being used in industrial processes, in non-destructive testing and in medical research, and that plutonium-run batteries were operating instruments sending back data from the moon. Scientists hope one day to use radioactive cesium to kill germs and viruses in treated sewage sludge, making it safe for use as fertilizers and cattle feed.

Perhaps the most significant pending decisions concerning nuclear waste management relate to the commercial reprocessing of spent nuclear fuel. Reprocessing is a procedure that converts uranium fuel that has been burned in reactors into a liquid and separates remaining uranium and plutonium from wastes. The recovered uranium and plutonium can be used in reactors as fuel.

"The basic technology," writes Sarah Miller, editor of *Nucleonics Weekly*, an industry newsletter, "was developed in the weapons program, and the plan was for industry gradually to build up civilian capacity in rhythm with the increase in the number of nuclear reactors."

There are three commercial reprocessing facilities in the United States: the Nuclear Fuel Services plant in West

Clinch River Reactor

The Clinch River breeder reactor in Tennessee, designed to produce endless fuel, seemed like the perfect answer to the world's energy problems. Environmentalists didn't see it that way and made the proposed project the symbolic centerpiece of the national fight over nuclear power.

Since Congress first authorized the program in 1970, more than $1 billion had been spent on the project. The estimated cost of the project grew from $700 million to at least $3.2 billion, and actual construction had not even begun by 1981.

The proposal had fallen on hard times during President Carter's administration. Throughout his term, Carter tried to kill the project, claiming the plutonium it created could result in the spread of atomic weapons. Carter was aided by strong opposition from environmental and taxpayer groups. But he never was able to overcome the alliance of nuclear advocates, Tennessee lawmakers and utility lobbyists; each year Congress appropriated funds for Clinch River. By 1981, the battlelines were clearly drawn and the issues well known on both sides. But powerful friends, heavy lobbying and a confused congressional budget process combined to keep Clinch River alive.

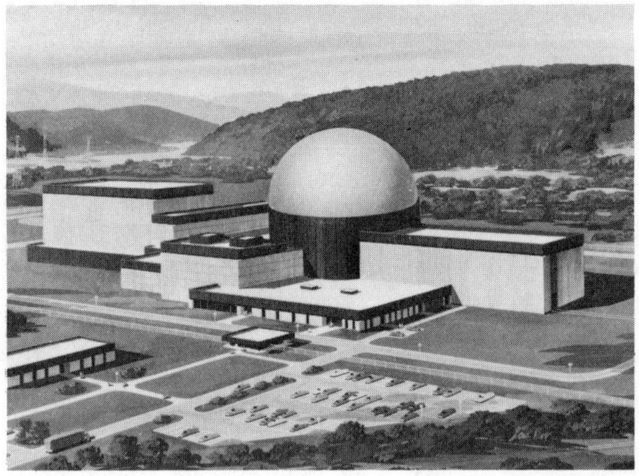

The Stockman Shock

The nation's utilities and the nuclear industry expected the Reagan administration to move ahead quickly on programs important to them, including Clinch River. But Reagan's choice of David A. Stockman to be director of the Office of Management and Budget sent shivers through Clinch River supporters. As a first-term congressman from Michigan in 1977, Stockman had prepared a study concluding that the federal government should abandon the project on economic grounds.

Stockman's initial draft of the fiscal 1982 budget did not include Clinch River funding. However, when Reagan presented the budget in March 1981, $254 million for the project was included. The president had inserted the funding, over Stockman's objections, at the request of Senate Majority Leader Howard H. Baker Jr., R-Tenn., a vigorous supporter of the project for his state.

Clinch River opponents, led by lobbyists Renee Parsons of Friends of the Earth and Jill Greenbaum of the National Taxpayers Union, focused their efforts in 1981 on the House Science Committee, which had 13 new members and had lost two of its most ardent nuclear supporters.

Parsons and Greenbaum, working with Rep. Claudine Schneider of Rhode Island and other freshman Republicans, put together a coalition of junior Republicans and liberal Democrats. The Republican members were subjected to heavy pressure from the Reagan administration. But in an unusually chaotic committee meeting May 7, 1981, with lobbyists lining the walls, Schneider's proposal to kill the project was approved 22-18. Of the committee's 13 new members, 10 voted with Schneider.

In the Senate Clinch River opponents convinced their allies — Edward M. Kennedy, D-Mass., and Dale Bumpers, D-Ark. — not to offer a proposal killing Clinch River. With Baker's potent opposition, they felt certain to lose.

But opponents of the project did not get a chance at that time to find out if the Science Committee's position was shared in the House at large. The issue was submerged in a larger debate in the spring and early summer over federal spending. In a battle over reconciliation legislation, a device designed to force Senate and House committees to comply with congressionally approved spending ceilings for the federal government, Clinch River never came to a separate vote. One version of the reconciliation legislation, produced by Reagan's White House, added money for the Clinch River project to attract the vote of Southern Democrats. House Democratic leaders sought to obtain a separate vote on this and other controversial parts of the White House plan, but failed. The House, without debating the Clinch River issue, approved the Republican budget plan, which included $230 million for Clinch River. As a result, no direct Clinch River vote occurred at that time.

Nevertheless, both sides were primed for the fight. A month later, though, on July 24, 1981, environmental and taxpayer groups learned that the industry and its friends were still in the driver's seat as they had been when the House several times in the previous four years voted to build the reactor. This time the House voted 186-206 against an amendment to cut funding for the project.

Valley, N.Y.; General Electric's Midwest Fuel Recovery Plant at Morris, Ill.; and the Allied-General plant in Barnwell, S.C. But all three had been plagued by technical and financial difficulties, and none was operating in mid-1981. The West Valley plant, the only one of the three ever to operate, opened in 1966 but had to close in 1972 for repairs because radioactive leaks were contaminating workers and the environment.

Politically Explosive Problem

What to do with nuclear garbage has become a politically explosive issue. The debate is "30 percent fact and 70 percent emotion," said one environmental lobbyist involved in the issue.

Environmentalists have been calling public attention to the problem, making life more difficult for the nuclear power industry that was already beleaguered following the March 1979 accident at Three Mile Island, Pa. Beyond the scientific problem of how to safely contain highly radioactive wastes, Congress must grapple with a number of other contentious issues, such as the rights of the states to refuse nuclear dumps, the application of federal environmental restrictions, and the federal government's responsibility for the burned fuel being generated by private nuclear plants.

The combination of these factors has produced a political thicket that has entangled and battered the several bills being pushed by various interests to solve the problems.

The most immediate problem is the burial of "low-level" nuclear wastes, which are generated in every community in the United States. Low-level wastes include contaminated paper, plastics, construction materials, tools, protective clothing, industrial wastes and contaminated trash produced by nuclear production.

Of the 100,000 cubic meters of low-level wastes produced annually, about 43 percent comes from nuclear power plants, 25 percent from hospitals, 24 percent from industry and 8 percent from the federal government. The Energy Department also buries about 50,000 cubic meters of this waste each year in its own dumps.

In a first step toward federal control of waste, the government in September 1980 assumed responsibility for

Nuclear Waste Storage Sites

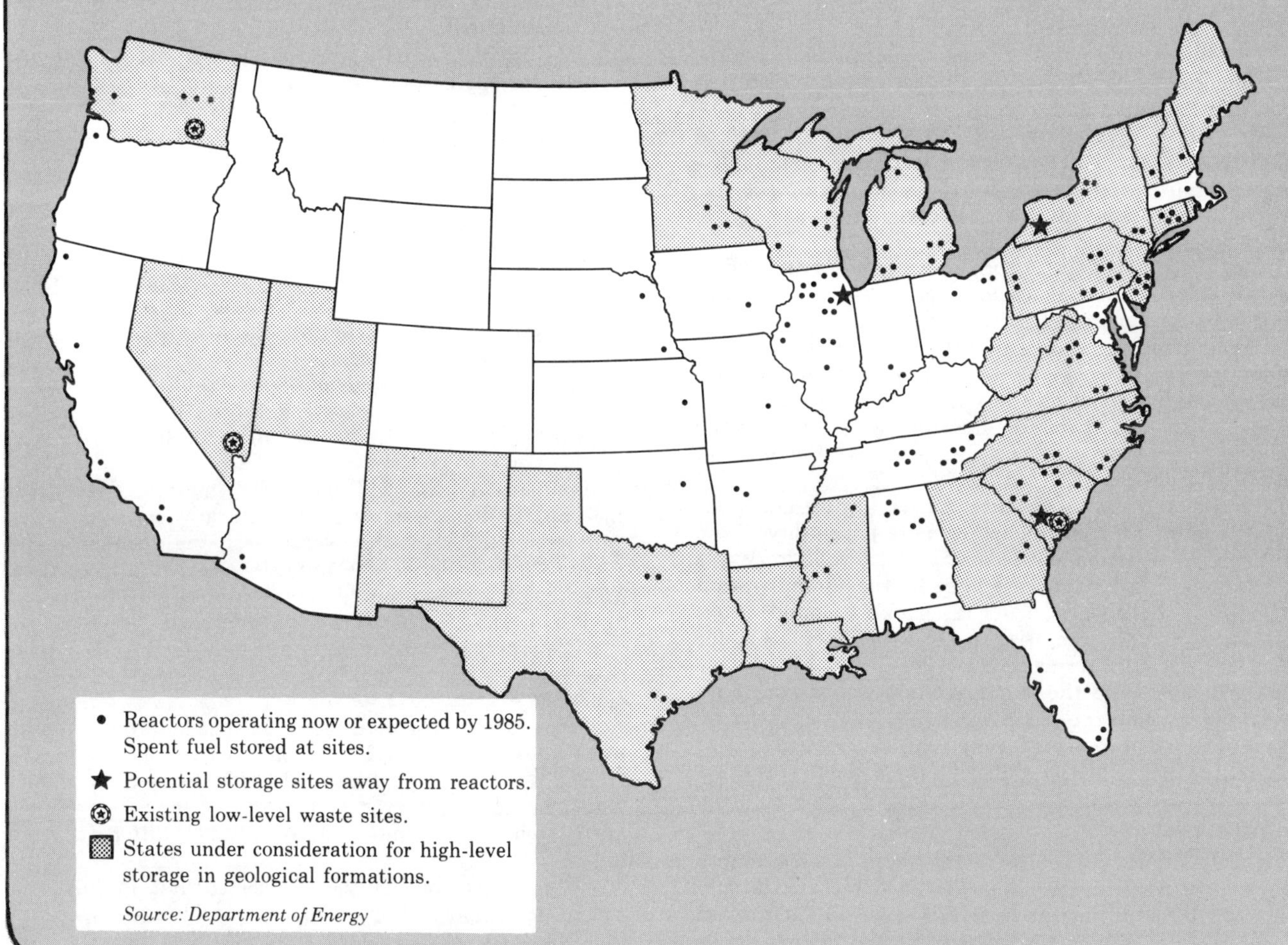

removing high-level radioactive waste at the defunct nuclear reprocessing plant in West Valley, N.Y. The law authorized the federal cleanup and removal of approximately 600,000 gallons of highly radioactive liquid waste at the Western New York Nuclear Service Center at West Valley. The cost of the cleanup, then estimated at $300 million, was to be split, with 90 percent paid by the federal government and 10 percent paid by New York. In May 1981, several congressional committees were investigating the agreement signed by the Carter administration to clean up the plant.

1980 Action

Congress and the executive branch made their first serious attempts to deal with the waste disposal problem during the 96th Congress in 1979-80. Congress, working independently of the executive branch, passed bills in both the Senate and House. But the two chambers were unable to reach a compromise and no final bill was passed. Critics blamed the administration's inability to sell its proposals to Congress for the plan's failure.

Carter Proposal

In 1978, President Carter established an Interagency Review Group to examine the nuclear waste problem. Based on its March 1979 recommendations, he issued what the White House called a comprehensive national policy on nuclear waste management.

According to Carter, the primary objective of his program was to effectively isolate radioactive waste resulting from both military and civilian activities from the biosphere so that they would pose no significant threat to public health and safety. "The effort," he said, "must proceed regardless of future developments within the nuclear industry — its future size, and resolution of specific fuel cycle and reactor design issues."

Carter's plan called for permanent geologic disposal of nuclear wastes. Following the requirements of the National Environmental Policy Act (NEPA), the federal government would evaluate four or five potential sites in a variety of different types of rock formation, selecting one site for development by 1985 with a goal of having it operational by the mid-1990s. Carter insisted that nuclear garbage dumps would be licensed by the Nuclear Regulatory Commission (NRC).

To the delight of environmentalists, Carter said spent nuclear fuel would continue to be the responsibility of the utilities until a permanent federal geologic repository was built. To their dismay, however, he said the administration would press for passage of its legislation to build away-from-reactor (AFR) facilities to store the spent fuel for which utilities do not have room.

Carter also said the administration would work with the states through the planning council to establish a regional network of low-level waste disposal sites. He asked Congress to permanently authorize the council.

Senate Bill

Carter's formal proposal came more than a month after the Senate Energy Committee had reported a substantially different nuclear waste bill in early 1980. Instead of emphasizing permanent geologic storage of radioactive wastes, the committee bill called for putting high-level wastes in above-ground vaults for as long as 100 years or more. The wastes could be monitored and even retrieved, if necessary or profitable. Geological investigations were to continue.

The Senate passed the bill July 30, 1980, by a vote of 88-7, five days after another Senate panel, the Environment Committee, reported a bill emphasizing permanent disposal. The Environment proposal would have set a specific timetable for the government to follow to have a permanent disposal site in operation by the year 2000. If the site were not established by then, the NRC could not issue construction permits or operating licenses for new nuclear power plants.

The final version of the bill provided for AFR storage of spent fuel for utilities, as proposed by the administration, in 1979. The government would take over the responsibility for storing spent fuel until a permanent geologic site was available. The utilities would pay a one-time fee, but would retain rights to the spent fuel if reprocessing were latter allowed.

The storage vaults for high-level waste were exempted from NEPA provisions that require an environmental impact statement before a site is decided upon. The impact statement eventually written would not have to consider alternative facilities, and the NRC in its licensing process also could not review alternatives, as it normally does.

The measure also authorized the state planning council. It said the states would participate in decisions on where to store wastes, but left details to be handled by floor amendment.

The Senate added a provision giving states authority to veto storage of nuclear wastes within their borders if their objections were upheld by either the House or Senate. However, this section would not apply to AFR spent fuel facilities.

House Bills

In the House, leaders of two of the three committees involved in the legislation reached a last-minute compromise in mid-November 1980. Though they managed to get their comprehensive waste bill through the House, the legislation died in conference.

The issue that proved most intractable to the conferees was the question of state authority over disposal of nuclear wastes from military activities. Although the Senate had voted to give states limited authority over military waste disposal, Energy Committee Chairman Henry M. Jackson, D-Wash., refused to allow any state say over military wastes. Jackson, a second-ranking member of the Senate Armed Services Committee, feared a precedent would be set for a state role in other military decisions. His unyielding position doomed the conference.

Congress did pass a separate bill enacting the relatively non-controversial title dealing with low-level wastes. *(Low-level wastes, box, p. 75)*

The compromise agreement between Interior Committee Chairman Morris K. Udall, D-Ariz., and John D. Dingell, D-Mich., chairman of the Commerce Subcommittee on Energy and Power, had by-passed the Science Committee, which had drafted its own, much different waste bill.

The Science bill had been reported first, in July, and called for demonstration of underground waste disposal at four sites by 1990. Under the bill, the projects were

Nuclear Wastes Vary in Danger, But Nobody Wants to Take Responsibility

Nuclear waste comes in a variety of forms that present varying degrees of danger.

High-level Wastes. High-level wastes are highly radioactive liquids generated when used nuclear reactor fuel is reprocessed. Presidents Ford and Carter both banned commercial reprocessing of fuel, but the government continues to reprocess fuel for military uses. About 75 million gallons of these high-level wastes had been generated through 1979. They were stored at sites in Washington state, Idaho, South Carolina and New York.

Transuranic Wastes. These are produced in the reprocessing of nuclear fuel and the production of nuclear bombs. While not as intensely radioactive as high-level wastes, transuranic wastes take far longer — many thousands of years — to decay to a safe form.

Low-level Wastes. Low-level wastes are generated from all activities using radioactive materials. They include protective clothing, hand tools, rags, vials and a variety of solutions, many from medical uses. It is this category that may become the most politically volatile in the near future, as the only three states with disposal facilities for commercial low-level wastes had closed them down as of September 1981.

Uranium Tailings. This waste from mills and mines contains naturally occurring radioactive materials. Huge piles of these tailings, in the form of fine sand, have been dumped at abandoned mills and mines in 11 states.

Spent Nuclear Fuel. Spent nuclear fuel is not classified as waste because it still contains minerals that could be reused, but if it were classified, it would be a high-level waste. Because of the ban on reprocessing, utilities must keep racks of spent fuel assemblies in pools of water near their reactors, and some of those pools are filling up. While the nuclear waste bills before Congress dealt primarily with high-level wastes, the problem of what to do with spent nuclear fuel from commercial reactors has drawn much political interest.

Even though the federal government has always had responsibility for handling military wastes from nuclear weapons programs and since 1954 has been responsible for wastes generated by commercial nuclear power, Congress has never passed detailed legislation concerning the problem. After four decades of waste generation, no permanent disposal sites have been provided for the hazardous materials, some of which remain radioactive for more than a thousand years. Instead, by the late 1970s the federal government had built a poor record of waste management.

Gus Speth, a member of the White House Council on Environmental Quality, summed up concerns about the government's track record in a September 1977 speech: "Perhaps the waste problem is manageable in theory; perhaps not. I hope it is. But many things that are theoretically doable never get done. Certainly the sorry history of radioactive waste management in this country to date provides no basis for confidence that things will work out."

Congress has not gone that far in linking waste disposal with continued nuclear development. But nuclear advocates had begun to realize by the late 1970s that inaction on nuclear waste was becoming a serious liability to the nuclear industry. The Carter administration held the same view, and its officials concluded that public opposition was a bigger problem than the remaining technical questions about isolating materials from air, water and human contact for several centuries. The solution they proposed was a methodical exploration of possible waste sites, with federal officials cooperating fully with the state and local governments.

In Congress, though, the sentiment has been for a better defined state role. The majority sentiment appeared to favor state authority to veto waste disposal if Congress went along with that action. Then, the problem of having all of the states refuse would be avoided and a federal role would be retained. But if a state truly did not want the radioactive waste, it is not likely a vote by Congress could force the citizens to accept it.

exempted from requirements of the National Environmental Policy Act and from NRC licensing. No public hearings were required on site selection. Environmental groups warned that the demonstration projects could be converted later to full-scale repositories, without having undergone full environmental and safety reviews.

Commerce and Interior reported their versions of the waste bill in August and early September. Commerce provided for the four demonstration sites, but required they be closed in the year 2000.

Interior rejected the idea of unlicensed test sites and set out a detailed schedule for the Energy Department to follow in developing a licensed, full-scale geologic waste repository, to be operational by about 1996. The committee argued that test sites could not demonstrate the ability to safely isolate wastes for more than a few years, a very short time considering the long period that nuclear wastes remain dangerous. Meanwhile, the emphasis on these demonstration sites would delay work on permanent repositories. That work, primarily the testing of different geologic formations to isolate the waste from man and the environment, should proceed, the panel said.

In addition to reporting a companion to the Science Committee bill, Commerce also reported legislation emphasizing permanent disposal, as a companion to the Interior approach. Interior had put its provisions in two different bills: one to accompany the Science bill, which had been referred to Interior and Commerce, and one of its own that was referred only to Commerce.

The November compromise fashioned from the Commerce and Interior versions, dropped the idea of underground demonstration projects and abandoned any provision for surface, vault-type storage. A sticking point was the question of state veto rights over waste sites. Commerce required both houses to agree with a state on blocking a waste dump within its borders. Interior said if either house went along, the state veto would be upheld. The November compromise adopted the Interior position, giving states more authority.

On the House floor in early December 1980, the question of state rights was the most controversial. An amendment was offered by Peter H. Kostmayer, D-Pa., to let a state's veto of a disposal site stand unless both houses of Congress voted to override it. But the amendment failed, 161-218, leaving intact the compromise in favor of one-house approval of a state veto.

The approach by the House bill was much closer to the Senate Environment Committee's proposal than the Senate Energy Committee's bill that had been approved by the Senate. The House Interior and Commerce compromise had left out any provision for away-from-reactor storage, which was included in the Senate bill and sought by the nuclear industry and the Carter administration.

Reagan Stance

The Reagan administration, led by Department of Energy Secretary James B. Edwards, had promised to make the establishment of permanent storage sites for highly radioactive wastes a priority issue. Edwards, according to a report in *The Washington Post* in February 1981, said that he did not believe state governors should have the power to veto the location of a site.

Sheldon Meyers, deputy assistant secretary for nuclear waste at the Energy Department, announced the administration's proposals before a House Energy Research and Production Subcommittee hearing in June 1981. Meyers said, "We strongly believe that the ultimate goal of the [department's] program must remain a system of licensed full-scale repositories to handle all high-level nuclear waste that will be generated."

Meyers listed three areas in which the Reagan administration planned to deal with the waste disposal problem:

- Plans to store commercial spent fuel at federally-owned away-from-reactor facilities would be discontinued.
- A terminal isolation program would be reoriented to help gain information for decisions on where to construct licensed waste storage repositories. Exploratory shafts would be sunk at several sites for underground investigations concerning site suitability.
- A waste isolation pilot plant project would provide research facilities for demonstrating safe disposal of waste from defense activities. The revised 1982 Reagan budget provided for the placement of radioactive materials in a research and development facility before 1990.

6

Food: Is It Safe to Eat?

One of the most difficult issues before government officials is drawing a line between protecting the public health and permitting consumers access to potentially dangerous substances that offer some apparent benefit or satisfaction.

This challenge, which has troubled Congress and federal regulators for some time, has also been placed increasingly before the private companies that manufacture or prepare the substances and offer them in the marketplace.

Reports have become commonplace during the last two decades about the potential hazards of popular U.S. habits such as eating processed foods, smoking cigarettes and even drinking beer. But public reaction to health warnings is unpredictable. When the dangers of agricultural pesticides were publicized in the 1960s, most people applauded government efforts to control their use. More recently, however, when regulators attempted to ban the artificial sweetener saccharin, they met with widespread opposition. The problem is magnified because regulatory decisions — such as whether or not saccharin is safe — sometimes must be based on uncertain scientific data.

Most of this chapter is devoted to a discussion of food and food additives. Three federal agencies have primary responsibility for regulating the contents of food Americans eat. The Food and Drug Administration (FDA), a part of the Department of Health and Human Services, sets standards for the safety of food and additives. An independent agency, the Environmental Protection Agency (EPA), establishes tolerances for the amount of pesticide residues left in or on food. The Department of Agriculture monitors the safety of meat. Jurisdictions may overlap. For example, a regulatory move to ban nitrite in meats involved both the FDA and the Agriculture Department. On Capitol Hill, the House and Senate Agriculture Committees, the House Energy and Commerce Committee and the Senate Labor and Human Resources Committee all have been involved in regulating food additives.

Delaney Clause

Much of the debate over food safety has centered on the 1958 Delaney clause, which flatly prohibits any food additive that "induces" cancer in humans or animals. The clause was named after its sponsor, Rep. James Delaney, D-N.Y. (1945-47, 1949-78). Representatives of the food industry have questioned reports linking common foods and beverages to cancer and other illnesses and expressed doubt about the scientific methods employed to detect health hazards. The food industry has lobbied for a revised clause that would allow regulators to take into consideration any benefits provided by a suspect substance. Consumer groups, meanwhile, have charged Congress and agencies authorized to protect the U.S. food supply with failure to subject food to sufficiently close scrutiny. These groups also claim that loopholes in the Delaney clause permit dangerous substances to remain on the market.

The saccharin ban proposed by the FDA in 1977 gave a major push to the debate about changes in food safety controls. Although Congress forbade the FDA to ban saccharin, no major overhaul of food safety legislation was begun by the middle of 1981. The Reagan administration vowed to offer a replacement for the Delaney clause.

Federal regulatory standards for food range from the unqualified ban of the Delaney clause, which applied to substances added by food manufacturers, to a two-step process applicable to pesticides and drugs given to animals. Preliminary approval of a substance was followed by monitoring for unacceptable levels in food and confiscation if food were contaminated. Tolerance levels for pesticides were set by the EPA. Manufacturers of animal drugs used to prevent disease and fatten livestock were required to show that technology existed to detect traces of the drug in animal carcasses. The Commerce Department handled contaminated fish; responsibility for monitoring meat and produce was shared by the FDA and the Department of Agriculture. Substances that had been sanctioned for use by the FDA before 1958 were exempt from both Delaney and tolerance settings, having been "grandfathered" in the food law revision of that year. They remained subject to a general safety requirement, however.

Distrust and Approval

The history of food legislation mirrors public distrust that has cut two ways, against both manufacturers and federal regulators. Constituents sometimes have pressured Congress to protect them from apparent hazards. But industry lobbyists and constituents also have persuaded members to block the FDA when it has tried to remove popular substances from the market.

For example, a battle along the same lines as the saccharin fight erupted in 1976, three years after the FDA proposed to set potency limits for vitamins and minerals and to regulate as drugs any diet supplements that exceeded those limits. Opponents, including health food and pharmaceutical groups, argued against "diet dictation" and "Big Brotherism," and Congress responded by severely curbing FDA authority over vitamins and minerals.

History of Regulation

Congress first authorized regulation of the food industry in 1906, following muckraking press reports of watered milk (with chalk added to restore white color), canned green beans whose color was maintained with copper, unsanitary meat processing and other disturbing food industry practices. Additional pressure on Congress arose from reports about the "Poison Squad," a group of volunteers who, under the supervision of the Department of Agriculture, were fed small doses of poisons similar or identical to substances found in then-common food preservatives. The 1906 law, the basis of the existing Food, Drug and Cosmetic Act, prohibited manufacture of or interstate commerce in adulterated or misbranded foods.

A 1938 modification of the law tightened labeling requirements and broadened the definition of prohibited additives to anything that was injurious to health, but it was not until 1958 that Congress required manufacturers to prove the safety of an additive before putting it into food. For pesticides, mandatory pre-market testing was enacted in 1954. Color additives, treated separately, were brought under mandatory pre-market testing and the Delaney clause in 1960.

The limits of scientific knowledge have been a key topic in the congressional debate on food safety. Pressures for decisions on saccharin and other additives pushed Congress and federal regulators into the murky world of scientific hypothesis where certainties are rare — and almost always challenged.

Key technical questions remained unanswered in arguments over how far federal regulators can go to remove from the food supply suspected carcinogens or other substances that may damage fetuses, impair the body's immune system or cause genetic damage. For example, no one appeared to know with certainty:

- How environmental exposure, genetic makeup, the disease process and personal habits mix to cause the approximately 100 types of cancer.
- How to predict the magnitude of risk to humans from a substance that causes cancer in laboratory animals.
- How to set a safe level for consumption of, or other human exposure to, substances that cause cancer in laboratory animals.

Affected industries have resisted regulatory efforts growing out of such an uncertain scientific base, but pressures for decisions despite scientific uncertainty remained strong.

Animal Testing

Much of the debate over carcinogenic substances turned on the accuracy of testing, with spokesmen for affected industries arguing that producing cancer in animals simply was not the same as producing it in humans. One industry group, the Calorie Control Council, criticized the data from the saccharin study, emphasizing the enormous quantity of the sweetener that was fed to small laboratory animals to produce a heightened incidence of cancer.

Cancer researchers responded that the sizable doses compensate for built-in shortcomings of animal tests and that test results are valid. Rats are smaller, their lives are far shorter and their cells multiply more rapidly than those of humans. Dosage differences must compensate for those disparities, researchers argued. Moreover, low-level risk such as that attributed to saccharin meant that relatively few cases of cancer would show up in an exposed population. Even if test animals could perfectly duplicate human life span and size, no one could test a substance on 220 million animals, thus duplicating the size of the U.S. population. Concentrated dosage is needed to reveal the probability of risk in smaller test "populations," the researchers claimed.

There are problems in using animal data to predict human susceptibility to a carcinogen, but ethics bar duplicating animal results by deliberately exposing humans to a cancer-causing substance. However, all but two substances known to cause cancer in humans similarly affect laboratory animals, according to researchers. An additional problem facing cancer scientists is how to determine from animal test data the number of humans who would develop cancer from exposure to a carcinogen.

The Vanishing Zero

A second related testing issue involved the dramatic improvement of methods for detecting the presence of chemicals. Scientists can now measure quantities as minute as a nanogram — a billionth of a gram; a gram is about a thirtieth of an ounce. And detection techniques may be refined even further.

The capacity to measure ever-diminishing quantities means that scientists may never be able to rule out the possibility that a troublesome substance is present at very small, trace levels. Researchers refer to this as "the search for a vanishing zero." The Delaney clause forbids any carcinogens in food, no matter how small the amount. Scientists fear that they may be incapable of guaranteeing the total absence of harmful substances.

The questions surrounding suspected carcinogens apply as well to other potential health hazards. Alarms have been raised concerning dangers associated with salt, sugar, lead in foods and caffeine. Some researchers are convinced that these and other substances contribute to a welter of ailments, among them heart disease, genetic malformation, and high blood pressure. Other researchers are not so sure. One topic on which almost the entire scientific community agrees is the danger presented by smoking. An estimated 54 million Americans continue to smoke, despite evidence linking the habit to various kinds of cancers.

Food Safety Legislation

Congress has discussed food safety reform for several years, but no cohesive legislative program has emerged, as legislators and regulators prefer to take what has been termed the "carcinogen of the month" approach to deal with such substances as saccharin and nitrite. A promised reform of food safety legislation by President Carter's administration failed to appear. President Reagan's interest in reducing government regulation suggested that his administration was willing to work for less food safety regulation.

An agriculture subcommittee in the U.S. House of Representatives in June 1981 began a series of hearings on food and pesticide safety issues. The focus of the hearings was a bill, HR 638, that would establish a National Science Council to decide questions of scientific fact arising out of regulatory actions. The hearings also reviewed risk-benefit systems, a process that requires regulators to weigh the risks and benefits of proposed regulations. According to Rep. George Brown, D-Calif., chairman of the House Agriculture Subcommittee on Department Operations, Research and Foreign Agriculture, "What we are seeking in these oversight hearings is a review of the decision-making policies used by federal agencies which regulate pesticide use and food production, processing and marketing. We must insure that our laws are flexible enough to keep abreast of the impacts of technology on human health while not impeding promising new advances in agricultural and marketing systems which could lead to significant public benefits."

SACCHARIN: A BAN THAT NEVER CAME

Officials of the Food and Drug Administration created a furor in March 1977 when they announced plans to prohibit the use of saccharin as a food additive. The decision was based on laboratory tests, conducted in Canada, in which rats fed large doses of saccharin showed an increased tendency to develop bladder cancer. The FDA also proposed to permit the sale of the popular artificial sweetener as an over-the-counter drug — temporarily, and with a warning label. Manufacturers would have six months to prove that the substance was an effective drug for diabetics and the obese.

Reaction from diet food and drink manufacturers and the diet-conscious American public was swift. Opponents of the ban ridiculed the Canadian tests, claiming that a human would have to drink 800 12-ounce cans of diet soda daily to match the saccharin intake of the laboratory rats. The Calorie Control Council, an industry group, argued that banning the sweetener threatened the health of diabetics and people who needed to control their weight. People would brush their teeth less with unsweetened toothpaste, opponents warned, and children would refuse to take unsweetened medicines.

The opponents of the saccharin ban made their opinions known on Capitol Hill. Some members of Congress claimed that the ban provoked more mail and telephone calls from constituents than any other issue in recent memory. In response, Congress in November 1977 adopted legislation ordering the FDA to postpone the ban for 18 months. The bill also asked the National Academy of Sciences to conduct a study of saccharin and food safety policy. Congress, however, let stand an FDA requirement that products containing saccharin carry a label warning: "Use of this product may be hazardous to your health. This product contains saccharin, which has been determined to cause cancer in laboratory animals." The FDA also required stores to post warning notices about saccharin.

NAS Report Part I

The first part of the National Academy of Science report requested by Congress was released in November

Saccharin Ban Delay

As signed into law, the 1977 bill delaying the proposed Food and Drug Administration (FDA) ban on the artificial sweetener saccharin contained the following major provisions:

- Prohibited the secretary of Health, Education and Welfare (HEW, now Health and Human Services) from banning or restricting for 18 months the sale or distribution of saccharin or any product containing it on the basis of studies or tests available before the date of enactment of the bill.
- Required that any food product containing saccharin introduced into interstate commerce beginning 90 days after enactment of the bill would be considered misbranded under the Food, Drug and Cosmetic Act if it did not contain the following label in conspicuous and legible type: "USE OF THIS PRODUCT MAY BE HAZARDOUS TO YOUR HEALTH. THIS PRODUCT CONTAINS SACCHARIN WHICH HAS BEEN DETERMINED TO CAUSE CANCER IN LABORATORY ANIMALS."
- Authorized the secretary to revise or remove labeling and information requirements if new information about saccharin warranted it.
- Required manufacturers of products containing saccharin to provide retail stores selling those products with warning signs informing consumers of the health risks associated with saccharin.
- Required the secretary to prepare information on the saccharin controversy to be displayed and distributed by retail establishments selling those products with warning signs informing consumers of the health risks associated with saccharin.
- Required the secretary to prepare information on the saccharian controversy to be displayed and distributed by retail establishments selling saccharin products.
- Authorized the secretary to require vending machines containing saccharin products to display in a conspicuous place on the machine a warning of the health risks associated with saccharin usage.
- Required the secretary to conduct studies and report to Congress within 15 months on a number of subjects, including the health benefits and risks to humans from carcinogenic substances in food.
- Required the secretary to report to Congress within one year on the chemical identity of any impurities found in saccharin, their toxicity and carcinogenicity, and the health benefits resulting from the use of artificial sweeteners in general and saccharin in particular.
- Directed the secretary to ask the National Academy of Sciences to conduct the studies; if it declined, authorized him to contract with another public or nonprofit entity.

1977. Saccharin, the report said, was by itself or in combination with other substances a relatively weak carcinogen in rats. Saccharin itself, not impurities in the substance, was the carcinogen. Other findings of the report:

- It was scientifically valid to conclude that if a substance caused cancer in animals, it would cause cancer in humans, but animal tests could not be relied upon to gauge the risk of cancer in humans.
- There were no acceptable epidemiological (population) studies linking cancer directly to human consumption of saccharin, perhaps because investigatory methods lacked the necessary sensitivity to detect the incidence of cancer from a weak carcinogen or distinguish between the effects of saccharin and those of stronger carcinogens.
- The benefits of saccharin use by diabetics and the obese had not been determined in clinical studies.
- Although the cancer risk of saccharin was probably low, "even low risks to a large number of exposed persons may lead to public health concerns."
- Children and women of child-bearing age consumed more saccharin than other groups.

The alleged saccharin-cancer link was disputed by three additional studies released in 1980. Prepared by the National Cancer Institute, the Harvard University School of Public Health and the American Health Foundation, the reports found little or no connection between saccharin and cancer and claimed that the dangers of saccharin use may have been overstated.

Congress twice has extended the moratorium on the FDA's saccharin ban. The most recent legislation, passed in 1981, prohibited the FDA from taking any action to remove the sweetener from the nation's food supply until 1983.

The saccharin ban highlighted the problem facing public health agencies: regulating substances proved harmful in tests but that also benefited some segments of the population. The ban also prompted calls for an overhaul of food safety legislation. Opponents of the Delaney clause have charged that the law is too rigid because it recognized neither the benefits of the suspect substances nor the fact that scientists had developed the ability to measure quantities of those substances far smaller than anyone had imagined in 1958.

NAS Report Part II

In the second half of its study ordered by Congress in 1977, the National Academy of Sciences (NAS) urged a reform of food laws to do away with the restrictive Delaney clause. The report urged Congress to allow regulators to consider health or economic benefits when a ban on suspected carcinogens is under consideration. The NAS report said Congress should rewrite federal food laws to permit a variety of regulatory opinions for carcinogenic and other food additives, depending on how risky they were for human health. The FDA would be empowered to classify a substance as high-, moderate- or low-risk and fashion an appropriate regulatory action: outright ban, restricted sales, continued sales with warning labels, or no regulatory intervention. Decisions, the report said, concerning classification and regulation of suspect substances should be based primarily on health considerations, but "perceived" benefits, such as those attributed to saccharin by diabetics, should be given due consideration.

In an unusual development, there was a minority report attached to the NAS study. In a strongly worded statement, dissenting members of the study panel said that

Cancer Death Rates, 1930-77

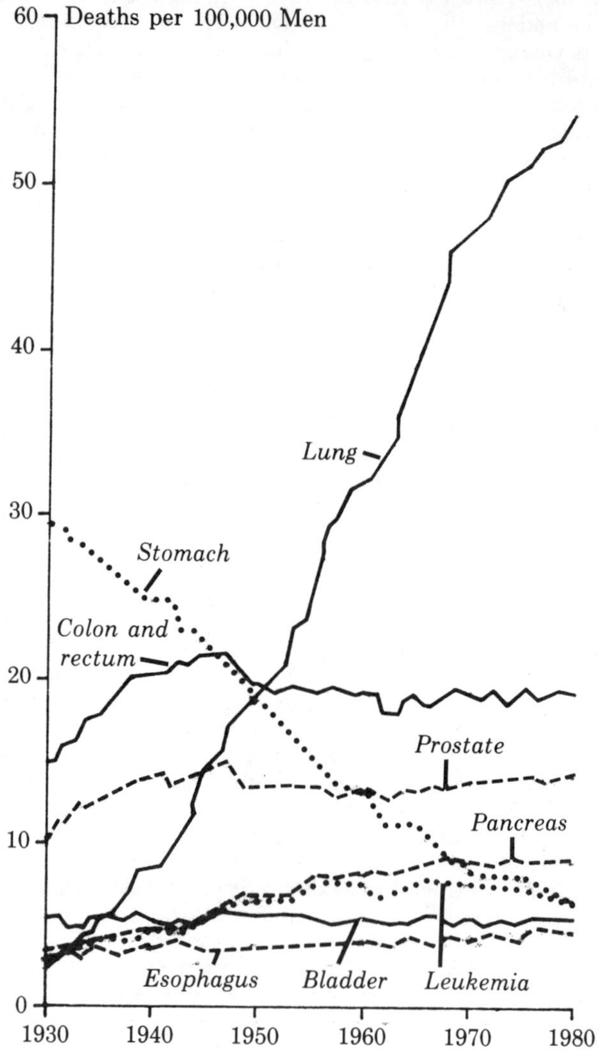

Source: Council on Environmental Quality

there was still no "scientifically defensible way to divide carcinogens" or other substances with irreversible health hazards into different risk categories. The dissenters also said that food regulation should be particularly strict, because of the "enormous" number of persons exposed to potential hazards and because the method of exposure — chronic ingestion — represented the "optimal" way to cause cancer.

Too Little Protection?

While the diet food and drink industry opposed the Delaney clause because it was too rigid, consumer groups faulted the clause for its laxity. The law exempted from testing apparently safe additives that were on the market before 1958. Those generally recognized as safe (GRAS) substances included, among others, salt, sugar and common spices that had been used for centuries with no apparent ill effects. But food safety activists have charged that widespread and long-term use of a substance does not necessarily prove its safety and point to cyclamate as an example of the law's spotty protection.

In 1969 it was discovered that cyclamate, an artificial sweetener on the FDA's GRAS list, caused cancer in laboratory animals. It was subsequently banned by the FDA, despite opposition from manufacturers (who switched from cyclamate to saccharin, also on the GRAS list, to sweeten their low-calorie products). The FDA periodically has been petitioned to lift the prohibition on cyclamates; an FDA administrative law judge last upheld the ban in February 1980, declaring that manufacturers have failed to prove that cyclamate is safe.

GRAS Evaluation

The cyclamate controversy caused President Nixon to order the FDA to evaluate the safety of all additives on the GRAS list. The study, undertaken for the FDA by the Federation of American Societies for Experimental Biology (FASEB), was completed in late 1980. The results, according to then FDA Commissioner Jere E. Goyan, were "generally reassuring to the American consumer."

The researchers broke down 415 substances into five categories. Class 1 — 305 items determined to be safe for use at current levels — included vegetable oils and hydrolyzates (flavor enhancers primarily used in meats). The researchers placed 68 substances in Class 2, which carried a designation that the substances were safe for use at current levels of consumption but potentially hazardous at higher levels. Substances in Class 2 included iron, sucrose and vitamins A and D. The FASEB panel recommended that the FDA permit the continued use of the 19 substances in Class 3, but urged the agency to fund additional studies to determine their safety. Caffeine and the widely used preservatives BHA (butylated hydroxyanisole) and BHT (butylated hydroxytoluene) were included in this category. The FASEB report placed five substances — salt and four modified starches — in Class 4 and urged the FDA to set stricter standards for their use or prohibit their addition to food. The 18 substances in Class 5 were left unclassified because of a lack of sufficient data.

The FASEB subsequently began an evaluation of GRAS substances that were approved after 1958. Included were malt syrup and extract, collagen (a protein used in sausage casings) and char-smoke flavoring. Results of the second phase evaluation were expected by the end of 1982.

New Sweetener

The FDA approved a new artificial sweetener, aspartame, in July 1981 for use in dry foods. Although the manufacturer received initial approval to market aspartame, FDA withheld final approval because the sugar substitute was suspected of causing brain damage. Subsequent tests conducted at the Massachusetts Institute of Technology found no link between aspartame and brain damage. But the MIT study recommended a new round of lengthy animal tests of aspartame before final approval and stated that the sweetener could pose a risk to persons suffering from phenylketonuria, an inherited illness characterized by an inability to correctly metabolize phenylalanine, an amino acid. One of the two amino acids that make up aspartame is a form of phenylalanine.

The FDA rejected the recommendation for further study, satisfied that the MIT tests were sufficient. But the agency required the manufacturer to monitor aspartame consumption levels and mandated that aspartame containers bear the label: "Phenylketonurics: contains Phenylalanine."

Aspartame, which the manufacturer planned to provide to the food industry by late 1981 and to consumers in tablet and granular form in 1982, was suited to replace saccharin only in certain cases. The new sweetener could not be used for cooking or baking because it broke down at high temperatures. And after long-term contact with water, it lost its sweet taste, although the manufacturer said that it retained its sweetness for about as long as the average shelf life of low-calorie beverages. The initial application for approval in 1973 did not cover the use of aspartame in beverage, but the manufacturer said it soon intended to request FDA permission for its use in liquid products.

The knotty problem of determining food safety persists. Science cannot establish with any certainty safe levels for human consumption for suspect substances. And consumers appear to have mixed feelings about how far Congress and federal regulators should go to protect them from the potential dangers of food additives. FDA moves against popular additives like saccharin aroused widespread anger. But, according to a 1978 FDA report, consumers felt that "the American public needs protection from the food industry."

PESTICIDES: A DOUBLE-EDGED SWORD

Pesticides — chemical pest killers — largely were responsible for boosting U.S. agricultural production to unprecedented levels in the 20th century. According to the Department of Agriculture, the average corn yield increased about three times between 1940 and 1972 and rice yields more than doubled.

But the good reputation pesticides had enjoyed for most of this century was sullied in the 1960s. Government and independent researchers discovered that buildups of pesticides in animals were connected with several ailments, including severe reproductive disorders. Fears arose about possible hazards to human beings. The government fashioned stricter regulations concerning pesticides, and Congress enacted legislation. But the controversy remained, supporters claiming that pesticides were the keystone of U.S. agriculture, critics alleging that their known hazards outweighed any benefits. The question of balancing benefits and costs — a process known variously as cost-benefit analysis or risk-benefit analysis — fell to the Environmental Protection Agency (EPA), the agency responsible for establishing tolerance levels in or on food. According to an EPA scientist, the task of comparing a pesticide's risks and benefits is "incredibly difficult."

Since 'Silent Spring'

Americans first became aware of the possible hazards of widespread pesticide use with the publication in 1962 of *Silent Spring* by Rachel Carson. In the book, which became a national bestseller, Carson argued that many pesticides in use on farms and timberlands had unknown and

Defining Pesticides

Pesticide is a general term for any substance or mixture of substances intended for preventing, destroying, repelling, or mitigating any pest (insect, rodent, nematode, fungus, weed, etc.). This includes any substance intended for use as a plant regulator, defoliant, or dessicant.

Between 35,000 to 40,000 pesticides products are registered with the Environmental Protection Agency (EPA). They are all made from one or more of approximately 600 basic chemical compounds. There are also approximately 1,200 active ingredients registered with the EPA.

Farmers use by far the largest volume of pesticides produced in this country, but a little less than half of registered pesticide products are intended for home, institutional or industrial use. All sterilizing, disinfecting, sanitizing, germicidal and bacteria killing chemicals (if they make pesticidal claims and are not sold exclusively for use in or on the living bodies of men or animals) are classified as pesticides and must be registered.

The three major families of pesticides are:

- Chlorinated hydrocarbons, or organochlorines — "Hard" pesticides, which break down chemically quite slowly and can remain in the environment for some time. Pesticides of this type include: DDT, DDD, DDE, dieldrin, chlordane, toxaphene, aldrin, endrin, helptachlor, and lindane.

- Organic phosphates, or organophosphates — Not persistent in the environment, but highly toxic to human beings. They include: parathion, malathion, chlarethion, thimet, phosdrin, methylparathion and trichlorphone.
- Carbamates — Of low toxicity to human beings.

The three major functions of pesticides are as:

- Herbicides — killing weeds
- Insecticides — killing insects
- Fungicides — killing fungus.

cumulative toxic effects that could be gauged only after many years of tests. Because so little was known about the effects of these chemicals on plants, animals and humans, Carson said, their use should be curtailed. She also criticized the U.S. Department of Agriculture's endorsement of increased pesticide use and contended that farmers often exceeded permitted tolerance without detection.

The use of agricultural chemicals began in the mid-19th century, when the trend toward intensive farming and specialized crop production created imbalances in nature that frequently led to drastic increases in pest populations. As agriculture became a commercial production industry, pesticides began to play an increasingly central role.

There are about 35,000 pesticides currently in use; they are derived from approximately 1,200 basic ingredients. An estimated 1 billion pounds of pesticides are applied annually in the United States, an increase of 40 percent over the past decade. Pesticide manufacturing is a $2 billion-a-year business.

Congress in 1947 enacted the Insecticide, Fungicide and Rodenticide Act. Designed to replace the Insecticide Act of 1910, the new law required registration of economic poisons and chemical pesticides prior to their sale in interstate or foreign commerce. Manufacturers were ordered to document claims made for their products' safety and effectiveness; the Agriculture Department was authorized to deny registration if a pesticide were mislabeled, ineffective or excessively dangerous to organisms other than those it was designed to control. The 1947 law also specified that labels include poison warnings (or other warnings of possible hazards) and instructions for use. Subsequent amendments in 1954 and 1959 required pretesting of pesticides used on food crops and widened the definitions of pesticides. Another law, adopted in 1964, bolstered the Agriculture Department's authority to remove unsafe pesticides from the market.

Pesticide Effects

After *Silent Spring* raised the issue, warnings of the potential dangers of pesticide use mounted. Their effects on wildlife were documented in scores of research projects. By the late 1960s, harmful buildups of DDT (dichlorodiphenyl trichloroethane) and other chemicals were discovered in bald eagles, fish, peregrine falcons and other animals.

Research also revealed that some pesticides move up the food chain through a process called biological magnification, in which minute quantities of chemicals stored in the body fat and tissues of creatures low in the food chain — plankton, for example — are transferred in constantly growing amounts to predators higher in the food chain.

Scientists also began examining the accumulation of pesticides in human beings. They found that Americans carried in their bodies an average of 12 parts per million of pesticide residues, nearly twice the level allowed for most foods in interstate commerce. Evidence presented in 1970 showed that even very small quantities of DDT could affect human metabolism. The National Cancer Institute reported in 1969 that 11 of 123 pesticides tested caused increased incidence of tumors in laboratory animals.

Responsibility for regulation of pesticides was transferred from the Agriculture Department to the EPA when the agency was created in 1970. The EPA's regulation and enforcement powers were enlarged with the passage of the Federal Environmental Pesticide Control Act of 1972. The legislation required that all pesticides be registered with the EPA and empowered the agency to control the manufacture, distribution and use of pesticides. It also freed the EPA to ban hazardous chemicals and imposed penalties for their improper use.

Pesticides were divided into two categories: general and restricted use by qualified applicators, depending on the hazards involved. Under the law, pesticide manufacturers or retailers were entitled to federal indemnity payments if their products were declared an imminent hazard by the EPA and removed from the market. No payments would be made, however, if the pesticide owners knew in advance that their products were hazardous but continued to use or produce them. The controversial indemnity provision was in the original House-passed version of the bill but was deleted by the Senate. It was re-inserted, due to pressure from the pesticide industry and agriculture interests, during a conference called to iron out the differences between the House and Senate versions of the bill.

Pesticide Bans

In 1969, the Departments of Agriculture, Interior and Health, Education and Welfare joined forces to impose limitations on the use of DDT. The EPA enlarged the prohibition in 1973, announcing a ban on almost all remaining uses of the chemical. EPA banned the pesticides aldrin, dieldrin, chlordane and heptachlor in 1975; the following year, manufacturers voluntarily ceased production of four other chemicals — mirex, Kepone, stribane and BHC. A controversy surrounding Kepone erupted in 1975 after employees of a small Kepone manufacturing plant in Virginia were discovered to be suffering from brain and liver damage, tremors and other ailments *(see Water chapter, p. 52)*.

EPA Critics

The EPA's efforts to regulate pesticides have left the agency open to criticism from farmers and the pesticide industry on one side and from environmentalists on the other. Farm and chemical industry spokesmen have charged that environmentalists have exaggerated the pesticide threat and argued that the nation relied on pesticides to provide its abundant supply of food and fiber. One EPA opponent charged that "The Environmental Protection Agency has started a trend that will turn our farms back to the insects, weeds and fungi . . . reduce output and quality . . . and accelerate food shortages." Environmental groups, on the other hand, have demanded that the EPA's regulation of potentially dangerous pesticides be strengthened.

The agency's pesticide programs were attacked in a 1977 report issued by the staff of the Senate Judiciary Subcommittee on Administrative Practice and Procedure. The report faulted EPA for accepting uncritically in most cases the animal test data submitted by pesticide manufacturers in support of registrations and tolerances allowing residues on or in food marketed in the United States. As an example of what it considered the agency's failure to regulate pesticides, the report cited the EPA's 1974 approval of tolerances for the pesticide leptophos in and on food shipped to the United States, despite evidence that the substance could cause nervous system disorders. (Tolerances for leptophos were revoked in 1976.) The pesticide came to public attention in December 1976 when news reports revealed that federal officials were investigating an outbreak of severe nervous disorders among workers at a Bayport, Texas, plant where leptophos was manufactured for export between 1971 and January 1977. "EPA's approval in 1974 of residue tolerances for leptophos in and on lettuce and tomatoes did much to encourage the use of the pesticide in other countries, such as Mexico and Egypt, since much of the world looks to the United States as the leader in science," the report said. "The result is that American consumers, as well as consumers of other nations, have been exposed to a demonstrably hazardous material."

The EPA's diligence in protecting consumers was questioned in another report, issued in December 1978 by the House Commerce Subcommittee on Oversight and Investigations. The report charged that the EPA, in setting tolerances for pesticide, was increasing public health risks by "veering away from the health-oriented language [of federal food law] toward the 'risk-benefit' balancing language of federal pesticide statutes."

The Federal Environmental Pesticide Control Act of 1972 saddled the EPA with a considerable administrative burden. It instructed the agency to register and classify some 50,000 pesticides that had come on the market during the previous 30 years. In the monumental task of screening these substances and classifying them for "general" or "restricted" use the agency had bogged down. As a result, Congress in 1978 adopted legislation designed to simplify registration and marketing procedures. The law permitted the EPA to register pesticides according to their chemical composition instead of product name, a change known as "generic" registration. The revised procedure allowed EPA to focus its efforts on about 1,400 basic substances.

Legislative Veto

The House of Representatives in 1979 endorsed legislation that would have made EPA pesticide regulations subject to a veto from either chamber of Congress. The Senate balked at the legislative veto provision, however, and the bill died. (President Ford vetoed a similar bill in 1976.) But in 1980, Congress approved legislation (PL 96-539) that included a provision allowing a legislative veto of EPA pesticide rules; under the provision, however, both houses of Congress had to approve any veto barring a regulation. Senate opposition to the legislative veto dissolved after the House agreed to provide for expedited judicial review of any case challenging the provision's constitutionality. Under the veto provision (similar to the power over Federal Trade Commission regulations Congress granted itself in May 1980), any regulation proposed to implement the Federal Insecticide, Fungicide and Rodenticide Act could be killed if both chambers passed a resolution of disapproval within 90 days after EPA proposed the rule. The law further required the EPA administrator to submit to the Scientific Advisory Panel, an outside board set up to review EPA's pesticide decisions, any data the agency used to order the emergency suspension of a pesticide and to permit peer review of the design of scientific studies conducted to regulate pesticides.

Pesticide Scares

Public fears of widespread pesticide use were aroused in July 1981 when the governor of California, Edmund G. Brown Jr., decided to allow pesticide spraying from airplanes of almost 120 square miles of the state to combat an infestation of Mediterranean fruit flies, hardy pests that render fruit and vegetables inedible. In an attempt to avoid aerial spraying, Brown earlier had ordered residents in the infected areas to destroy all fruits and vegetables and to apply the pesticide malathion on the ground. But the U.S. Department of Agriculture intervened, threatening to impose a quarantine on all California produce if Brown refused to order aerial spraying. Despite local opposition to spraying, Brown gave in to the federal threat and the spraying began. The justification for the spraying was two-fold: to prevent the spread of the flies to other parts of the country and to save California's $14 billion agriculture industry.

Other recent pest eradication programs have caused alarm. Citizens in New England and New York metropolitan areas have objected to the use of chemicals to fight the

Caffeine Content of Foods and Drugs

Product	Caffeine (mgs)
Coffee *(5 oz.)*	
Regular Brewed	
Percolated	110
Dripolator	150
Instant	66
Decaf Brewed	4.5
Instant Decaf	2
Instant or Brewed Tea *(5 oz.)*	45
Soft Drinks *(12 oz.)*	
Dr. Pepper	61
Mr. Pibb	57
Mountain Dew	49
Tab	45
Coca-Cola	42
RC Cola	36
Pepsi-Cola	35
Diet Pepsi	34
Pepsi Light	34
Cocoa *(5 oz.)*	13
Milk Chocolate *(1 oz.)*	6
Drugs *(per tablet)*	
Vivarin Tablets	200
Nodoz	100
Excedrin	65
Vanquish	33
Emperin Compound	32
Anacin	32
Dristan	16.2

Source: Center for Science in the Public Interest

gypsy moth. In New England, neighbors argued bitterly in town meetings about whether to allow chemical sprayings to protect vegetation. In 1981, gypsy moth caterpillars attacked more than 500 species of plants. Democratic Representative Edward J. Markey, who represents Medford, Mass., where the gypsy moth first appeared in the United States late in the 19th century, cautioned against massive applications of pesticides. "We can't forget that what may seem like a prudent and expedient action now can have drastic implications for the general public far into the future."

Integrated Pest Management

In the wake of dozens of allegations during the 1960s and 1970s that pesticides caused severe damage to humans, plants and animals and in light of mounting evidence that insects quickly develop resistance to the poisons, the EPA has attempted to persuade farmers to replace pesticide use with a system of pest control called Integrated Pest Management (IPM). Designed to battle pests without resorting to chemicals, IPM utilizes parasites, predators, viruses, traps, sterile male insects and crop rotation to reduce pest populations. Despite heavy promotion of IPM, it has not yet been widely implemented by farmers and other growers.

Congressional Action

Like other areas of food safety, pesticide control offers no easy answers to questions concerning safety and ill health. The White House in mid-1981 endorsed a legislative proposal to shift the regulatory burden of the Federal Insecticide, Fungicide and Rodenticide Act from the EPA to the Department of Agriculture. The proposal, if enacted, was expected to lead to increased production and use of pesticides, especially in commercial applications. That would likely keep the pesticide debate active for some time.

CAFFEINE: FROM COFFEE TO COLAS

In September 1980, Dr. Jere E. Goyan, then commissioner of the Food and Drug Administration, issued a warning to pregnant women to avoid the use of caffeine because the drug was suspected to be teratogenetic (causing birth defects). Goyan said, "So while further evidence is being gathered on the possible relationship between caffeine and birth defects, a prudent and protective mother-to-be will want to put caffeine on her list of unnecessary substances which she should avoid."

The commissioner's warning came after an FDA study found that pregnant rats that had been force-fed large quantities of caffeine produced offspring with birth defects. The amounts administered to the rats were proportional to the caffeine ingested by a medium-to-heavy coffee drinker. The FDA proposed in October 1980 to remove caffeine from its list of substances generally recognized as safe (the GRAS list) and place it on the agency's "interim" GRAS list. Interim status meant that new uses of caffeine would not be allowed while manufacturers conducted further tests to determine the safety of the drug. At the same time, the FDA offered new regulations permitting soft-drink manufacturers to use the names "cola" and "pepper" to describe caffeine-free beverages. Under current food standardization regulations that insure that generically named foods contain certain ingredients, all cola and pepper beverages must contain caffeine. FDA spokesmen anticipated that the revised caffeine regulations would take effect in early 1982.

FDA Criticism

Reaction to the caffeine controversy followed a course established by the proposed saccharin ban, with advocates and opponents taking predictable positions. Industry representatives castigated the FDA, saying that the agency based its warning to pregnant women on questionable evidence. Consumer groups said that the agency was too cautious. The Center for Science in the Public Interest, a food activist organization, petitioned the FDA to order manufacturers to put health warning labels on packages of coffee and tea.

The results of the FDA caffeine tests came under criticism from an unexpected source. Three FDA inspectors reported in October 1980 that the laboratory in which the caffeine tests were conducted was "dirty and disorganized," according to *The Washington Post*. The inspectors' criticisms of the lab's procedures led the FDA to appoint a panel of government scientists to re-evaluate the tests. The panel reported in June 1981 that although caffeine appeared to be related to birth defects, it was not clear that caffeine was directly teratogenetic.

Widely Used Drug

Caffeine, a drug that stimulates the central nervous system, is a main ingredient of coffee, tea, cola and pepper drinks and chocolate. It is contained in some prescription drugs and such over-the-counter remedies as headache, cold and allergy pills. Caffeine also is added to pills that fight fatigue and it is a component of some non-cola beverages.

The immediate effects of caffeine in the body are well documented. Minutes after the drug is ingested, the heart and lungs quicken their pace, the kidneys produce more fluid, the stomach's excretion of acid increases. Caffeine clears the mind and fends off drowsiness.

As a result of the questions surrounding the safety of caffeine, more coffee drinkers are switching to decaffeinated brands. Yet the methods used to remove caffeine from coffee beans have been cited as potentially hazardous. The two most widely used procedures apply a chemical solvent directly to the beans or use hot water to remove the caffeine and a solvent to separate the caffeine from the water. The hot water is then reused. Both methods leave traces of the solvent on the beans, according to some researchers. A third, more costly method, using pure water to extract the caffeine, is not widely employed.

In 1975, the National Cancer Institute advised makers of decaffeinated coffee that large doses of Trichloroethylene, a common caffeine-extracting agent, caused cancer in laboratory mice. The FDA, after hearing of the problem, began tests of the substance. Decaffeinated coffee makers voluntarily banned its use and switched to methylene chloride, a substance currently under study at the National Cancer Institute.

FDA's warning about caffeine focused on birth defects. Other studies have pointed to caffeine as a possible cause of bladder cancer, breast disorders in women and hyperactivity among children. The evidence implicating caffeine as a contributor to bladder cancer remains inconclusive. Other studies, with similarly inconclusive results, suggest a connection between caffeine and non-cancerous fibrocystic breast disease in women, a disorder characterized by breast lumps and pain occuring before menstruation. Some researchers suspect that caffeine contained in the cola drinks, chocolate milk and candy that constitute a considerable part of the diet of many young Americans may bring on restlessness and insomnia in youngsters. Still other studies have concluded that three cups of coffee drunk quickly can modify verbal performance and higher levels of consumption can cause symptoms similar to those of anxiety neurosis.

Further FDA moves to restrict the sale of caffeine-containing products was certain to encounter stiff opposition from the coffee and soft-drink industries. Both are big business. The United States imports more coffee than any other agricultural product; coffee is the second biggest commodity in international trade, surpassed only by petroleum. And cola drinks dominate the $13-billion-a-year U.S. soft drink market.

American Coffee Consumption

Type	Cups Per Person Per Day 1962	1977	1979	1980
Regular	2.45	1.30	1.42	1.39
Instant	0.67	0.64	0.62	0.62
Decaffeinated	—	0.27	0.33	0.34
All coffee	3.12	1.94	2.06	2.02

Source: International Coffee Organization

SMOKING: A KEY LINK TO CANCER

Smoking — inhaling tobacco smoke into the lungs — is now considered by most scientists to be the main cause of lung cancer in the United States, killing 85,000 Americans annually.

The federal government periodically has mounted campaigns to publicize the health risks of smoking, and legislation requires that cigarette packages and advertisements carry health warnings. But the tobacco industry and its friends in Congress representing tobacco-growing states so far have prevented the government from taking any further action — action that would reduce tobacco price supports, is one example — that would hinder cigarette sales.

Tobacco smoke is a mixture of gases, liquids and compounds. Among the most hazardous compounds in cigarette smoke are tar, nicotine, carbon monoxide, cadmium, nitrogen dioxide, ammonia, benzene and formaldehyde. Tar is the particulate — solid — matter in the tobacco blend that is vaporized as the tobacco burns. Nicotine is an addictive and poisonous substance.

In addition to lung cancer, smoking has been connected with heart disease (some researchers claim it is responsible for one-fourth of all annual heart attack deaths) and cancers of the esophagus, pancreas, larynx, mouth and bladder. It also is estimated to cause 70 percent of the chronic bronchitis and emphysema suffered nationwide.

Researchers have discovered that the carbon monoxide in the cigarette smoke may replace as much as 12 percent of a smoker's red blood cells, impeding the supply of oxygen to the heart. The American Medical Association has estimated that 320,000 Americans die each year as a result of smoking-related illnesses; the doctors' group says that smoking is the leading preventable cause of death in the United States.

Surgeon General's Report

The connection between tobacco smoke and ill health officially was recognized in the much-discussed 1964 Public Health Service report released by the surgeon general. The report, titled "Smoking and Health," concluded that "cigarette smoking is a health hazard of sufficient importance in the United States to warrant appropriate remedial action." Cigarette sales fell off sharply after the release of the report, but rebounded by the end of the year. Since the mid-1960s, the proportion of Americans who smoke has dropped, while cigarette consumption has increased.

Although smoking long had been suspected of causing cancer, the Public Health Service did not engage in official research until June 1956. The surgeon general suggested that a scientific study group, established by the National Cancer Institute, the National Heart Institute, the American Cancer Society and the American Heart Association, review studies of smoking conducted abroad. The panel concluded that there was a cause-and-effect relationship between heavy smoking and lung cancer. The surgeon general agreed with the conclusion.

In 1961, the heads of various health promotion organizations — the American Cancer Society, the American Public Health Association, the American Heart Association and the National Tuberculosis Association — urged President Kennedy to establish a commission to study the "widespread implications of the tobacco problem." Representatives of these groups subsequently met with the surgeon general who, in April 1962, proposed that the Public Health Service conduct its own investigation into tobacco use. Additional pressure to undertake a study was provided by the release of a 1962 report of the Royal College of Physicians of London on smoking and its relation to cancer and other diseases. The report said that "cigarette smoking is a cause of lung cancer and bronchitis, and probably contributes to the development of coronary heart disease and various other less common diseases."

In July 1962 the surgeon general met with representatives of the American Cancer Society, the American College of Chest Physicians, the American Heart Association, the American Medical Association, the Tobacco Institute, the Food and Drug Administration, the National Tuberculosis Association, the Federal Trade Commission and the President's Office of Science and Technology. Out of this meeting came a consensus that a special Scientific Advisory Committee should undertake a two-part study. The result of the first part of the study was the report, "Smoking and Health."

Warning Labels

The "remedial action" urged by the surgeon general's report eventually was translated into legislation and regulation. The Federal Cigarette Labeling and Advertising Act went into effect Jan. 1, 1966. It required all cigarette packages to bear the statement, "Caution — Cigarette Smoking May Be Hazardous To Your Health." The law barred, until July 1, 1969, any requirement of a health warning in cigarette advertising.

The Federal Communications Commission ruled June 2, 1967, that, under the fairness doctrine, broadcasters were required to make available free air time for anti-smoking messages because the pro-smoking messages contained in cigarette advertisements were deemed a controversial matter of legitimate public importance. As a result of the commission's ruling, thousands of messages — warning of the dangers of smoking — appeared on radio and television over the next 40 months. The messages had a temporary effect: cigarette sales in 1969 dropped by 12 billion.

Congress enacted legislation in 1970 barring all cigarette advertisements on radio and television, effective Jan. 2, 1971. The FCC subsequently ruled that broadcasters no longer were required to run anti-smoking messages and the practice was cut back sharply. Cigarette sales continued to grow, hitting an estimated 611 billion in 1980. The 1970 law also changed the wording of the health warning on cigarette packages to read: "Warning: The Surgeon General Has Determined That Cigarette Smoking Is Dangerous To Your Health." But it prohibited the Federal Trade Commission from requiring health warnings on printed cigarette advertisements before July 1, 1971.

Tar, Nicotine Disclosure

Faced with the possibility of regulation by the Federal Trade Commission, U.S. tobacco companies in February 1971 agreed to disclose the tar and nicotine content of the cigarettes they advertised in print.

The following November, the Interstate Commerce Commission restricted smoking to the rear five rows of seats on interstate buses, and strengthened rules against smoking on trains. The commission said "second-hand" smoke was an "extreme irritant to humans, particularly . . . upon eyes and breathing" and judged it "capable of adversely affecting the adequacy and availability" of interstate carrier service.

The Civil Aeronautics Board in July 1973 required commercial airlines to provide seats in non-smoking sections. A 1981 modification required airlines to provide no-smoking seats if passengers requested them within a prescribed period of time (usually 30 minutes) before departure. Airlines no longer were required to arrange no-smoking seats for standby passengers and other passengers who boarded planes just prior to takeoff.

Passive Smoking

Some researchers claim cigarette smoke harms nearby non-smokers as much as the smoker, causing reactions in individuals suffering from emphysema, asthma, bronchitis, sinusitis, hay fever and chronic heart disease. These researchers say healthy "passive smokers" can suffer headaches, coughing, wheezing, eye irritations, sneezing, hoarseness, nausea, sore throat and dizziness.

Deadlier consequences have been reported among non-smokers who spend considerable time near smokers. A research report published in March 1980 claimed that non-smoking workers regularly exposed to smoke from their fellow employees' cigarettes suffered a marked deterioration of the small air tubes and sacs in their lungs. In January 1981, the results of a study conducted in Japan revealed that the non-smoking wives of men who smoked ran an increased risk of developing lung cancer, estimated to be one-third to one-half the risk incurred by smokers. However, this claim was disputed in a June 1981 report issued by the American Cancer Society which found little connection between smokers and the incidence of lung cancer among their spouses.

Tobacco itself — unsmoked — also has come under suspicion as a possible carcinogen. A study released in March 1980 claimed that tobacco chewing and snuff dipping (holding tobacco between the gum and the cheek) increased the risk of cancer of the mouth and throat.

Millions Still Smoke

Despite all the evidence linking cigarettes to cancer and other illnesses, approximately 54 million Americans continued to smoke almost 20 years after the surgeon general's report on the dangers of the practice.

Health officials were encouraged, however, by signs that the proportion of American smokers was dropping. In 1955, almost 55 percent of the men living in the United States smoked and 24.5 percent of the women. By 1966, male smokers had decreased to 50 percent of the male population, but the figure for women had risen to 32.3 percent. In May 1981, it was reported that 28.9 percent of U.S. women smoked in 1981 and 36.7 percent of the men. Among the entire adult population (17 years and older), 32.6 percent smoked in 1980. According to the Department of Health and Human Services, by 1980 33.3 million Americans had broken the smoking habit.

Health officials especially were pleased with the figures outlining the decline of smoking among women. In recent years, as the number of smoking women — particularly teenagers — rose, officials voiced fears that cancer of the lungs would overtake breast cancer as the leading form of cancer afflicting females. Moreover, the surgeon general warned in 1980 that pregnant women who smoked ran an increased risk of miscarriage and spontaneous abortion. The surgeon general's report also provided evidence that smoking during pregnancy could harm the fetus's physical and intellectual development.

Anti-smoking Campaigns

Since 1964, the federal government has mounted various campaigns designed to educate the public about the hazards of cigarette smoking. In March 1978, the Office on Smoking and Health was created as the government's primary unit to conduct an anti-smoking campaign and placed in the Department of Health, Education and Welfare. (The department's name was changed to Health and Human Services when an independent Education Department was established in 1979). The office enjoyed the support of then HEW Secretary Joseph A. Califano Jr., himself a reformed smoker.

In spite of these efforts, the Federal Trade Commission reported in 1981 that the public remained misinformed about the potential health risks of smoking. The FTC staff report said that 30 percent of the public was not aware that smoking can lead to heart disease, that 50 percent of the women did not know that smoking during pregnancy can harm the fetus and that fewer than 3 percent of the people exposed to cigarette advertisements read the health warnings that accompany all ads. The staff report recommended that the commission mandate more strongly worded warnings for advertisements.

Reaction to widespread publicity surrounding smoking and health has taken two notable directions. Non-smokers have become increasingly successful at avoiding exposure to cigarette smoke by banning smoking in many public places. And smokers have been switching to low-tar and low-nicotine brands.

Lobbying by non-smokers offended by exposure to cigarette smoke has resulted in the passage in most states of legislation restricting smoking in public areas. In addition, anti-smoking rules have been imposed by hundreds of local communities. In May 1973 Arizona became the first state to enact statewide smoking restrictions. The law barred lighting up in elevators, indoor theaters, libraries, art galleries, museums, concert halls, physicians' waiting rooms, school buildings and on buses. Minnesota's 1975 law became the model comprehensive legislation affecting smoking. In all enclosed indoor public areas, including offices and retail stores, smoking was flatly prohibited or allowed only in segregated smoking areas. Unrestricted smoking was permitted only in places not frequented by the public, for example, factories closed to the public.

Sources of Lead Intake, 1980

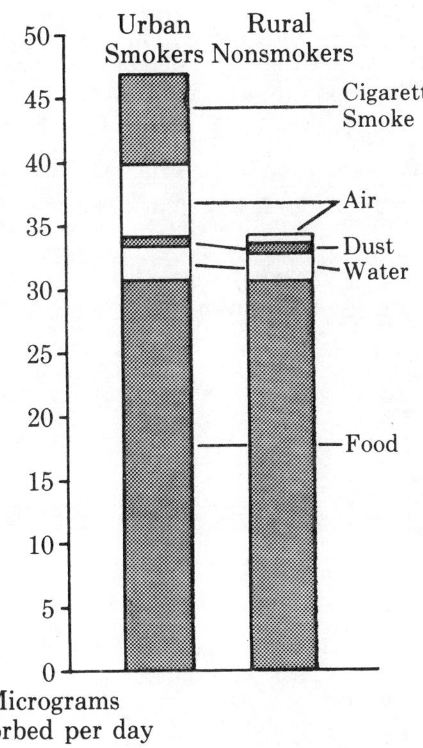

Source: National Academy of Sciences

Switch to Milder Cigarettes

Low-tar and low-nicotine cigarettes account for 43 to 50 percent of the nation's $18 billion-a-year cigarette industry. As more smokers have changed from higher tar and nicotine brands to cigarettes with smaller amounts of these substances, the industry has flooded the market with new brands. As a result, the average tar content of cigarettes has dropped 32 percent since 1968, the average nicotine content, 26 percent.

Low-tar smokers took some comfort from the 1981 surgeon general's report which stated that switching to low-tar cigarettes caused a slight reduction of the risk of lung cancer. However, the report cautioned that there was little evidence that the milder brands reduced the incidence of cardiovascular diseases, emphysema, and chronic bronchitis or lowered the threat to pregnant women. The report also warned that some of the flavoring agents manufacturers add to low-tar and low-nicotine brands to boost flavor — shellac, caramel, eugenol and other chemicals — may produce carcinogens when they are burned.

Price Supports

Tobacco price supports came under fire in mid-1981 as Congress sought to shape legislation in line with President Reagan's austere budget.

Long considered sacrosanct, the price supports appeared vulnerable in 1981. During Senate budget debate May 2, Sen. Howard M. Metzenbaum, D-Ohio, lost on his effort to simply eliminate funding for the tobacco supports, but the surprisingly close vote, 56-42, suggested that there was more sentiment for a cutback in this program than had been believed. The announcement that the United States could lose as much as $123 million in 1981 on the tobacco it held as collateral for loans did little to improve the program's prospects.

OTHER HAZARDS: A COMPREHENSIVE LIST

Several times in the past decade, federal agencies or independent researchers have called attention to possible health hazards posed by food or food additives. The list of substances thought to be dangerous was growing: nitrosamine in beer became a suspected carcinogen, cholesterol intake was connected to heart disease, salt was linked to high blood pressure, food additives were suspected of causing hyperactivity, the preservatives BHA and BHT became suspect, and nitrites, nitrates and artificial food colors were viewed as possible carcinogens. There were fears among scientists that other additives may cause birth defects, genetic damage and other health problems.

Chemical additives were contained in many foods that were a regular part of the American diet. They were added to perform various functions: preservatives prevent spoilage, anti-oxidants ward off rancidity and stabilizers maintain consistency; artificial flavors and colors enhance taste and appearance; and acidulants counteract tart tastes. Other chemical additives were used to firm, harden, dry, leaven, sweeten (non-calorically), cream and sterilize. And some natural products — the most common are salt and sugar —were added during some food processing.

Additive Bans

Food additives have been credited with keeping the nation's food supply bountiful and inexpensive. Moreover, additives have played a critical role in efforts to wipe out scurvy, rickets, goiter and botulism. But some observers fear that hazards associated with chemical additives outweigh their benefits.

The most celebrated cases of potentially harmful additives in recent years have focused on the non-caloric sweeteners saccharin and cyclamate. Another controversial case concerned the artificial coloring Red dye No. 2. The most widely used artificial color in the manufacture of food, drugs and cosmetics, Red dye No. 2 was banned by the FDA in 1976, five years after Soviet scientists reported that it caused cancer in laboratory mice. It was estimated that 1.3 million pounds of Red dye No. 2 were produced in 1975 and added to such foods as ice cream, processed cheese, cookies, pie crusts, cake mixes, mayonnaise and jam; it also was added to lipsticks and pill coatings.

Although the food-coloring industry opposed the ban, most food processors switched to Red dye No. 40, a substance developed by the Allied Chemical Corp. It too was cited as a possible carcinogen by food safety activists, but the FDA permitted it to remain on the market after subjecting it to a battery of tests.

Animal Feed Antibiotics

The FDA provoked congressional hostility in 1977, when it suggested a ban on antibiotics and other drugs routinely added to animal feed to prevent disease and promote growth. Congress has since, in the agriculture appropriations bills, directed the FDA to postpone the ban until research and public hearings on the issue are completed.

Cattlemen and other meat producers claimed that the drugs — the two most widely used are the antibiotics penicillin and tetracycline — were essential to prevent illness among confined animals in crowded feedlots. But experts in infectious diseases argued that the practice of regularly adding antibiotics to animal feed is part of a general pattern of overuse that is reducing the effectiveness of drugs as humans build up a tolerance for them. Officials at the U.S. Public Health Service Center for Disease Control reported that antibiotics were losing their efficacy against such serious diseases as gonorrhea, typhoid and childhood meningitis.

About 40 percent of the antibiotics manufactured in the United States are used for animals. According to a report issued in 1979 by the Office of Technology Assessment, nearly all poultry, 90 percent of hogs and veal calves and 60 percent of beef cattle bred in the United States consume antibiotics in their feed.

Experts claimed that in European nations where cattle feed antibiotics were banned, the effectiveness of the drugs was on the rise. But officials of U.S. pork, beef and poultry associations insisted that the European results were mixed and argued that antibiotics make a small but critical difference in livestock weights and enable producers to raise more animals in confined quarters. The antibiotics issue was closely monitored in 1981 by Rep. John D. Dingell, D-Mich., chairman of the House Commerce Committee and a vocal advocate of restricting antibiotics.

Proposed Nitrite Ban

The FDA and the Agriculture Department created a stir in 1978 when they proposed a gradual phasing out of the widely used meat preservatives sodium nitrite and sodium nitrate. The proposed ban involved the FDA and the Agriculture Department because these two agencies share jurisdictions: FDA for additives, the Agriculture Department for meats. Nitrites and nitrates — added to most processed meats — retard the formation of health-threatening micro-organisms, including bacteria spores that can cause botulism. Nitrite also helps cooked hams and hot dogs retain their reddish/pink color. Meats that contain sodium nitrite and sodium nitrate include ham, bacon, bologna, corned beef, salami and hot dogs.

The federal agencies acted after researchers at the Massachusetts Institute of Technology reported that nitrites and nitrates in cooked food sometimes form nitrosamines, substances that have induced cancer in laboratory animals. The Agriculture Department did not formally propose a nitrite ban, but simply asked the Justice Department whether it could choose a phase-out of the substance rather than a flat ban if the cancer studies proved conclusive. The Department of Justice replied in March 1979 that under existing law the phasing approach was illegal. In response, the Carter administration introduced legislation to defer any agency action banning the preservative for about one year; after a year, nitrites would be phased out as safe substitutes were developed. An FDA spokesman said the bill did not contradict the administration's advocacy of a reform of food safety laws because nitrite was a "unique" substance requiring special treatment and added that it would not set a precedent for breaching the Delaney clause.

The meat industry, which uses sodium nitrite to preserve an estimated $12.5 billion worth of food annually, expressed doubts concerning the dangers of nitrites. The MIT study also was criticized by a 1979 General Accounting Office report which questioned the researcher's diagnosis of cancer in laboratory animals. After a review of the MIT study, the FDA and the Agriculture Department announced in August 1980 that there was insufficient data to ban nitrites.

The FDA raised another controversy when it reported in September 1979 that several brands of U.S. and imported beer contained traces of nitrosamines, chemicals known to cause cancer in animal tests. The FDA cautioned that although the amounts of nitrosamines were relatively small, safe levels of exposure to carcinogenics never have been determined. The nitrosamines were believed to be formed during the drying of barley malt, a key ingredient of beer. Beer manufacturers subsequently altered the drying process and the FDA reported in 1980 that nitrosamine levels were well within the agency's limits of 5 parts per billion parts of beer. Beer drinkers received some good news in 1979 from the American Heart Association. The health group reported that studies indicated that mild intake of alcohol, notably beer, appeared to reduce the risk of heart attack.

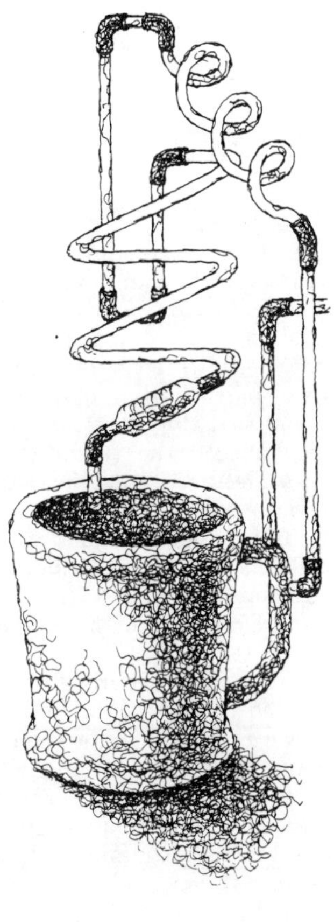

Salt, Sugar, Other Additives

Researchers have pointed to possible health hazards associated with the most common of food additives, including sugar and salt. Health guidelines issued by the Agriculture Department and the Department of Health and Human Services in February 1980 warned consumers to avoid excessive consumption of fat, cholesterol, sugar, salt and alcohol, which have been linked in studies to heart disease, diabetes, tooth decay, high blood pressure and some cancers.

These recommendations paralleled the conventional advice offered by food activists and health-promotion organizations. However, another report, issued by the National Academy of Sciences in May 1980, came to some surprising conclusions. Echoing one of the government's guidelines, the NAS report recommended limiting salt use to reduce the likelihood of high blood pressure. But its authors added that they had uncovered no evidence linking an individual's health to his intake of cholesterol and fat.

Food researchers long have regarded excessive amounts of salt in the diet to be dangerous to health and well-being. It has been estimated that each American consumes 15 pounds of salt annually, much of it contained in processed foods such as soups, cured meats, potato chips and crackers. Studies of animals raised on diets high in salt have detected a connection between salt and high blood pressure and an increased risk of heart attack and stroke.

A possible link between cancer and diet habits was hinted at in the results of a study of Mormons conducted by a scientist at the University of California at Los Angeles. He found that Mormons — members of the Church of Jesus Christ of Latter-Day Saints — enjoyed a low rate of cancer mortality. Dietary restrictions prohibit the use of coffee, alcohol and tobacco and caution against excessive consumption of meat. Utah, where Mormons make up nearly three-fourths of the population, has a cancer death rate 25 percent below the national average.

Some researchers think that food additives may cause hyperactivity in children. A California doctor, Benjamin F. Feingold, has popularized an additive-free diet that he claims can improve the behavior of the estimated one million to five million hyperactive children in the United States. Although its efficacy has been questioned by some food experts, the additive-free diet has been used widely.

Research into food additives again underscores the pitfalls of public health policy. The potential hazards are many — cancer, birth defects, heart disease, high blood pressure — yet scientists fail to agree on which substances are harmful, and Congress, industry groups and food activists cannot reach a consensus on how they should be regulated.

Lead in Food

Lead is a key raw material of industrial society. Yet fears are mounting among scientists that the amount of

Lead Emissions, 1980

Source	Total Production*	Emission*
Natural		
Wind blown and volcanic dust	200,000	2
Sea spray	1,000,000	<1
Forest foliage	100,000	<0.1
Volcanic sulfur	6,000	0.001
Total		2
Man-made		
Lead alkyls	400	280
Iron smelting	780,000	47
Lead smelting	4,000	24
Zinc and Copper mining	15,000	42
Coal burning	3,300,000	15
Total		400

*10^6 kg per year

Source: Council on Environmental Quality

Among the chief sources of lead emissions are industrial facilities. Exposure to lead, even at low levels, can cause fatigue, headache, poor appetite, clumsiness and diminished mental capacity.

lead in the environment — and particularly in food — may be reaching dangerous levels.

The ill effects of long-term exposure to lead are well documented. Symptoms include loss of appetite, clumsiness, headache, fatigue, convulsions and coma. Recent studies indicate that lead can cause serious physical and psychological harm.

According to a report on environmental topics issued in 1980 by the Council on Environmental Quality (CEQ), "Boston school children who at three years of age had blood levels slightly above 30 micrograms [of lead] per 100 milliliters [of blood], the level defined as undue lead absorption by the Center for Disease Control, showed noticeable intellectual and behavioral deficiencies at age seven. Children with elevated levels of lead in their baby teeth also showed behavioral deficiencies." Other studies suggest that high concentrations of lead can cause chromosomal abnormalities, harm fetuses and increase the risk of miscarriage and stillbirth.

A major, though declining, source of lead exposure for children is lead-based paint in older, deteriorating housing. Paint chip poisoning received attention in the late 1960s when it was revealed that poor children in run-down neighborhoods were eating the paint flaking off tenement walls. Congress passed the Lead-Based Paint Poisoning Prevention Act in late 1971 and instructed the Department of Housing and Urban Development (HUD) to implement it. Since then, HUD has spent nearly $9 million on lead-paint research in an effort to curtail poisonings. Other programs — public and private — have had some success removing lead paint from older housing.

The issue of lead in the environment was the subject of a 1980 report prepared by the National Science Foundation. It concluded that control of lead remained an important public health priority.

Researchers have identified several major sources of lead in the environment. These include the air, which contains lead from automobile exhaust (this source of lead has been cut back substantially since the Environmental Protection Agency began restricting the lead content of gasoline in 1973), smelters and coal burning furnaces, lead-based paints, cigarette smoke and food. It is used in the manufacture of batteries and some ceramic glazes.

The cleanest areas in North America enjoy lead concentrations in the air of about 10 nanograms per cubic meter (ng/m^3; a nanogram is one-billionth of a gram). The air in urban areas contains about 500 to 10,000 ng/m^3; the air quality standard established by the EPA is 1,500 ng/m^3. Most of the lead in the atmosphere comes from auto exhausts and industrial emissions.

Food, according to the CEQ, is the major source of public exposure to lead. The National Academy of Sciences has estimated that food accounts for 65 to 92 percent of the lead ingested by the average adult American.

Lead enters the food chain in various ways: lead in the atmosphere is deposited on plant leaves, and plants also absorb the metal from the soil. Some lead may be transferred from machinery to foods during the preparation of processed foods. A particularly widespread source of lead is the solder used to seal the seams on cans of food. Some researchers have alleged the tuna fish packed in lead-soldered cans has a lead concentration 10,000 times greater than natural concentrations. Canned foods comprise about 20 percent of the average U.S. diet; scientists have suggested that lead-soldered cans contribute 50 percent of the average lead intake.

The Food and Drug Administration has begun to study the issue of lead contamination with an eye toward restricting lead content in food. Standards for lead levels in baby foods were expected by the end of 1981. An FDA spokesman claimed, however, that manufacturers are aware of the potential dangers of lead exposure and have made progress in cutting back lead levels in foods. Measures taken include reducing the lead content of solder used to seal can seams and switching to seamless containers. It will be years, experts believe, before it can be determined if these regulatory actions have reduced appreciably the amount of lead in the average American diet.

More Regulation or Less?

The reports and warnings of the past two decades regarding the hazards of modern life have had a measurable impact on U.S. smoking and eating habits.

Fewer Americans smoke cigarettes and more are drinking decaffeinated coffee. The increasing number of "natural" and "health food" stores and restaurants attests to the shift among Americans to unprocessed foods. A portion of the population appears to want the government to increase its authority to regulate the safety of food. Yet the impressive Reagan election victory in 1980 seems to indicate the voters prefer less government intrusion in their lives. And there is little enthusiasm on Capitol Hill to undertake a full-scale reform of the welter of laws covering food safety. As has occurred frequently in the past, the impetus to alter food safety laws likely will follow a revelation linking a commonly used substance to a disease.

7

Dangers of the Workplace

'Tis a sordid profit that's accompanied by the destruction of health. . . . Many an artisan has looked at his craft as a means to support life and raise a family, but all he has got from it is some deadly disease, with the result that he has departed this life cursing the craft to which he has applied himself.

Bernardino Ramazzini, an Italian physician, considered the founder of occupational medicine, 1705

There are approximately 100 million American workers — many of them exposed to some kind of occupational health hazard: carcinogenic agents, toxic chemicals, radiation and dust that cause physical disease; or job-related pressures of noise, crowding, stress or boredom that can have adverse psychological effects.

Each year 100,000 Americans die from occupational illnesses and almost 400,000 new cases of occupational disease are recognized, according to estimates by the National Institute for Occupational Safety and Health (NIOSH). And the 1979 Surgeon General's Report on Health Promotion and Disease Prevention asserts that the actual extent of occupational disease is probably much greater because the link between job and disease is often unrecognized or unreported.

"Occupational health" once referred only to the attempt by management or unions to limit the number of limbs lost to machinery, eyes damaged by chemical sprays or lives lost in explosions or mine cave-ins. In *Crisis in the Workplace,* a 1971 study of occupational health prepared for the Ford Foundation, Nicholas Ashford of the Massachusetts Institute of Technology (MIT) calculated that more than one in 40 industrial workers in the United States died or suffered a reportable injury on the job. In that year, reported accidents at non-agricultural workplaces caused more than 14,000 deaths, more than 100,000 permanent disabilities and upwards of two million temporary injuries, according to Ashford, who in 1980 was assistant director of the Center for Policy Alternatives at MIT and chairman of the National Advisory Committee on Occupational Safety and Health.

In recent years, in addition to the usual kinds of injuries or fatalities caused by falls, fires and machinery, many new occupational hazards and illnesses have come to light. Toxic substances associated with work — and either imperceptible to the worker or ignored — have been taking a severe toll, sometimes not until years after exposure. These newer forms of occupational hazards are the byproducts of technological advancements and are far more difficult to overcome than the older, more obvious kind.

The severity of many occupational illnesses that strike robust workers in their prime adds an element of tragedy to the situation. In addition, each new revelation of a hitherto unsuspected health hazard arouses fear that there may be other harmful substances, as yet undetected.

Another factor arousing public interest is that a dangerous condition in the workplace may menace the health of the population at large. The worker may bring the unseen contamination home, possibly in his clothing, and thus spread the infection. Erik P. Eckholm in *The Picture of Health,* a study jointly sponsored by the United Nations Environment Program and Worldwatch Institute, provided several examples of this dangerous phenomenon. Asbestos fibers carried home from factories on clothes and bodies have caused cancer among families of asbestos workers. From washing their husbands' clothes years earlier, some women are dying of asbestos-induced cancer. The same fate has struck asbestos workers' children who had close contact with their fathers.

According to Eckholm, examinations in the United States have revealed dangerous levels of lead in the blood of lead workers' children, chiefly a consequence of inhaling lead dust brought home on clothes. A worker exposed to mercury can easily carry the substance home on clothing, on the hands and under the fingernails. The mercury can then vaporize, or be eaten, adding to worker exposure and possibly endangering his family as well.

Eckholm also explained that residents of areas where copper, lead or zinc smelters are located get lung cancer more often than the average person, apparently because they inhale airborne arsenic emitted by the plants. "The carcinogenic hazard of arsenic may cross plant boundaries into the general community," National Cancer Institute researchers said. Angiosarcoma, a rare liver cancer linked to vinyl chloride exposure, has been diagnosed among people living near vinyl chloride polymerization and fabrication plants.

Many studies show that the substance the worker deals with in high concentration at work often may be found in a product widely distributed for consumer use. A familiar example is an agricultural pesticide that makes farm workers ill and also contaminates crops sent to market.

Occupational diseases represent a major public health challenge because they affect so many workers. But these diseases also carry a broader social significance. Studies show that often health hazards first discovered in workplace environments are later found in lower concentrations in society at large.

Under careful review, according to the 1979 Surgeon General's Report on Health Promotion and Disease Prevention, is a recent estimate that if the full consequences of both current and recent past occupational exposures are taken into account, perhaps 20-40 percent of all cancers may be related to carcinogens encountered in the workplace. As Eckholm illustrated in his study, industrial workers have served as "toxic-substance early warning signals." Thus, much of our knowledge about carcinogenic materials has been learned by studying the unusual patterns of disease and death among workers. "Humans, rather than rodents, have been society's guinea pigs," he wrote.

LAWS TO PROTECT AMERICAN WORKERS

The need for government action to protect the health and safety of the worker became apparent as industrial activity expanded during the 19th century. The Massachusetts Department of Factory Inspection, established in 1867, was the first state agency to deal with job safety. Ten years later Massachusetts became the first state to enact a law imposing safety standards on industry; the standards applied only to the operation of spinning machinery in textile plants.

Other states followed with various types of job-safety laws. Though the protection was limited, the laws encouraged injured workers to bring damage suits against employers for negligence. This, in turn, encouraged support for proposals to establish an insurance system that would not only guarantee indemnity to an injured worker but relieve the employer of the expense of litigation and the risk of having to pay damages.

The principle of compulsory insurance was not readily accepted, however. Several early state laws to this effect were declared unconstitutional. Beginning with New Jersey in 1911, the states enacted workers' compensation laws that stuck. Mississippi in 1948 became the last of the 48 states then in the Union to enact such a law.

A big argument for workers' compensation was that it would encourage employers to maintain safe conditions to reduce their payment for casualty insurance. Studies over the years have not agreed on the effectiveness of the system in actually reducing work-connected injury and illness, although most studies have taken it for granted that the overall effect was beneficial. Some indicated that the accident rate dropped immediately after a compensation plan was adopted but the effect tended to level off as the years passed. Others attempted to show that the plans became increasingly effective as benefits were liberalized and worker-coverage extended.

Until the late 1960s the federal government was quite modest in its demands on private industry for the protection of employees. Nor was the issue of worker health and safety given prime attention by the public except briefly in the wake of a particularly sensational disaster. The Office of Industrial Hygiene and Sanitation had been established in the U.S. Public Health Service in 1914, but its work was (and remained over the years) mainly research and investigation. The agency had no enforcement duties. Except for legislation pertaining to mines and railroads, the only direct intervention into private enterprise for worker safety was provided by the Walsh-Healey Act of 1936, which mandated health-safety standards for companies holding government contracts for more than $10,000.

The situation changed during the 1960s. By this time the public had become sensitized to the issue of environmental pollution, and there was general recognition that what harmed workers on the job could affect the well-being of the entire population. A sharp upturn in the number of reported industrial accidents led to enactment of the Coal Mine Health and Safety Act of 1969.

By 1970 job-related accidents accounted for more than 14,000 worker deaths, nearly 2½ million workers were disabled, 10 times as many person-days were lost from job-related disabilities as from strikes and the estimated new cases of occupational diseases totaled 300,000. In the early 1970s Congress passed two more bills to regulate job health and safety: the Federal Railroad Safety Act of 1970 and the Occupational Safety and Health Act of 1970, which created the Occupational Safety and Health Administration (OSHA).

Congress, in that same act, ordered that a special commission be set up to look into "the fairness and adequacy" of workers' compensation laws. Among the reasons for congressional concern, the act cited "the growth of the economy . . . increases in medial knowledge . . . [and] new technology creating new risks to health and safety." The presidentially appointed body, known as the National Commission on State Workmen's Compensation Laws, undertook an exhaustive review and issued a great deal of data and analytical material before it was disbanded July 31, 1972. It did note that accident rates were not necessarily lower in states where benefits were relatively high.

A 1976 review, prepared by Lee Ellis, a research analyst on occupational health under a government grant, was even more skeptical. While a study of available data showed the risk of serious work accidents had been appreciably reduced between the late 1920s and the early 1970s, it also showed the rate had declined for home accidents as well. Until definitive data became available to buttress their claims, he said, others should stop talking about "the beneficial effects of workmen's compensation on the occupational safety movement. . . ."

OSHA: Key Agency

The most significant development in the protection of worker health and safety was passage of the Occupational Safety and Health Act on Dec. 29, 1970. The agency administering the act, OSHA, has had several reorganizations and changes of leadership, and its activities have met with criticism and controversy. But the act succeeded in introducing a new principle into American life — that the worker has a legal right under federal law to a safe place to work. Moreover, the employer is now required, under penalty of law, to meet government-imposed standards of safety. This principle seems to have become firmly entrenched. Under the act, it is illegal for an employer to punish, discriminate against, fire or demote an employee for reporting a safety or health hazard, requesting an OSHA inspection or participating in union safety and health activities.

The act established OSHA as a new agency in the Department of Labor and created a new post of assistant secretary of labor for occupational safety and health to run it. In one way, the act represented a compromise between those who thought responsibility for worker safety should remain where it traditionally had been, with the states, and those who thought the time had come for the federal government to take a firm hand. The act provided that any state could develop its own occupational health and safety program, but the plan and its operation would be subject to the federal agency's approval.

If a state plan is approved, the state may enforce it. But the federal office will evaluate the state effort for at least three years and may withdraw approval during that period. When a state plan is approved, OSHA agrees to pay up to 50 percent of the cost of operations. By 1981, 24 states had OSHA-approved programs.

The act covers 5 million employers and some 60 million employees in such varied fields as construction, longshoring, agriculture, law, medicine, charity and disaster relief, organized labor and private education. Coverage includes religious groups to the extent that they employ workers for secular purposes. Self-employed persons, family-owned and operated farms and workplaces already protected by other federal agencies are not covered. Since federal agencies are exempt from OSHA regulations and enforcement provisions, each agency is required to maintain its own job safety and health program.

The House in 1979 passed a bill to extend federal occupational safety standards to the U.S. Postal Service. But the full Senate did not act on it and it died at the end of the session. The legislation was spurred by the Postal Service's on-the-job injury rate, the highest of all federal agencies. In 1977 the Postal Service accounted for 34.4 percent of all illnesses and injuries reported for the federal work force. Opponents of the legislation feared that it would be the first step toward equating the federal government with private industry for regulatory purposes.

The Occupational Safety and Health Administration:

- Encourages employers and employees to reduce hazards in the workplace and to implement safety and health programs.
- Establishes "separate but dependent responsibilities and rights" for employers and employees for the achievement of better safety and health conditions.
- Maintains reporting and recordkeeping procedures to monitor job-related injuries and illnesses.
- Develops and enforces mandatory job safety and health standards.
- Encourages the states to assume the fullest responsibility for establishing and administering their own occupational safety and health programs, which must be "at least as effective" as the federal program.
- Monitors federal agency safety programs and receives an annual report from each agency about its job safety and health efforts.
- Establishes advisory committees when necessary to assist in developing standards.
- Imposes temporary emergency standards when workers are in grave danger due to exposure to new toxic substances or hazards.
- Grants variances for special circumstances.
- Provides consultation services to small businesses to assist them in meeting OSHA standards.

Adoption of Standards

One of OSHA's major tasks is developing standards to protect workers. Before the act became effective, no centralized and systematic method existed for monitoring occupational safety and health problems. Statistics on job injuries and illnesses were collected by some states and by some private organizations; national figures were based on projections that were not always reliable. With OSHA standards came the first basis for consistent, nationwide procedures.

When it began operating, OSHA adopted many of the consensus standards that had been developed over the years by the American National Standards Institute Inc. and the National Fire Protection Association. These standards, however, frequently were either outdated or represented minimum rather than ideal standards. According to OSHA, the agency has worked since 1970 to update, revise and add to these standards to cover as many potential workplace hazards as possible. The legislation creating OSHA stressed that the standards developed should be feasible and should be based on research, experiments, demonstrations, past experience and the latest available scientific data.

Inspections and Investigations

To enforce its standards and regulations, OSHA is authorized to conduct workplace inspections. Before 1978 OSHA compliance officers were allowed to enter a workplace at any time without advance warning or a search warrant. However, in May 1978 the Supreme Court ruled that an employer has the right to refuse admission to an OSHA inspector who does not have a warrant. The ruling has not had a dramatic effect on the agency; most employers are willing to admit the compliance officers without a warrant. When they refuse, a warrant can be obtained from

Occupational Injury and Illness in American Industry

Year	Total Cases	Rate Per 100 Workers	Number of Fatalities for Employers with 11 or More Employees
1979	6,105,700	9.5	4,950
1978	5,799,400	9.4	4,590
1977	5,460,300	9.3	4,760
1976	5,163,700	9.2	3,940

Source: U.S. Bureau of Labor Statistics

a federal court relatively quickly. Because of the limited number of inspectors available to cover more than 5 million workplaces (1,200 staff inspectors in 1981, according to OSHA head Thorne Auchter), OSHA gives top priority to industries that have the greatest potential for worker injury. Generally, inspectors are concentrated in five target industries that have more than double the national average of occupational deaths and injuries: meat and meat products, lumber and wood products, longshoring, roofing and sheet metal, and miscellaneous transportation equipment (chiefly mobile homes, campers and snowmobiles). Additional emphasis has been placed on five health hazards that pose relatively high risk of injury and death: carbon monoxide, silica, lead, asbestos and cotton dust.

Most violations result in civil fines of up to $1,000. A willful or repeated violation carries up to a $10,000 penalty. For failure to correct a cited violation within the time prescribed, a penalty of $1,000 per day may be imposed.

Recordkeeping

OSHA requires employers of 11 or more employees to maintain records of occupational injuries and illnesses. An *occupational injury* is defined by OSHA as any injury such as a cut, fracture, sprain or amputation that results from a work-related accident in the work environment. An *occupational illness* is defined as any abnormal condition or disorder, other than one resulting from an occupational injury, caused by exposure to environmental factors associated with employment. Included are acute and chronic illnesses that may be caused by inhalation, absorption, ingestion or direct contact with toxic substances.

Health and Safety Committees

OSHA encourages the formation of health and safety committees in workplaces. Many such committees make regular job-site tours to help monitor general conditions. They also make spot inspections to check out worker complaints or keep tabs on particularly hazardous areas. If hazards have been cited by OSHA, the committee may be able to help make sure the conditions are corrected within the time period OSHA has established. Through collective bargaining, many committees have obtained a role in finding solutions to health and safety disputes.

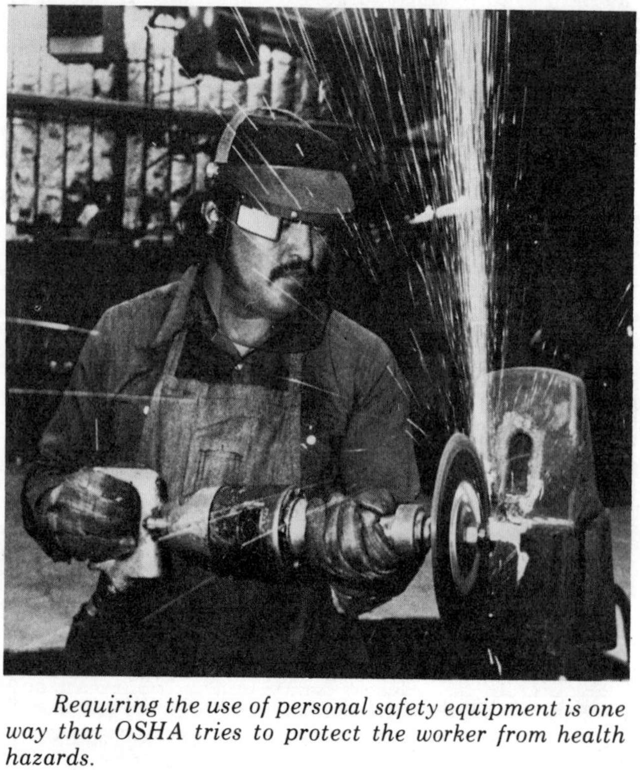

Requiring the use of personal safety equipment is one way that OSHA tries to protect the worker from health hazards.

OSHA asserts that health and safety committees are an effective way to improve workplace conditions because they are becoming more popular. Department of Labor surveys show that the number of union contracts providing for health and safety committees is increasing.

Independent Review Commission

Enforcement activities are the responsibility of the Occupational Safety and Health Review Commission, an independent agency not connected with OSHA, although the two work together closely. The Occupational Safety and Health Review Commission functions essentially as a "court" where employers may seek relief whenever they disagree with one or more aspects of an enforcement action. There are three members of the review commission, appointed by the president by and with the advice of the Senate for staggered terms of six years each.

NIOSH

The law also provides for safety research, training of personnel and employee education. The research function is vital because standards on toxic substances are dependent on scientific findings. Responsibility for research is placed in the hands of the National Institute for Occupational Safety and Health (NIOSH), established by the act. The law orders the institute to develop "criteria dealing with toxic materials and harmful physical agents and substances which will describe exposure levels that are safe for various periods of employment, including . . . exposure levels at which no employee will suffer impaired health or functional capacities or diminished life expectancy as a result of his work experience." This standard-setting function has been the source of much controversy.

Early History of OSHA

At its birth, OSHA enjoyed solid congressional support — the 1970 legislation that established it passed by overwhelming votes in both the House and Senate. Enthusiasm for the agency quickly waned, however, as members of Congress began to hear from businesses affected by the first actions implementing the act. Many businesses — especially small businesses — have been unrelenting in their criticism of OSHA.

Within one month of its creation, OSHA adopted some 4,400 standards from existing federal regulations, industry codes and the American National Standards Institute. Labor groups complained that the agency's enforcement activities were sporadic and weak, that its administration of the act was poor and that it failed to significantly reduce workplace hazards. Union leaders criticized OSHA for acting slowly in the face of thousands of potential hazards. In 1977, seven years after its establishment, OSHA had set only four standards in the health field (for asbestos, vinyl chloride, 14 carcinogens and coke-oven emissions). But during 1978 OSHA promulgated six more standards. Units of the Ralph Nader consumer-interest organization in Washington, D.C., kept up a steady flow of pamphlets berating OSHA — saying it was not fulfilling its mandate or was going soft on industry.

At the same time, critics, especially chemical manufacturers and other industrial interests, charged that OSHA standards were difficult to understand and frequently were unreasonably rigid. They complained that penalties for first violations were often unfair and that the cost of compliance was at times too burdensome. The paperwork requirements imposed on employers also were attacked. *Business Week* called OSHA the agency "hardest to live with," and members of Congress reported more complaints about OSHA than any other agency.

Some Steps Following an OSHA Inspection

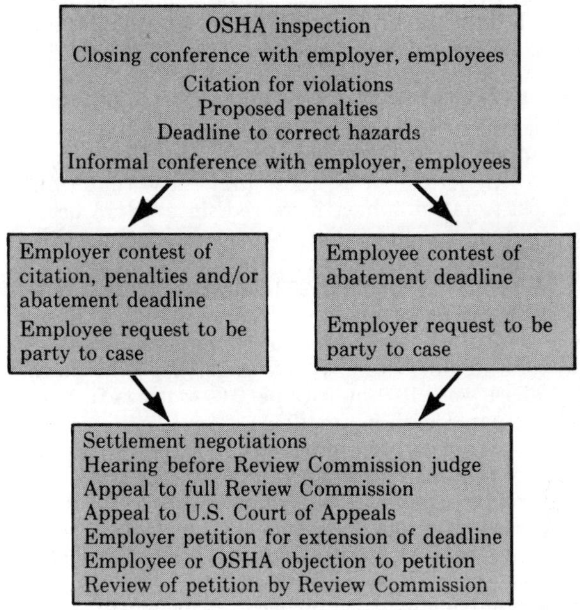

Source: Occupational Safety and Health Administration

Inspection Complaints

One of the most pervasive complaints in the early years was that OSHA's inspection and enforcement staff concentrated on job safety as opposed to job health. The factory or shop inspector traditionally was more attuned to accident prevention than to the more subtle hazards to health. Even worse were complaints that inspectors were issuing citations for minor technical deviations from standards — what became known as the "broken toilet seat violation."

A kind of folklore grew up about absurd "violations" cited against places of business. In addition, businessmen and shop owners complained about the officiousness of inspectors. Richard P. O'Brecht, director of labor law for the U.S. Chamber of Commerce in 1976, told a congressional committee that criticism of the agency reflected not an absence of commitment to worker safety but the "frustration and often outrage caused by what many employers view as the heavy-handed application of the OSHA program."

The tension reflected a conflict inherent in almost any worker protection program. While everyone applauds the goal of reducing the risk of worker injury, illness or death, there are large areas of doubt as to whether some of the safety measures — actual or proposed — are worth the cost. Inevitably, opinion differs on what action should be taken.

All regulatory agencies of government inspire a certain amount of resentment. Safety regulations touch an even more sensitive nerve than most. To the business operator, a citation for a violation is at best a nuisance. It is likely to be expensive and to be personally offensive for implying that the employer may be heartlessly indifferent to the welfare of the employees. The owner of a small business, in particular, is likely to bristle at the sudden appearance of a government inspector armed with authority to look around the shop.

In his study of occupational health, Nicholas Ashford observed that "inherent difficulties [are] encountered whenever the law is used as the predominant mechanism for social control of science and technology." He found this to be especially true of the OSHA program, which he said "cannot be successfully implemented if we continue to ignore the fundamental conflicts and tensions which exist between various groups of people and between various institutions in our society."

It is generally agreed, even within the agency itself, that OSHA made a clumsy start and was ill-equipped, both in funds and qualified personnel. President Richard Nixon, on signing the OSHA bill, praised it as "one of the most important pieces of legislation . . . ever passed by the Congress." Nixon said it represented "the American system at its best: Democrats, Republicans, the House, the Senate, the White House, business, labor, all cooperating in a common goal — the saving of lives, the avoiding of injuries, making the place of work for 55 million Americans safer and more pleasant." His choice of OSHA administrator, George Guenther, however, was regarded as a political appointee lacking special qualifications needed to marshal united support from the diverse forces mentioned by Nixon. Guenther's problem was compounded by a small budget and an inadequately trained staff.

In 1975 the AFL-CIO drew up a list of proposed reforms. "It is time the federal government lived up to the promise . . . of a safe and healthy workplace for every American worker," the statement said. Among the "specific actions" it recommended were:

- More money for the agency, more qualified manpower and more facilities, including a laboratory.
- "Full federal preemption of promulgation and enforcement of occupational safety and health standards in all states."
- Coverage for all workers, including state and local government employees.
- Authority for compliance officers to issue on-the-spot orders that employees leave places of "imminent danger."
- Transfer of NIOSH, the occupational health research agency, from the Department of Health, Education and Welfare (now Health and Human Services) to the Department of Labor and also transfer of health and safety responsibility for miners and railroad workers to Labor.

Support for Both Sides

Job injury statistics can provide ammunition for both critics and supporters of the Occupational Safety and Health Administration (OSHA) that Congress established in 1970. Depending on what figures are used, OSHA has either increased or reduced the job-related dangers to American workers.

Serious injuries, those that cause time to be lost from work, have increased since OSHA began keeping reliable safety records in 1972, critics point out. In 1972 there were 3.3 such injuries for each 100 workers. By 1979 that statistic had grown to 4.3 injuries.

But while serious injuries have increased, the total number of all work injuries has gone down. There were 10.9 injuries per 100 workers in 1972, compared with 9.5 in 1979.

Some experts argue, however, that overall injury rates are not a good indicator of OSHA performance, because the number of accidents is greatly affected by factors beyond OSHA's control. For example, according to OSHA policy analyst Frank Frodyma, increased workers' compensation benefits since the early 1970s have made it financially easier for injured workers to take time off before going back to work. The longer they stay home, the worse it makes the accident statistics look.

And certain injuries go through fads. Back strain, for example, has been growing considerably as a reason for taking time off. But much of that increase has occurred in service industries such as retailing and banking, and the injuries happen for reasons, such as tripping over a file cabinet, that OSHA could not be expected to prevent.

Changes in the economy also affect injury rates. During economic upswings companies buy new equipment, which workers might not be familiar with, and hire relatively less experienced new workers. In addition, economic good times lead to more construction — a particularly dangerous occupation.

Actions by government agencies other than OSHA also affect injury rates. For example, a substantial percentage of worker fatalities occurs in motor vehicle accidents. This helped to explain a sharp decline in worker fatalities after Congress set a nationwide speed limit of 55 miles an hour.

To these criticisms have been added others from the General Accounting Office, an arm of Congress, in a series of reports. The GAO noted that OSHA permitted states, while developing their programs, to maintain lower safety standards than are required by the federal government. Federal agencies themselves have been criticized in these reports as having inadequate worker-protection programs. The House Government Operations Committee, after several days of hearings, said in a report on Sept. 27, 1976: "In its five years of operation, the OSHA administration has failed to provide adequate protection for the health of American workers." But the committee was "encouraged" by the commitment for improving the program that was shown by Morton Corn, a University of Pittsburgh professor and specialist in industrial hygiene, who took over as agency director in 1975.

Small Business Exemptions

The first big wave of limitations on OSHA came in 1976. That year Congress decided that some businesses should be exempt from regulation because of their small size. Over the next few years this issue would recur, with business arguing that small businesses should not have to put up with the burden and expense of inspections, and labor responding that a small business was not inherently safer than a large one.

Small business operators argued that rules and regulations were often so wordy and technical that they had difficulty understanding them. "How can he [the employer] determine whether his wooden ladders are properly constructed and in compliance by being referred to 11 pages of fine print on the subject which includes everything from algebraic equations to the fiber stress characteristics of more than 50 different types of wood?" O'Brecht of the Chamber of Commerce asked.

In earlier years, the small businessman had no one to turn to. Unlike the big corporations, he had no technical specialists to handle such problems. If he asked the agency to send an inspector to see if he was in conformity and to advise him on correcting any deviations from the standard, he stood in jeopardy of being cited for a violation. Now, OSHA provides a free on-site consultation service for employers in every state. Consultants from the state government or a private contractor help employers identify hazardous conditions and determine corrective measures. This service is available upon employer request, but priority is given to smaller businesses, which generally are less able to afford private sector consultation. The emphasis of this service is placed on highly hazardous jobs.

Streamlining and Consolidation

In early 1977 President Carter appointed Eula Bingham assistant secretary of labor for occupational safety and health. In an effort to reduce the complaints about OSHA, Bingham pledged to adopt a set of "common sense" priorities and to make fundamental changes in administration and policy. She promised to focus attention on the most dangerous industries and devote less time to inspecting small businesses (except those with a higher-than-average rate of serious injury). Bingham also announced development of an expanded educational program and the abolition of what she characterized as nit-picking and out-of-date regulations.

Under Assistant Secretary Bingham, streamlining and consolidation became the key words in OSHA's efforts in the area of safety standards development. Nearly 1,000 safety standards were revoked during the first month of fiscal year 1977. OSHA staff members also worked particularly to simplify the rules and regulations in construction, fire protection and electricity.

Despite the changes Bingham initiated, OSHA continued to come under attack. As OSHA was attempting to

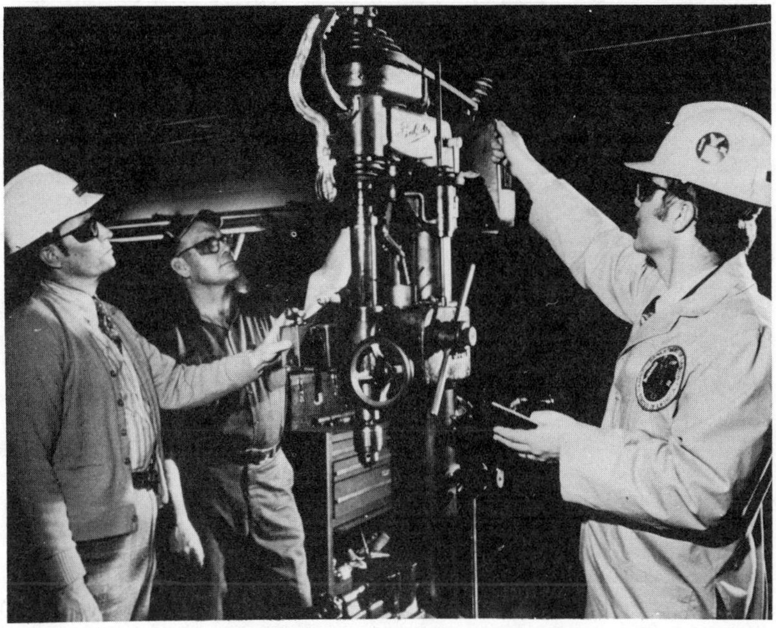

An Occupational Safety and Health compliance officer points out an alleged violation of the safety standards to the employee and employer representatives accompanying him on an inspection.

increase its effectiveness through internal changes, legislators were at work devising plans to change OSHA through external measures. The agency also faced serious challenges from the courts.

The first OSHA exemption based on a business' size, added to the fiscal 1977 Labor-HEW appropriation bill, applied only to companies with 10 or fewer employees. The other amendment approved that year prohibited inspectors from fining a business for health and safety violations the first time they were detected, unless the violations numbered 10 or more, or involved serious hazards to the workers.

The next challenge to OSHA came in 1978 when Sen. Dewey F. Bartlett, R-Okla. (1973-79), proposed an amendment to the Small Business Administration (SBA) authorization that based exemptions on businesses' previous safety records. Bartlett's amendment, approved by the Senate but subsequently deleted in conference, would have allowed an exemption for businesses with 10 or fewer employees provided they were in a category of business that, on average, had fewer than seven job injuries a year for every 100 employees.

The same idea reappeared in 1979, this time as an amendment to the fiscal 1980 Labor-HEW bill. The amendment prohibited OSHA from making general safety inspections of businesses with 10 or fewer employees if they were in industries with injury rates of less than seven per 100 employees.

However, OSHA could still inspect those businesses to investigate health hazards, workers' complaints or serious accidents. (A controversy over federal funding of abortions prevented final passage of the Labor-HEW bill; however, the OSHA provisions were attached to the fiscal 1980 continuing appropriations resolution, H J Res 440 — PL 96-123.)

Another limitation contained in PL 96-123 prohibited OSHA from inspecting businesses that already had been inspected by a state safety and health agency in the preceding six months.

Schweiker Bill

The first major attempt to legislate changes in OSHA occurred in 1980 and created expectations that the agency would face continuing legislative challenges. Business owners had been getting a sympathetic response from members of Congress about their complaints against OSHA almost since the agency was founded. But until 1980 they never had any realistic hope of winning a major legislative battle against their foe.

According to Sen. Richard S. Schweiker, Pa. (House 1961-69; Senate 1969-81), then ranking Republican on the Labor and Human Resources Committee, the much-criticized agency should concentrate on businesses with bad safety records. To that end, he introduced legislation that would exempt an estimated 90 percent of businesses from OSHA safety inspections. Over the years, limitations on appropriations had whittled the OSHA jurisdiction down — but the Schweiker bill was the first to provide a statutory exemption from coverage for whole groups of businesses. Its sponsor, Schweiker, became secretary of health and human services in the Reagan Cabinet.

The bill had the support of Labor Committee Chairman Harrison A. Williams Jr., D-N.J., one of the principal authors of the Occupational Safety and Health Act of 1970 and formerly an opponent of any attempt to strip OSHA of its authority. The Schweiker bill differed from Bartlett's earlier amendment in two important respects. Instead of providing exemptions only to small businesses, it would give them to all businesses, regardless of size, provided they met safety requirements. And, instead of basing the exemptions on industry-wide injury statistics, it would make each business qualify on the basis of its own safety record.

Although the Schweiker bill was not enacted, it raised a basic question about the future direction of federal job safety efforts: Should regulation concentrate on the workplaces where injuries were most likely to occur, or should it protect all workers, through the threat of inspection of every business, no matter how safe? One basic idea

Occupational Injury and Illness by Industry

Type of Work	1978	1979	Type of Work	1978	1979
Construction	16.0	16.2	Wholesale and retail trade	7.9	8.0
Manufacturing	13.2	13.3			
Agriculture, forestry and fisheries	11.6	11.7	Services	5.5	5.5
Mining	11.5	11.4	Finance, insurance and real estate	2.1	2.1
Transportation and public utilities	10.1	10.2			

Source: U.S. Bureau of Labor Statistics

behind the Schweiker bill was that OSHA was spread too thin — approximately 1,200 agents to inspect about 5 million workplaces. That was too few, supporters of the bill argued, to waste on inspecting businesses with good safety records, when they could focus instead on the most dangerous jobs.

An indication of the weakness of existing inspection policies, according to Schweiker, was that serious accident rates had risen since OSHA was established. One statistic that measures accidents, the number of job-related injuries that lead to lost time from work, increased 38 percent between 1972 and 1978.

Even more important politically was the frustration felt by business owners who had to submit to repeated safety inspections no matter how injury-free their workers had been in the past. Inspections cost businesses time and money even when no fines are handed out for safety violations.

For example, one company in Georgia that makes fruitcakes lost thousands of dollars in production when it had to shut down for inspections twice in two years. Yet the company claimed that it had never had a serious accident in 40 years of operation.

"After nine years under the act's present safety regulatory scheme, we are left with no demonstrable record that it works and with a bad taste all around from the experience," Schweiker argued.

The solution to both these problems, backers of the Schweiker bill said, was to replace the "stick" of inspections and fines against employers with the "carrot" of exemptions for businesses that were successful in protecting workers through their own efforts. Under the bill, businesses that reported a low rate of injuries for a year would be free, in most cases, from the threat of a routine safety inspection during the next year. On the one hand, supporters of the bill asserted, the new approach would allow inspectors to spend all their time on the 10 percent of businesses that were most dangerous to their workers. On the other hand, it would also relieve most business owners from the trouble and expense of inspection. The bill would not make changes in health inspections. Those mainly involved checking possible exposure to dangerous chemicals, the effects of which frequently do not show up for a number of years.

Labor unions and OSHA officials attacked the bill as both wrong in theory and unworkable in practice. Actually, OSHA already had begun to adopt one of the ideas underlying Schweiker's bill — that inspections should concentrate on the most dangerous types of businesses. Since taking office in 1977, OSHA Administrator Bingham had sought to steer agency efforts away from its former "nit-picking" regulation of minor safety violations, and toward major problems likely to cause serious injuries.

Many OSHA standards had been simplified and clarified. More than 11,000 safety and health rules had been critically assessed, and nearly 10 percent had been revoked as obsolete, overly detailed or irrelevant. In addition, 95 percent of all discretionary safety inspections were being targeted on larger workplaces and more hazardous industries.

But, Bingham told the Labor Committee, the existing orientation still retained the "all-important" principle that all businesses remain under OSHA's legal authority. The threat of inspection, no matter how unlikely, made every business conscious of safety, she said — just as the faint possibility of an audit made most taxpayers file an honest return.

A statutory exemption, however, would leave many workers without any protection, Bingham argued. "The bills before you would create two classes of workers — one entitled to full protection under the law, the other relegated to second-class status," she said.

Moreover, opponents of the bill pointed out, there was no way to assume on the basis of one year that a business would be safe the next. Many businesses experienced considerable fluctuations in their injury rates from year to year because of the installation of new equipment, for example, or the hiring of relatively unskilled new workers. "No statistical analysis yet devised of past experience can assure workers that their work places are safe while they are working in them," Bingham said.

From a practical standpoint, critics contended, the bill would base its exemptions on inadequate information. Businesses could prove their safety either with their reports to state workers' compensation systems, or by filing affidavits with OSHA. However, state systems varied widely and often collected inadequate information. Bingham said that, even with federal financial help, few if any of the state systems could supply OSHA with all the information it needed to separate safe from unsafe businesses. And employer affidavits would be subject to falsification, unions worried, even though the affidavits would have to be posted in the workplace.

The intense lobbying at an early phase may well have stifled the bill. While the sponsors knew labor opposed it, they were not prepared for what followed — an outpouring of mail, visits from anguished labor leaders and articles in the labor press marking defeat of the bill as one of the top priority issues of the year. Peggy Taylor, an AFL-CIO lobbyist, said defeating the bill was the top legislative priority of the United Steelworkers of America and the Oil, Chemical and Atomic Workers, and was a principal lobbying concern of groups such as the Amalgamated Clothing and Textile Workers and the building trades unions. The bill died before the end of the 96th Congress in 1980.

OSHA Supreme Court Cases

Since 1978 there have been several important Supreme Court decisions affecting OSHA's health and safety regulations to protect workers.

In May 1978 the court ruled in *Marshall v. Barlow's Inc.* that an employer has the right, based on the Fourth Amendment, to refuse to allow an OSHA inspector to enter and inspect his or her premises unless the inspector has a search warrant. Only about 1 percent of the businesses that OSHA attempted to inspect in fiscal year 1979 invoked this right and demanded a warrant.

In July 1980 the court ruled in two cases that OSHA's benzene exposure standard was invalid because the rule was unsupported by sufficient evidence that it was necessary to protect the health of workers. A "safe" workplace need not be completely "risk-free," the court declared. However, other 1980 and 1981 Supreme Court decisions upheld OSHA actions to protect workers.

Benzene Decision

The OSHA benzene regulation would have reduced the permissible exposure to benzene from 10 parts per million to one part per million.

By a 5-4 vote the court struck down the OSHA benzene standard, finding that OSHA had not met its responsibility of providing substantial evidence to show either that workers exposed to the higher level *would* contract cancer or that workers exposed only to the proposed lower level *would not* contract cancer.

The court's decision in the cases of *Industrial Union Department, AFL-CIO v. American Petroleum Institute,* and *Marshall v. American Petroleum Institute* made clear that such a standard might be valid if supported by such evidence, a qualification that rendered the ruling less a blow to OSHA's power than was initially thought.

As Justice John Paul Stevens explained for himself and three other members of the majority (Chief Justice Warren E. Burger and Justices Potter Stewart and Lewis F. Powell Jr.), OSHA is required by law "to find, as a threshold matter, that the toxic substance in question poses a significant health risk in the workplace and that a new lower standard is therefore 'reasonably necessary or appropriate to provide safe or healthful employment and places of employment.' "

OSHA had not made such a finding in the case of the benzene standard, which therefore could not be upheld, ruled the court. The court did not address the question, raised before a lower federal appeals court, of whether there must be a reasonable correlation between the benefits that such a standard would produce and the costs it would entail.

OSHA had indicated that only 35,000 employees would benefit from the new lower benzene standard. Most of these were in the rubber manufacturing industry, which could comply with the new standard without undue expense. But other workers who would be affected were in the petroleum refining and petrochemical industries where the cost of compliance was estimated to run as high as $82,000 per worker. OSHA estimated the total initial cost of compliance at $500 million. The American Petroleum Institute, representing the latter two industries, brought the suit challenging the benzene standard as unjustified.

The fifth member of the majority, William H. Rehnquist, agreed with the result of Stevens' reasoning, but not with the reasoning itself. Rehnquist, consistent with his strict constructionist reading of the Constitution, concluded that Congress' delegation to OSHA of the standard-setting authority was so broad and undefined as to be an unconstitutional delegation of legislative power to the executive branch. He argued that Congress had improperly delegated to OSHA the decision whether to protect human life above all other concerns in regulating workplaces or whether, instead, to strike some balance between "statistical lives and industrial resources."

"If we are ever to reshoulder the burden of ensuring that Congress itself make the critical policy decisions, this is surely the case in which to do it," he wrote. "It is difficult to imagine a more obvious example of Congress simply avoiding a choice which was both fundamental for purposes of the statute and yet politically so divisive that the necessary decision or compromise was difficult, if not impossible to hammer out in the legislative forge."

In a lengthy and bitter dissent, four justices attacked the majority's decision as being a complete misinterpretation of the Occupational Safety and Health Act, as well as an improper attempt by the court to substitute its judgment for the agency's findings.

Justice Thurgood Marshall, writing for himself, Justices William J. Brennan Jr., Byron R. White and Harry A. Blackmun, criticized the court's decision as usurping the power of Congress. The reasoning set out in Stevens' opinion, wrote Marshall, had no support in the language, structure or legislative history of the 1970 Occupational Safety and Health Act.

The "threshold finding" that the plurality of the justices would require OSHA to make was their own invention, he continued. "[I]t can be understood only as reflecting the personal views of the plurality as to the proper allocation of resources for safety in the American workplace."

A probable effect of the benzene case was that OSHA in the future would conduct more elaborate studies and provide more compelling evidence before promulgating carcinogen studies. In 1981 OSHA modified its cancer policy to reflect the benzene decision.

OSHA's original cancer policy went into effect in April 1980. The policy did not regulate specific substances but established criteria for classifying carcinogens and set forth efficient procedures for future rulemaking involving specific carcinogens. By 1980 OSHA estimated that at least 500 substances were suspected of causing cancer in the workplace.

Under the OSHA policy, such substances would be separated into two categories: those that present a clear and present danger (Category I) and those that show only a "suggestion" of carcinogenicity (Category II). The cancer policy had required the automatic setting of the lowest feasible level for Category I potential carcinogens. That requirement was modified in January 1981 so that consideration must be given to the significance of the risk before a carcinogen standard could be issued.

When the cancer policy was instituted by OSHA, business leaders opposed it, claiming that OSHA was forcing companies to spend billions of dollars without enough evidence to show that the improvements would save lives or prevent injuries. OSHA officials argued that its cancer policy provided better protection for the worker by speeding up the process of regulating carcinogens. The 1981 modification appeared to strike a compromise between these two groups.

Refusal of Unsafe Jobs

Another 1980 Supreme Court decision strengthened some of OSHA's powers. On Feb. 26 the court ruled in *Whirlpool Corp. v. Marshall* that workers may refuse to perform tasks they consider unsafe without fear of recrimination from their employers. The federal job safety regulations that allowed such refusal — if there was a real danger of death or serious injury and if there was not enough time to correct the situation through ordinary channels — were vigorously opposed by industry representatives. The case originated at an Ohio Whirlpool Corp. appliance plant where a worker fell to his death in June 1974 while cleaning off a metal screen 20 feet above the floor. Subsequently, two other workers, Virgil Deemer and Thomas Cornwell, refused to perform the same job, claiming that corrective measures taken by the company had not been sufficient. They were sent home, not paid for the shift and officially reprimanded.

The 1970 Occupational Safety and Health Act prohibited employers from discriminating against workers who asserted any of the rights that the act guaranteed. The act itself did not guarantee a right to refuse to work in unsafe conditions. But a regulation promulgated by Secretary of Labor F. Ray Marshall under the act did grant workers such a right when there was no available alternative way of dealing with hazardous conditions. Marshall subsequently sued Whirlpool for discriminating against Deemer and Cornwell in retaliation for their refusal to work under conditions they believed to be unsafe. Whirlpool challenged the regulation as inconsistent with the law.

Just six weeks after hearing arguments in the *Whirlpool* case, the Supreme Court unanimously upheld the regulation. The limited "right to refuse to work" that it provided was clearly in line with the objective of the 1970 law — to prevent death or serious injuries in the workplace, the court held.

The justices were not persuaded by Whirlpool's arguments that Congress, in the process of approving the 1970 Act, had rejected such a right. Writing for the court, Justice Potter Stewart emphasized the limited nature of this right. The law set up an elaborate mechanism through which workers could seek correction of unsafe conditions by their employer, through OSHA or through the federal courts.

Thus, "as a general matter, there is no right afforded by the Act which would entitle employees to walk off the job because of potential unsafe conditions at the workplace," Stewart wrote. But the court upheld the power of OSHA to protect an employee against retaliation when he refuses an order to work under conditions that he reasonably believes pose an imminent risk to his safety, providing there is no opportunity to seek corrective action.

Employers were protected from abuse of the regulations by retaining the right to challenge in court the good faith of the employee and by seeking the discharge or reprimand of the employee if such good faith was lacking.

Cotton Dust Standard

In 1981 the Reagan administration sought to reduce the federal presence in the field of occupational health and safety. Thorne G. Auchter took over as head of OSHA with the conviction that his agency had over-regulated industry. He also wanted to cut down on the number of OSHA inspections. Auchter, however, was not brought in specifically to dismantle OSHA. Even OSHA's greatest critics generally conceded that in its 11 years of existence the agency had increased the awareness of the country regarding occupational safety and health matters. The conservative Heritage Foundation recommended to Reagan that the statutory framework of the Occupational Safety and Health Act, although imperfect, contained enough flexibility to allow for deregulation without enacting new legislation.

It was clear by the early spring of 1981 that President Reagan's desired emphasis upon cost-benefit analysis, expressed in Executive Order 12291, also had become Auchter's emphasis. The executive order, issued February 1981, required federal agencies to assess the costs and benefits of major regulations.

In March 1981 OSHA, in reaction to Reagan's order, announced that it would reconsider its controversial cotton dust regulations with a cost-benefit approach in mind. In the cotton dust announcement, OSHA said it would "use its reexamination of this particular standard to explore the usefulness of cost-benefit analysis in setting worker health regulations generally." It was "time to reexamine the traditional resistance to cost-benefit analysis," Auchter said. The Reagan administration then asked the Supreme Court to delay its ruling in two cotton dust cases, which had been argued Jan. 21, while it reassessed the economic impact of the OSHA standards. But the justices brushed aside the request.

On June 17, 1981, the court rejected arguments by the textile industry that OSHA be required to demonstrate that benefits to workers outweigh costs to industry before promulgating a cotton dust standard. By a 5-3 vote in the cases of *American Textile Manufacturers Institute v. Donovan* and *National Cotton Council v. Donovan,* the court upheld the stringent OSHA cotton dust standards.

Writing for the majority, Justice Brennan declared that economic and technical feasibility constitute the only limits on OSHA's power to adopt worker health and safety standards. And in this case, OSHA found the cotton dust standard feasible on both counts.

"Congress itself defined the basic relationship between costs and benefits, by placing the 'benefit' of worker health above all other considerations save those making attainment of this 'benefit' unachievable," Brennan wrote. He noted Congress had specifically required the use of cost-benefit analyses in certain other laws, but did not include such language in the 1970 OSHA law. The majority was unequivocal in its belief that only Congress could undo in 1981 what it did in 1970.

Justices Rehnquist and Stewart and Chief Justice Burger dissented. Stewart said OSHA failed to justify its conclusion that the new cotton dust standard was economically feasible, while Rehnquist and Burger said the "feasibility" test was no standard at all. It simply served to mask an unconstitutional delegation of legislative power to an executive branch agency, they said.

The 5-3 vote in favor of the cotton dust standard reflected a shift by Justice John Paul Stevens, who had voted against OSHA in the 1980 benzene case. Justice Lewis Powell, who also voted against OSHA in that decision, did not participate in the cotton dust case.

To protect workers from byssionsis ("brown lung") and other respiratory diseases, OSHA in 1978 required textile manufacturers to install machines to clean cotton dust from the air and, in areas where such ventilators were ineffective, to order workers to wear masks containing respirators. OSHA also required that permissible cotton dust levels be brought down from 1,000 micrograms per cubic meter of air to 200 micrograms for the most hazardous sections of the mills. That level is said to be the equivalent of a grain of salt in a box of air a meter (39.37 inches) long on each side.

The textile industry immediately challenged the standard, arguing that the giant vacuum devices and elaborate duct work required to meet the cotton dust standard were too expensive and that the burden would drive some companies out of business. The American Textile Manufacturers Institute complained that the standard's benefits were uncertain and that there were cheaper ways of reducing the incidence of disease, such as careful medical screening. These same arguments had been made by industrial users of benzene when they tried to get their exposure standards softened in 1980.

Textile manufacturers also argued that workers often mistake brown lung for other respiratory problems that are not linked to the industry. They asserted that textile firms should not be expected to pay compensation to workers suffering from asthma, chronic bronchitis or other breathing difficulties that may result from smoking.

Historically, textile workers have been smokers. Studies on the subject have reached contradictory conclusions on whether lung damage can be uniquely attributed to smoking or exposure to cotton dust.

The court's cotton dust ruling was considered one of the most significant in the recent history of regulatory law. *Business Week* said on July 6, 1981:

> The high court's review of OSHA's legislative history could spell trouble for the [Reagan] Administration's reliance on cost-benefit tests in other areas as well. The decision is forcing the Administration to review several regulatory statutes, especially those that — like the OSHA law — make no direct mention of weighing costs and benefits. These include major portions of the Clean Air Act, Safe Drinking Water Act, Water Pollution Control Act, Federal Mine Safety & Health Act, and National Motor Vehicle & Traffic Safety Act. The Supreme Court's cotton-dust decision will almost certainly be used as a precedent by opponents of regulatory cutbacks, and the mere threat of such challenges could head off the use of cost-benefit tests in some areas.

The court did not rule out cost-benefit analysis as part of health standards but did say it was not specifically required by law. Textile industry lawyers said that this ruling left room for use of cost-benefit analysis in determining which chemicals should be regulated. Assistant Labor Secretary Auchter agreed, saying that the court "did not specifically exclude cost/benefit analysis" in areas other than health standards.

Critics of industry's approach contend that cost-benefit analysis undermines regulation and obstructs and delays an already cumbersome procedure for establishing standards. The hearing and decision-making process for the cotton dust standards took two years, not including court time. The industry critics also question the morality of suggesting that there is a dollar figure, beyond which it ought to be considered unreasonable to save a life.

A further problem with cost-benefit analysis is who does the analysis. Cost-benefit critics point to contradictory studies to illustrate this point. At the request of Congress, the Labor Department performed a cost-benefit study and estimated that 83,610 workers or 14 percent of those exposed to cotton dust could get brown lung. The OSHA standards would cost industry about $655 million to implement, or about $8,000 per case avoided.

But industry, using its own studies, estimated that only 1 percent of the workers exposed to cotton dust were likely to get byssionsis. Implementation of the standards under these estimates might cost $1.1 billion, instead of $655 million. By industry's analysis, each case avoided would cost over $100,000.

Assistant Labor Secretary Auchter, in an August 1981 interview with *Nation's Business* magazine, addressed the analysis problem. "You know the old saying: There are lies, damned lies and statistics," he said. "You have people on one side with a bunch of statistics and people on the other side, saying those statistics are wrong, ours are right. And you even have people wandering around in the middle saying here's a bunch of statistics and you can do what you want with them."

Cost-Benefit Analysis

Behind all the arguments on legislation to preserve the environment or protect the worker lies the basic question of cost. It has become customary to apply the concept of a cost-benefit ratio to questions of policy in this area. To some it seems crass to balance a dollar figure against the health or life of a human being. It helps to consider the balance as between cost and risk, a more acceptable frame of reference, familiar to all in the form of insurance.

Philip Handler, president of the National Academy of Sciences, told a scientific forum in 1973: "There is no escape from the need, somehow, to equate dollars and lives, to agree to the dollar value of an average human life in the population at risk. . . ." In a 1975 extension of his remarks, Handler said: "[W]hen the government contemplates regulatory activity to diminish the risk associated with some technology . . . an attempt is required to state both the cost and the benefits in quantitative form."

Generally speaking, the employer is more interested in the cost of instituting a safety or health-protection measure and the employee is more interested in getting the maximum amount of protection. It has been pointed out, however, that if the risk is not too great, the worker may prefer to forgo a safety measure in favor of some other benefit — higher wages, for example. Some studies are critical of unions that for years pressed for other benefits as alternatives to health-protective measures.

Since Congress first enacted the Occupational Safety and Health Act, the business community has argued that it allows the federal government to set stringent health and safety standards without balancing the benefits to workers against the costs to employers. OSHA imposes stringent restrictions on exposure of workers to hazardous substances. Its decisions are based on the best available evidence about those hazards. That evidence, especially when the diseases take a generation to appear, sometimes is skimpy.

When not enough is known about a substance in the workplace, OSHA has been faced with the decision of holding back until more is learned or taking the maximum precautions. The agency has chosen the latter course and paid only minimal attention to how much it will cost the affected industries. All indications in 1981 were that Reagan administration officials wanted to reverse that trend and lend more sympathy to the business argument for cost-benefit analysis. Robert Stewart Smith of the New York State School of Industrial and Labor Relations at Cornell University complained about OSHA in 1976: "[T]he basic problem with the implementation of the act is that there is no fundamental agreement on the practical methods of balancing considerations of greater safety and health against considerations of cost."

Smith argued that "the government ... should not force more safety and health on society than workers would choose for themselves if they had to pay the costs ... In their private lives ... they smoke cigarettes, drive when they could walk, ski when they could read a book, and use power mowers when safer hand mowers would do."

The Cost of Protection

It is generally taken for granted that the cost of protection will be high. Nevertheless, a government program of the OSHA type appears to have become a permanent element in the nation's economic life. And some of the early suspicion of OSHA's motives has subsided.

A spokesman for the construction industry has remarked that "most of our original apprehension has proven groundless." The spokesman added OSHA "is neither as effective as some of its advocates thought it would be nor is it the obstacle to normal operations that was originally anticipated by industry." Of one thing he was sure: "OSHA is here and working and ... it is never going to go away."

It is not clear that the public or even industry would want OSHA to go away. Americans are becoming increasingly aware that workplace hazards can add to production costs and consumer prices. According to the National Safety Council, the total national cost of work-related injuries and fatalities incurred for 1979 was approximately $30 billion, including $19 billion for workers' compensation insurance.

According to OSHA, the added production costs derive from a variety of sources including medical payments and insurance, workers' compensation, lost productivity and buying power, welfare spending for survivors and the disabled, absenteeism, turnover, safety-related strikes, liability/fire/property insurance, low productivity, equipment damage and waste of materials.

Some 245 million workdays are lost each year to injuries — 10 times more than the average number of days lost each year in strikes. OSHA says that if improved conditions cut absenteeism by one day per worker per year, as much as $15 billion could be added to America's output of goods and services. Just one aspect of treatment for the 10,000 Americans with work-related kidney disease could cost an estimated $50,000 for each patient or $500 million annually.

OSHA maintains that the cost of workplace hazards can be reduced. Questor, a large conglomerate corporation with 68 plants making dozens of products, reduced its workers' compensation costs by one third by eliminating many health and safety hazards. Boise Cascade, a large timber and housing company, estimated in 1975 that each accident cost $7,275 in added medical expenses, workers' compensation, equipment damage, lost time and other expenses. Between 1973 and 1975, total accidents in Boise's operations were reduced by one-third, saving more than $12 million a year.

WORKPLACE DISEASES AND METHODS OF CONTROL

A cumulative listing of the multifarious hazards of the workplace would give so overwhelming an impression of danger that it might discourage all but the bravest to seek employment of any kind. Even artists, craftsmen and hobbyists are not free from occupational dangers. Samuel S. Epstein pointed out in his study, *The Politics of Cancer*, that artists often are exposed under poorly ventilated conditions to benzene in common materials, such as resin and fluorescent dye solvents, paint and varnish removers and silk-screen washes. And many of the hazards of the workplace are familiar in all circumstances of modern life — so avoiding work is not the answer. The odds of being injured on the job can be vastly reduced by taking ordinary precautions. To be successful, these safety measures must rely on employer efforts and support from employees, unions and government regulatory bodies.

The 1979 Surgeon General's Report on Health Promotion and Disease Prevention suggested several ways that occupational hazards can be controlled, such as requiring appropriate engineering controls and special protective equipment, training employees to work with hazardous equipment and monitoring workers' exposure to hazards. The problem with many prevention strategies, according to the report, is that hazard control technology has lagged behind the growth in industrial use of hazardous chemicals.

People in mining, agriculture (including forestry and fishing) and construction are six, three and three times, respectively, more likely to die from a work-related injury than other private sector workers. And work-related problems are reported by a wide variety of employee groups, including medical technicians, cosmetologists, flight attendants, dentists and air traffic controllers.

Safety Hazards

Workplace injuries have numerous causes. Arms, legs or fingers can be caught in unguarded machinery. Improper maintenance of electrical equipment can result in fatal shocks. Fires and explosions may claim many lives at one time. Nicholas Ashford cites the most frequent causes of accidents in *Crisis in the Workplace: Occupational Diseases and Injury, a Report to the Ford Foundation* (1971) are:

- Fires and explosions from chemicals, pressurized containers or transmission lines.
- Physical injury, possibly dismemberment, from unshielded parts of machinery that saw, mold, roll, cut, mix, flatten, bend, grind or simply move under mechanical power.
- Electrical hazards from improper grounding or shielding.
- Injuries to the eye from wood or metal chips discharged during cutting or grinding — or from the splashing or misting from liquid aerosols.
- Crushing and mangling injuries from moving and lifting equipment, especially prevalent in construction and stevedoring.

The workplace is a significant source of exposure to substances that may adversely affect pregnancy. This table lists occupations where the percentage of women employees is high. Some of the substances to which they are exposed are known to cause birth defects, stillbirths and miscarriages.

Occupational Exposures in Trades Employing Large Numbers of Women

Occupation	Exposure
Textile and related occupations	
Textile workers	Raw cotton dust, noise, synthetic fiber dusts, formaldehyde, heat, dyes, flame retardants, asbestos
Sewers and stitchers, upholsterers	Cotton and synthetic fiber dusts, noise, formaldehyde, organic solvents, benzene, toluene, trichloroethylene, perchloroethylene, chloroprene, styrene, carbon disulfide, flame retardants, asbestos
Hospital and health personnel	
Registered nurses, aides, orderlies	Anesthetic gases, ethylene oxide, X-ray radiation, alcohol, infectious diseases, puncture wounds
Dental hygienists	X-ray radiation, mercury, ultrasonic noise, anesthetic gases
Laboratory workers (clinical and research)	Wide variety of toxic chemicals, including carcinogens, mutagens and teratogens, X-ray radiation
Electronics assemblers	Lead, tin, antimony, trichloroethylene, methylene chloride, epoxy resins, methyl ethyl ketone
Hairdressers and cosmetologists	Hair spray resins (polyvinyl pyrrolidone), aerosol propellants (freons), halogenated hydrocarbons, hair dyes, solvents of nail polish, benzyl alcohol, ethyl alcohol, acetone
Cleaning personnel	
Launderers	Soaps, detergents, enzymes, heat, humidity, industrially contaminated clothing
Dry cleaners	Perchloroethylene, trichloroethylene, stoddard solvent (naphtha), benzene, industrially contaminated clothing
Photographic processors	Caustics, iron salts, mercuric chloride, bromides, iodides, pyrogallic acid, silver nitrate
Domestics	Solvents, hydrocarbons, soaps, detergents, bleaches, alkalies
Transportation personnel	Carbon monoxide, polynuclear aromatics, lead, and other combustion products of gasoline, vibration, physical stress
Clerical personnel	Physical stress, poor illumination, trichloroethylene, carbon tetrachloride and various other cleaners, asbestos in air conditioning
Opticians and lens grinders	Coal tar pitch volatiles, iron oxide, dust solvents, hydrocarbons
Printing personnel	Ink mists, 2-nitropropane, methanol, carbon tetrachloride, methylene chloride, lead, noise, hydrocarbon solvents, trichloroethylene, toluene, benzene, trace metals

Source: Council on Environmental Quality

• Falls from equipment or from high places of work, most frequent in farming and construction work.

On-the-job accidents kill about 13,000 Americans each year. Nine million more are so severely affected by work-related injuries that they require medical care or are at least temporarily unable to work.

Health Hazards

Hundreds of chemicals are suspected of causing cancer and millions of workers may be exposed to them. Since 1900, the U.S. cancer death rate has tripled, partly because of the increased use of new, untested substances.

OSHA, in its health and safety literature, lists areas of the body most directly affected by workplace substances:

Skin. Many workplace chemicals strong enough to dissolve, degrease, disinfect, harden, soften, fuel or lubricate are also serious threats to human skin. In fact, according to OSHA, skin disorders are the most commonly reported work-related health problems with hundreds of thousands of cases occuring every year.

Lungs. Dust, fumes, and mists can cause many health problems by clogging, burning or irritating the lungs. Some work-related lung diseases are incurable or fatal. Some chemicals can aggravate cases of bronchitis or emphysema.

Heart. It is believed that some substances speed up the body's formation of cholesterol fat. Over the years, cholesterol can stiffen and narrow the blood vessels that supply the heart with oxygen. If this "hardening of the arteries" becomes severe, the heart muscle is starved of oxygen and a heart attack may result. Lung damage can make the heart work harder to pump enough oxygen through the body. Physical stress from severe heat and cold also can put an added burden on the heart.

Hearing. Millions of workers face possible hearing loss from workplace noise. According to Ashford, excessive noise not only can impair hearing but "triggers changes in cardiovascular, endocrine, and neurological function." Some noises can cause tension, thus quickening pulse rate, increasing blood pressure and narrowing the blood vessels. Over a long period of time, these deleterious effects may strain the heart. Noise also can contribute to accidents by making it impossible to hear warning signals or approaching vehicles.

Nervous System. Some chemicals enter the blood stream by penetrating the skin. Others become vapors or fumes and enter through the lungs. Still others may be ingested into the stomach. Once in the blood, they may assault the central nervous system, injure the kidney or liver, cause bone marrow damage and anemia or induce psychological disorders. Some chemicals may cause headaches, insomnia or loss of coordination or feeling. Heavy exposure can cause paralysis or convulsions and may be fatal. Substances that attack the nervous system include lead, arsenic, carbon monoxide, benzene, inorganic mercury and chemicals known as "halogenated hydrocarbons."

Reproductive Organs. Some job health hazards threaten not only this generation of workers but unborn children as well. Birth defects, stillbirths, miscarriages and sterility can all result from exposure to certain chemicals or toxic substances. Some 200,000 children are born each year in the United States with serious birth defects — two-thirds of them having unknown causes. No one knows how many may be caused by workplace substances.

Increasingly, women are moving into industrial jobs traditionally held by males, and some factories and shops traditionally employ mainly female workers. Of approximately 100 million workers, 41 million are women, according to Samuel S. Epstein in *The Politics of Cancer.* In 1977, 49 percent of all U.S. women were in the work force, as opposed to 38 percent in 1960.

According to Eric Eckholm, at least one million American women of childbearing age are exposed on the job to chemicals and metals that might cause birth defects, cancer, miscarriages or, possibly, behavioral problems. He wrote in 1977, "While the developing fetus is probably far more sensitive than an adult to hazardous agents, sufficient knowledge on which to base allowable exposure standards for pregnant women is not available."

According to the 1980 annual report of the Council on Environmental Quality (CEQ), a growing body of scientific evidence shows that "environmental exposures to smoking, alcohol, and other chemicals can affect: the ability to conceive, by causing infertility in both males and females; the viability of the fetus, by causing spontaneous abortions, miscarriages, and stillbirths; and the health of the infant, by causing low birth weight or birth defects." Exposure to toxic substances also can affect heredity by acting directly on ova and sperm, creating defects that may be passed on for generations.

Controversy has arisen over whether to remove women from workplaces where substances could adversely affect them. Women's rights advocates charge that such wholesale discrimination is illegal and that not all women of childbearing age should be regarded as potential mothers. Yet, as Eckholm pointed out in his study, many women do not realize they are pregnant until many weeks after conception, during which time irreversible fetal damage could occur.

In 1978 a chemical maker, American Cyanamid, decided to remove all fertile women from jobs in the lead chromate pigment manufacturing section of its plant at Willow Island, W. Va. OSHA cited the company under the general duty clause of the Occupational Safety and Health Act, which requires an employer to provide a workplace free of hazards that might cause death or serious physical harm (instead of removing employees), and fined it $10,000. In early 1980 the Oil, Chemical and Atomic Workers Union and the American Civil Liberties Union sued the company under the 1964 Civil Rights Act on the ground that the company was discriminating unfairly against women.

According to the CEQ's 1980 annual report, a spokesperson for American Cyanamid stated: "In the real world [having the workplace safe for everyone is] totally unachievable without emasculating the chemical industry.... There is no way ... to always protect [the fetus]. In those instances where we cannot protect the fetus, we are required to move it away from the hazard, and that has to mean moving the mother as well."

Recent research also has suggested that some industrial influences on males' reproductive organs can cause birth defects in the children they father. The CEQ reported in 1980 that among the environmental agents known to affect male reproduction are lead, zinc, cadmium, dibromochloropropane (DBCP), vinyl chloride, anesthetic gases, chloroprene and a number of hydrocarbons and polycyclic hydrocarbons.

Construction Workers

Each year many workers on construction sites suffer electric shock while using portable electric tools and equipment. About 800 construction workers are killed annually. Construction workers have the most dangerous occupation, according to the Bureau of Labor Statistics. In 1979, 16.2 percent of occupational injuries and illnesses were in the construction industry while only 13.3 percent were in the manufacturing industry and 11.4 percent were in the mining industry. *(See chart, p. 95)* The nature of the job exposes construction workers to falls, dangerous machines and moving vehicles. But one of the more serious health hazards for construction workers is exposure to asbestos.

Asbestos and Its Dangers

Asbestos, known as the "magic mineral," is a widely used material that is resistant to heat and corrosive chemicals. Depending upon the chemical composition, fibers may range in texture from coarse to silky. The properties that make asbestos fibers so valuable to industry are their high tensile strength, flexibility, heat and chemical resistance, and good frictional qualities. Certain grades of asbestos can be spun or woven. Others can be laid and pressed to form paper or structural reinforcement material. It is used in the manufacture of friction products, textiles, insulation, cement, asphalt, plastic, wallboard, pipes, textiles, food and beverage processing, brake linings and countless other products. OSHA estimated that approximately 77 percent of asbestos products in 1972 were used in construction work. These products included floor tiles, roofing felts and shingles. If those products are cut, torn or broken, asbestos exposure can occur. Other products such as cement powders and acoustical materials contain asbestos in a loose form that can be spread throughout the workplace by air currents.

Asbestos fibers, carried into the body as airborne particles, are like fine glass slivers and can become embedded in the tissues of the lungs and digestive system. Once asbestos fibers become trapped in the lungs' alveoli (air sacs), they cannot be removed. Scientists around the world have demonstrated the link between asbestos and cancers of the lungs, stomach, large intestine, rectum and peritoneum (a lining of the abdominal cavity). According to Epstein's study, asbestos has led to approximately 50,000 deaths a year in the United States from cancer and other diseases.

Asbestosis. A well-recognized dust-origin disease that afflicts construction workers and other handlers of asbestos is asbestosis. After workers have been exposed to asbestos for many years, the inhaled particles will leave the lungs permanently scarred. Asbestosis, an emphysema-like condition, is similar to black-lung disease. Early symptoms may include coughing, shortness of breath, and broadening of the fingertips; crackling sounds in the lungs may be evident later. Chest pain and fatigue after slight exertion may also occur. The breakdown of the alveoli within the lungs will eventually make it impossible for the body to take in enough oxygen. Heart failure may result because of the increased effort required to pump blood through the lungs.

It was not until the 1940s that an association between the inhalation of asbestos and lung cancer was supported by epidemiologic evidence. By the early 1960s the evidence was overwhelming. In 1976 Dr. Irving J. Selikoff, director of Environmental Sciences Laboratory of Mount Sinai School of Medicine in New York City and a specialist in asbestosis research, estimated that 400,000 of the million Americans who work or have worked with asbestos will die of cancer by the year 2025 unless far better treatment is devised. In testimony before a Senate committee, Selikoff referred to asbestosis as a "hidden time bomb."

Lung Cancer. Lung cancer exacts the highest mortality of any asbestos-related disease. According to OSHA, lung cancer has caused up to 24 percent of all deaths in some groups of individuals heavily exposed to asbestos, compared with a risk factor of 4 to 5 percent for the general population.

After exposure to asbestos, lung cancer may take as long as 20 years to develop. Among workers using asbestos products, the total amount of lung cancer depends on exposure, age and duration of asbestos-related work.

The incidence of lung cancer increases dramatically among asbestos workers who smoke. Asbestos workers who smoke regularly have a 92 times greater risk of dying from lung cancer than do non-smokers who do not work with asbestos. When compared with the general smoking population, asbestos workers who smoke show an eight times greater risk of lung cancer. Industry has argued that these studies prove that smoking and not asbestos is the real problem for asbestos workers. However, Samuel Epstein points out that recent studies, including one by NIOSH in 1977, indicate that the smoking effect is less clear-cut than earlier reports suggested and that non-smoking asbestos workers also have excess risks of lung cancer.

Mesothelioma. Mesothelioma is a cancerous tumor that spreads very rapidly in the cells of membranes covering the lungs or abdomen. No successful treatment is yet known. By the time symptoms are diagnosed, death usually occurs within one year. Symptoms are a shortness of breath and chest or abdominal pain. Although evidence shows that even brief exposures — from as little as a few days — can cause mesotheliomas, the cancerous tumors may not develop for as many as 30 years. Although very rare in the general population, mesotheliomas account for about 10 percent of the deaths in asbestos workers.

Gastrointestinal Cancer. Asbestos that has contaminated food, beverages, cigarettes or anything put in the mouth can be swallowed and passed along the digestive tract. Increased rates of cancers of the stomach, colon and rectum have been observed in asbestos workers. There is also evidence that asbestos may cause cancers in the esophagus, the tube leading from the mouth to the stomach.

OSHA Exposure Standard

Asbestos has been observed to cause disease in workers, their families and even persons living near asbestos plants. According to OSHA, lung abnormalities have been seen in 38 percent of some asbestos workers' family members. As noted earlier, particles of asbestos may be carried into the home on the body, clothing or materials taken from the work site. Epstein illustrates this point in his study by explaining the case of a 45-year-old New Jersey woman who was dying of cancer. Her doctor was puzzled by the disease because the woman was a lawyer and her rare malignancy had been seen only in asbestos workers. But the origins of her disease became clear when the doctor examined the records of her past. Her father had spent 1947 working in an asbestos-insulation factory. When he came home each night, his clothes and hair had been covered with whitish fibers and his daughter had often laundered his work clothes. Her father had died of cancer two decades after his work in the factory.

Only recently has it been discovered that even low levels of asbestos can cause cancer. According to OSHA, asbestos-related disease has been observed in shipbuilding and ship repair workers who have had only brief or intermittent exposure to asbestos. Any time asbestos or an asbestos product is damaged or disturbed, asbestos fibers are released into the air. Even when asbestos dust is invisible, it poses a threat. In fact, the smallest asbestos particles present the most serious health hazard.

According to OSHA, cancer death rates of 40-45 percent have occurred among certain asbestos factory workers. On April 26, 1978, HEW Secretary Joseph A. Califano Jr. warned that as many as half of all workers exposed to asbestos could develop serious diseases such as cancer of the lung and gastrointestinal tract, mesotheliomas and asbestosis. Califano also estimated that from 8 to 11 million workers may have been exposed to asbostos since the start of World War II. OSHA estimates show that more than one-half million people in the United States work with products that contain asbestos.

While asbestos mining and milling operations employ a relatively small percentage of the American workforce, as many as 50,000 workers are believed to be involved in the primary manufacture of asbestos. The number of persons engaged in secondary manufacturing — making products using components that contain asbestos — raises the number of exposed workers considerably.

OSHA estimates that about 40,000 American insulation workers are exposed to asbestos dust from thermal, acoustical and electrical insulation products. The agency also estimates that secondary exposure to insulation materials may threaten another three to five million workers in building construction and shipyard trades.

Because of these facts and other scientific evidence, OSHA issued a standard to limit worker exposure to asbestos. The OSHA standard prohibits employee exposure to more than two asbestos fibers (longer than 5 micrometers) per cubic centimeter of air or 1 million fibers per cubic meter, averaged over an eight-hour period. This standard is still 20 times in excess of the level that NIOSH recommends, according to Epstein's study.

But when OSHA began hearings in 1972, representatives from industry argued against lowering the standard to 2 million fibers per cubic meter of air. According to Epstein, industry said that the original 5 million standard exposure level did not cause much disease and that to lower it further would create severe economic dislocation and unemployment. The OSHA standard also established a ceiling limit: At no time may an employee be exposed to more than 10 fibers (longer than 5 micrometers) per cubic centimeter of air. According to OSHA, once they issued their asbestos standard to help protect workers from cancer, companies undertook cleanup efforts that included the installation of enclosures, better ventilation and elimination of hazardous steps in the spinning of asbestos textiles.

Asbestos is another example of how disease among workers often provides the first hint that a material might be an unsafe product for society. Virtually everyone has been exposed to asbestos fibers at some time. Epstein explains in his study that the indestructibility of asbestos, its indiscriminate use, and the careless disposal of its waste products make it difficult to predict the extent and level of exposure to the general public.

Asbestos fibers are present in the streets, in water supplies and in offices. Asbestos has been used to insulate buildings and ships, to fireproof buildings, to line car brakes, and even to filter beers and wines. Another source of asbestos exposure is crushed stone containing unbound asbestos in roads and driveways. Epstein explains that counts of 10 million fibers per cubic meter of air have been found in the vicinity of construction sites during asbestos spraying and 3 million fibers have been found in public buildings treated with asbestos as a fire retardant. Yale University replaced all the ceilings in its 10-story school of art and architecture because dangerous numbers of asbestos fibers were flaking off.

Agriculture

Agricultural workers, like miners, face severe occupational diseases. When they constituted only 4.4 percent of the U.S. labor force in 1971, farm workers accounted for about 16 percent of the country's recorded occupational deaths and 9 percent of the recorded injuries, according to Eckholm's study. Only mine and construction workers have worse safety records. As Eckholm pointed out, migrants are

Occupations and Risk of Cancer, 1975

Site of Cancer	Carcinogen	Occupations
Liver	Arsenic, vinyl chloride	Tanners, smelters; vineyard workers; plastic workers
Nasal cavity and sinuses	Chromium, isopropyl oil, nickel, wood and leather dusts	Glass, pottery and linoleum workers; nickel smelters, mixers and roasters; electrolysis workers; wood, leather, and shoe workers
Lung	Arsenic, asbestos, chromium, coal products, dusts, iron oxide, mustard gas, nickel, petroleum, ionizing radiation, bischloromethylether	Vintners; miners; asbestos users; textile users; insulation workers; tanners; smelters; glass and pottery workers; coal tar and pitch workers; iron foundry workers; electrolysis workers; retort workers; radiologists; radium dial painters; chemical workers
Bladder	Coal products, aromatic amines	Asphalt, coal tar, and pitch workers; gas stokers; still cleaners; dyestuffs users; rubber workers; textile dyers; paint manufacturers; leather and shoe workers
Bone marrow	Benzene, ionizing radiation	Benzene, explosives, and rubber cement workers; distillers; dye users; painters, radiologists

Source: P. Cole and M. B. Goldman, "Occupation," chapter 11 in J.F. Fraumeni, Jr., ed., Persons at High Risk of Cancer *(New York: Academic Press, 1975), pp. 167-84.*

American workers are exposed to an increasing number of cancer-causing materials. More than 2,000 chemicals in the workplace have been reported to be potential human carcinogens. The range of industries involving exposure to occupational carcinogens is shown in this table.

usually worst off among farm workers since the ordinary hazards of the fields are often compounded for them by unsanitary living conditions, poor nutrition and extreme poverty.

Hundreds of farm workers are killed each year and tens of thousands are injured by machinery accidents and other hazards. The National Center for Health Statistics has reported approximately 1,000 accidental electrocutions annually since 1971 with about a fourth being industry and farm related.

Many other farm workers suffer health damage from exposure to pesticides, chemical fertilizers and other chemicals. According to the 1979 Surgeon General's Report on Health Promotion and Disease Prevention, workers engaged in manufacturing the pesticide dibromochloropropane have experienced an infertility rate two to three times as great as the general population. Farm worker poisoning by pesticides and herbicides is a widespread problem. Because pesticides intentionally kill insects, poisonings among some people who work amid them is inevitable. But a greater problem is the reckless use of chemicals. Pesticides frequently are overused, applied with improper equipment or used in unnecessarily dangerous combinations. Workers often are sent onto freshly sprayed fields before the greatest danger has subsided; sometimes they are inadvertently doused by spray planes or helicopters.

A serious problem cited by Eckholm is that many temporary pesticide-induced maladies are never brought to a doctor's attention, are inaccurately diagnosed by doctors or go unreported to public health officials. Many pesticide-caused deaths remain uncounted for the same reasons. Eckholm pointed out that when the California State Department of Public Health carried out a household survey of farm workers in Tulare County, it found that "during 1969, 25 percent of the farm workers had seen a doctor for pesticide-related illness, but official figures put the number at less than 1 percent." The unreported symptoms of pesticide poisoning included nausea, skin and eye irritations, chronic headaches and sleeplessness.

As is the case with so many occupational health threats, the pesticide problem can affect the population at large because there are "allowable" traces of pesticides in food supplies. No health consequences related to chronic, low-level consumption of pesticides have been detected yet.

Industrial Hazards

Industrial workers face serious occupational hazards, old and new. Each year in the United States about 1,000 new chemicals are produced in commercial quantities. American workers thus are exposed to an ever-increasing number of materials that may have cancer-causing potential. Nine of every 10 industrial workers are not adequately protected from exposure to at least one of the 163 most common hazardous industrial chemicals, according to the 1979 Surgeon General's Report. And the report concludes that of nearly 34,000 workplace chemicals that have reported toxic effects, more than 2,000 have been reported to be potential human carcinogens.

Job-connected illnesses of this kind are by no means a new discovery. More than 200 years ago, British physician Percival Potts identified among chimney sweeps a high incidence of scrotum cancer attributable to their overexposure to coal tar. Half a century ago, a number of young women who painted radium on watch dials became victims of cancer. Marie Curie, discoverer of radium, suffered radium burns and her death in 1936 was attributed to the cumulative effects of radium poisoning. Since then, many substances have been found to produce cancer among workers in a wide variety of industries. Workers in many factories today live with the threat of arsenic, carbon monoxide, coke-oven emissions, mercury and vinyl chloride poisoning. One problem is that safe exposure levels to industrial carcinogens often cannot be determined.

Studies of cancer incidences have shown that cancer rates for both sexes are highest in the most heavily industrialized areas. There are excessive lung cancer rates among males living in counties where paper, chemical, petroleum and transportation industries are located. The 1979 Surgeon General's Report said that the concentration of hazardous industries in certain geographic areas or in otherwise economically depressed communities, or their presence as the only industry in a community, gives workers no opportunity to choose a safer job. When the mobility costs outweigh the perceived health costs, workers often stick with their jobs.

Mercury

Mercury is one of the oldest metals known to man. Silvery white and liquid at room temperature, it was dubbed "quicksilver" in 350 B.C. Even the ancient Romans recognized it as a poison.

According to OSHA, the "Mad Hatter" in *Alice's Adventures* was not simply a figment of author Lewis Carroll's imagination. The character reflected an unpleasant reality in the 19th century hat industry. Felt hats, at that time, were produced by treating — or "carroting" — fur with a solution of mercury and nitric acid. Workers who inhaled the mercury vapor eventually suffered brain damage and went "mad." In fact, the fur and felt hat industries were a major source of occupational mercury poisoning in this country until about 1940, when a chemical substitute was found for treating furs.

There is no escaping mercury. Trace amounts are in the air, food and water. OSHA explains that many people occasionally are exposed to it through medical and dental treatments (dental fillings, for example, contain mercury). No one knows for sure what is a "normal" level of mercury in the human body, but scientists do know one thing: at high levels, mercury is dangerous and can cause a whole range of physical and mental problems. And exposure to it on the job or from contact with contaminated materials can add greatly to a worker's body burden of mercury.

Mercury is especially dangerous because it vaporizes at temperatures as low as 10 degrees Fahrenheit. This means that the colorless, odorless vapor may be present anywhere mercury is used. When spilled, liquid mercury breaks up into tiny beads that lodge in cracks and sink traps, mix with dust and penetrate porous materials such as wood, tile, iron pipe and firebrick. Enough mercury can accumulate on working surfaces, especially wooden floors, to cause a serious health hazard. Mercury also can cling to clothing — especially knitted fabrics — and to shoe soles, so a worker can easily take it home.

NIOSH estimated in 1975 that some 150,000 people may have been exposed to mercury at work. Today, the major industrial uses of mercury include the manufacture of electrical equipment such as fluorescent lights, hearing aid batteries and communications gear; and the production of chlorine and caustic soda — a process in which mercury is used as an electrode.

OSHA warns that workers in at least 56 different occupations risk exposure to mercury. They include mercury miners and refiners; embalmers; boilermakers; producers and users of disinfectants, insecticides, fungicides and bactericides; investment casting makers; electronic device makers; electroplating workers; measuring-instrument makers; makers and loaders of explosives and munitions; dentists; chemical and medical laboratory workers; paper, paint, ink and dye makers; amalgam makers; gold and silver extractors; leather and fur processors; taxidermists; wood preservative workers; photographers; and fingerprint detectors.

Mercury can enter the body through the lungs, the skin and the digestive system. But breathing the vapor is the most common cause of mercury poisoning. Short exposures to high levels can cause acute poisoning — characterized by tightness and pain in the chest, difficulty in breathing, inflammation of the mouth and gums, fever and headaches.

Acute poisoning, however, is rare. Much more common among workers is chronic poisoning caused by long-term exposure to lower levels of mercury. Symptoms of chronic poisoning include inflammation of the mouth and gums, weakness, an increase in saliva, loss of appetite and weight, and impaired digestive and kidney functions. Effects of mercury on the central nervous system often show up as tremor or shaking, particularly in the hands. Often attributed to other causes are personality changes — irritability, temper outbursts, excitability, shyness, indecision — that also can signal mercury poisoning.

In addition, scientists are finding that long-term exposures to very low levels of substances such as mercury can slow a worker's reaction time and interfere with the ability to perform delicate tasks. For example, OSHA reported in 1975 that a team of researchers at the University of Michigan tested 142 volunteers from four plants that use mercury in the manufacture of chlorine or electronic materials.

The workers, OSHA said, had an average of five years' exposure to mercury and were asked to perform precise motor tasks such as finger and toe tapping, button pressing, pencil flipping and following a maze with a stylus. The scientists also measured muscle tremor while the volunteers held weights slung over their wrists. The tests then were repeated with a control group that had not been exposed to mercury. According to OSHA, results showed that the exposed workers had more trouble performing small, fast, repetitive movements; had slower tapping rates; and had more frequent muscle tremors. OSHA concluded that these were indications that the mercury — even at low levels — was affecting the motor control centers of the brain.

The way to prevent any health damage from mercury is to limit exposure to it. OSHA explains that this can be done through ventilation of any area where mercury or mercury compounds are handled, through use of enclosed systems that isolate mercury processes, through regular monitoring of the work environment and of workers' health status, and through simple good housekeeping. One state official told OSHA of a laboratory where employees over the years had a strange history of mental problems. When the building finally was demolished, seven pounds of mercury were found under the laboratory floor.

OSHA claims that medical tests of more than 100 Maryland dentists and dental technicians showed that two-thirds had high levels of mercury in their blood — apparently as a result of inhaling vapors from mercury accidentally spilled during preparation of fillings. The mercury lodged in carpets or floor tiles in the dentists' offices and was not removed through normal cleaning. OSHA issued a standard that said no worker should be exposed to a ceiling limit of more than 0.1 milligram per cubic meter of air.

Studies have shown that it is possible for industry to limit airborne mercury to a level below the upper limit now set by OSHA. For example, in one jewelry plant the level of mercury in the air dropped dramatically — from 0.35 milligram per cubic meter of air to 0.03 milligram — after installation of a ventilation system, according to OSHA.

Vinyl Chloride

Most industrial health hazards — such as lead, mercury and silica — have been recognized for decades or centuries. But only since the 1970s has vinyl chloride, a colorless gas derived from chlorine and petrochemicals, been shown to be highly dangerous. Vinyl chloride (VC) is the basic ingredient in making polyvinyl chloride (PVC), which is used in about 55 percent of today's plastic products. These include phonograph records, wire and cable insulation, floor coverings, garden hoses, furniture, upholstery fabrics, car bodies, coating of fabrics and wallpaper, containers, bottles and food wrapping. The chemical has been produced on an industrial scale in the United States since 1933, but on a large scale only since the 1950s.

In the late 1960s unusual changes were noted in the hands of workers who cleaned polyvinyl chloride polymerization chambers. Through later administration of high concentrations of vinyl chloride to rats by inhalation, it was learned that the chemical produced not only vascular and bone changes, but also cancers. By 1973 much lower doses had been linked with a number of tumors in rats, including those of the liver, but no unusual tumors had been reported in exposed workers.

Until January 1974 the gas, which always had been handled with relative care because it is both explosive and highly flammable, was still generally considered of low toxicity. Then it was found to cause a rare form of cancer of the liver — angiosarcoma — which cannot be diagnosed until it is incurable.

The B. F. Goodrich Co. disclosed in 1974 that three workers in its Louisville plant had died of angiosarcoma, apparently from breathing air contaminated with vinyl chloride. Since then, more than 50 cases of this rare tumor in vinyl chloride workers — including four more related to the Louisville plant — have been located throughout the world.

Polyvinyl chloride is all around us. We may ride to work on a vinyl seat, walk across vinyl-tiled floors on PVC-soled shoes, eat sandwiches wrapped in PVC from a vinyl tablecloth, relax to the sound of PVC records. Infants suck on PVC pacifiers. Although studies are continuing in both government and private laboratories, no one has yet discovered any danger in these finished products. By the time the plastics reach this stage, most of the vinyl chloride has been chemically locked into the PVC and will not come out again.

The danger comes during the production process. At each stage of production, there are certain potential trouble spots where the VC gas may escape into the air and reach the workers through random leaks from pump seals, compressors, valves, gaskets and storage tanks. Plants also must deal with reducing the amount of the gas that escapes during the quality-control sampling. During loading or unloading, tank car workers may be exposed to high concentrations in the air. Because of the danger from fire and explosion, the plants usually are spread over sites of several acres, with the result that the VC gas is not confined to small areas, but often can be found in low levels throughout the plant.

The highest exposures in the entire industry apparently are those experienced by the workers who climb into the vats or reactors to chip out the PVC residue. In the past, these cleaners were surrounded by concentrations as high as 1,600 parts of VC per million parts of air. In 1975 OSHA said that exposure levels for reactor cleaners may have reached 500 parts per million. Fourteen of the 16 men who had died from VC-related angiosarcoma in the United States up to 1975 had, at one time or another, been vat cleaners.

In addition to the danger of angiosarcoma of the liver, studies of workers exposed to VC show that they have higher than normal rates of cancer of the lung, brain and bone marrow. Studies have shown that plastics workers exposed to vinyl chloride are at 200 times greater risk for liver cancer, four times greater risk for brain cancer and two times greater risk for lung cancer than the general population. Suicide rates were found to be twice the normal rate in one study of 161 workers in a Kentucky plant, according to OSHA. Vinyl chloride's attacks are slow; the cancers, for example, may not show any symptoms until 15 years after the beginning of a worker's exposure. Epstein pointed out in his study that it is difficult to get an accurate count of the number of U.S. workers included in all the stages of PVC production. He said that in 1978 there were about 17 VC manufacturing plants, employing about a thousand workers and 40 PVC plants employing about 6,000 workers. There were no figures available on the number of fabrication plants or on the number of their employees, which he estimated must run into the hundreds of thousands.

Epstein also pointed to the health hazards of those living near PVC plants. EPA has estimated that 4.6 million people live within five miles of VC/PVC plants. EPA also estimated that VC/PVC plants in 1975 were losing 220 million pounds of VC into the air annually, mainly from PVC plants. These statistics, along with reports of excess birth defects in Ohio women living near VC/PVC plants, prompted EPA in October 1976 to propose regulating VC a hazardous air pollutant. The public also has been exposed to VC from aerosol propellants in consumer products such as insecticides, hair sprays, disinfectants and furniture polishes.

The basic protection from VC must come from engineering controls: avoiding leakage of the gas into the air. OSHA established a new standard in 1974 reducing allowable exposure to the deadly chemical from 500 parts per million (ppm) of air to only 1 part per million, averaged over an eight-hour day, with a maximum peak of 5 ppm. If these limits are not met, employers must reduce exposures to "the lowest practicable level," and personal respirators must be made available to the employees who are exposed.

When the new standard was proposed, officials of the chemical and plastics industries said they doubted that it could be met. They cautioned that thousands of vinyl chloride workers might have to be laid off, and that the lack of a substitute could eliminate some two million jobs in industries that use vinyl chloride. "The plastics industry has been shaken to its roots," *The Wall Street Journal* commented.

But when the standard went into effect, the industry went to work finding ways to comply. More efficient methods were found to reduce vinyl chloride waste in the production process, and to keep the chemical from entering the work environment. Vinyl chloride production rose to record levels in 1976. New vinyl chloride plants were opened and the predicted layoffs in other industries never took place. By April 1978 OSHA sampling for vinyl chloride in 500 workplaces found 93 percent of them obeying the standard.

Carbon Monoxide

Carbon monoxide, a colorless, odorless, tasteless gas, is one of the most widespread and dangerous industrial hazards, according to OSHA. Mild poisoning can cause nausea, dizziness or headaches, while acute poisoning can result in brain or heart damage or even death.

The poisonous gas is produced by the incomplete burning of any material containing carbon, such as gasoline, natural gas, oil, propane, coal or wood. Forges, blast furnaces and coking ovens all produce carbon monoxide, but the most common source of exposure in the workplace is the internal combustion engine.

OSHA warns that the following types of workers are most likely to be exposed to harmful levels of carbon monoxide: acetylene workers, blast furnace workers, boiler room workers, brewery workers, carbon black makers, coke-oven workers, custom workers, diesel engine operators, dock workers, garage mechanics, metal oxide reducers, miners, organic chemical synthesizers, petroleum refinery workers, pulp and paper workers, steelworkers, toll booth and tunnel attendants, and warehouse workers.

Carbon monoxide can kill or cripple in a matter of minutes if large amounts of it are present in the air. The more carbon monoxide in the air and the longer a worker is exposed to it, the greater the danger. The poisoning can be reversed if caught in time. But even if a worker recovers, acute poisoning may result in permanent damage.

The OSHA standard for exposure to carbon monoxide prohibits worker exposure to more than 50 parts of the gas per million parts of air, averaged over an eight-hour workday. Exposures higher than 100 parts per million are serious violations of the OSHA rule and exposures 550 parts per million and higher constitute a state of imminent danger.

Formaldehyde

Formaldehyde is under consideration for regulatory action by OSHA and other agencies. In August 1981 Dr. Arthur C. Upton, chairman of pathology at the Institute of Environmental Medicine of New York University Medical Center and a former director of the National Cancer Institute, told regulatory and health officials that formaldehyde, a chemical to which an estimated 750,000 industrial workers are exposed, is "decisively" a cancer-causing agent in animals and a "likely" carcinogen in humans. Formaldeyde is used in resins that bind plywood, wallboard, particle board, furniture joints and carpet backings. It is also used in preserving corpses and putting

Sources of Benzene Exposure, 1977

Industries Causing Benzene Exposure to the Public

Source	Number of People Exposed to Various Concentrations of Benzene, parts per billion* (in thousands) 0.1-1	1-2	2-4	4-10	Over 10	Total Number of Exposed People
Petroleum refineries	6,529	64	4	—	—	6,597
Chemical manufacturing	7,497	970	453	644	319	9,883
Solvent operations	208	5	2	—	—	215
Coke ovens	15,726	521	50	2	—	16,299
Gasoline stations						
People using self-service	—	—	—	—	37,000	37,000
People living nearby	87,000	31,000	—	—	—	118,000
Urban exposures from autos	68,337	45,353	—	—	—	113,690

** Based on estimates of annual averages.*

Source: Center for Resources and Environmental Systems Studies

Workers in petroleum and petrochemical refineries, in chemical plants and in the steel industry are at particularly high risk from benzene exposure.

the permanent press in fabrics. Urea formaldehyde foam insulation is used to weatherize approximately 600,000 homes. A trade association, the Formaldehyde Institute, says products using formaldehyde or derived from it comprise 8 percent of the U.S. gross national product.

Upton said that 10 of 100 male rats developed highly destructive nasal cancers after 382 six-hour exposures, over 588 days, to formaldehyde. None was found in control rats or in rats exposed to hydrochloric acid gases. When exposed to a mixture of the gases and formaldehyde, nine of 100 rats developed tumors. Upton's study confirmed a 1979 study by the Chemical Industry Institute of Toxicology.

Even before the new study was released, Dr. Peter F. Infante, OSHA's top specialist in carcinogen identification, had argued that available evidence showed formaldehyde to be a carcinogen in animals and a cancer risk in humans. The Formaldehyde Institute challenged Infante's findings, arguing that data he relied on had been refuted by Harry B. Demopoules, an associate professor in Upton's department.

In September 1981 EPA discounted Infante's study as unworthy of immediate action and recommended against priority regulation of formaldehyde as a carcinogenic agent. The agency said that current studies implied no "significant risk" of serious harm to exposed people.

Lead

Lead, one of the most useful metals in modern industrial society, has long been known to be highly toxic. According to the 1980 Council on Environmental Quality (CEQ) report, Pliny the Elder, a Roman naturalist and writer in the first century A.D., warned against the poisonous effects of lead fumes. Charles Dickens referred in 1861 to lead's acute effects on human health including convulsions, coma and death. Symptoms of chronic exposure include fatigue, headache, poor appetite, clumsiness and diminished mental capacity. Lead can also damage the nervous system, the blood-forming system and the kidneys.

Americans are regularly exposed to low levels of lead, but cases of acute poisoning are infrequent. The chief sources of lead emissions are automobile exhaust and industrial facilities. Lead is used to manufacture batteries and seal "tin" cans and is an ingredient in many paints and gasolines.

Physicians and scientists are also concerned about the effect of lead on reproductive systems, according to the CEQ report. The substance has been shown to disrupt the ovarian cycle in women, and to produce impotence, impaired libido and decreased number and quality of sperm in men.

Dr. Philip J. Landrigan, director of epidemiology at NIOSH, has explained that lead is also particularly dangerous for young children because their nervous systems are still undergoing development and are thus vulnerable.

According to *Smithsonian* magazine (September 1981), Dr. Herbert L. Needleman and a research team at the Children's Hospital Medical Center in Boston studied 2,335 first- and second-graders in 1979 and found that the higher the lead concentration in the children's teeth, the lower their scores on intelligence and functional tests and the lower their ratings on classroom performance.

OSHA's lead standard protects workers from exposure to more than 50 micrograms per cubic meter of air averaged over eight hours. Permanent engineering controls instead of respirators are required. Union officials had argued that respirators were difficult to breathe through. Workers who accumulate lead above certain levels in their blood must be transferred to other jobs or be sent home for up to 18 months at no loss of pay, benefits or seniority.

Since 1978 this OSHA standard has been challenged in the courts. OSHA acknowledged when it issued the standard that it would be difficult for lead smelters to comply. Industry representatives argued that the cost of required engineering controls was unreasonable. Eula Bingham, then head of OSHA, argued that it was not "overregulating to say that a company should not make profits that a worker has to pay for with his kidneys or his lungs. . ." But in 1981 OSHA under Thorne Auchter was reviewing the lead standard to determine its cost effectiveness.

Benzene

Benzene is one of the 12 largest volume chemicals used by U. S. industries. According to Epstein's study, benzene production in 1977 was approximately 11 billion pounds, some 90 percent of which was produced in petroleum refining and petrochemical industries, and the remainder in the coke ovens of the steel industry.

Two centuries have passed since Percival Potts linked coal tars to the scrotum cancer that killed young chimney sweeps in England. Yet, thousands of workers in steel mills still inhale the same substance. OSHA estimated that in 1978 a coke-oven worker's chance of getting certain kinds of cancer was from two-and-a-half to more than seven times greater than that of other steelworkers. OSHA said that approximately 100 coke-oven workers needlessly died every year from job-related cancer. Many others were disabled.

Dr. Irving J. Selikoff of the Mount Sinai School of Medicine in New York addressed this issue:

> Starting in 1936 and at intervals thereafter, scientists reported that lung cancer was much more common among men working in [steel] plants like this. Yet for the last forty years, a period during which tens of thousands of American men were daily exposed to these cancer chemicals, decades in which they had every right to assume that their workplace was safe, no precautions whatever were taken to prevent their inhalation of these materials. They were not even told of the danger!
>
> ...[S]teel workers during the 1930s, 1940s, 1950s and 1960s surely had the right to expect that someone was seeing to it that cancer would not be their fate. *There was no someone.*

In 1975 Roosevelt Johns, one of 50 coke-oven workers who testified at Department of Labor hearings, told how he got lung cancer as a result of 25 years of the work. His doctors were unable to remove the cancer because his heart stopped during the operation. Johns then was given more than 40 cobalt treatments and went to the hospital every 90 days for a six-day stay to be injected with a new drug. He died in 1976.

According to Epstein's study, 60 million tons of blast furnace coke are produced from coal each year in 65 U. S. steel plants, most of them concentrated in four states: Pennsylvania, Indiana, Ohio and Alabama. For each ton of coke, about four gallons of "light oil," most of it benzene, are produced as a byproduct. Since coke ovens are old and "leaky," benzene is allowed to escape. Benzene levels are estimated to range as high as 50 parts per million inside the plants.In the past, benzene exposure ranged from 100 to 500 ppm. In 1971 OSHA set the benzene exposure standard at 10 ppm. In 1978 the agency changed the permissible level of benzene exposure to 1 ppm. Industry, led by the Manufacturing Chemists Association and the American Petroleum Institute, attacked the standard, arguing that there was a "threshold" below which it was safe to expose workers to benzene. The industry attack led to the July 2, 1980, Supreme Court decision invalidating OSHA's benzene exposure standard. The permissible level of benzene exposure returned to 10 ppm.

The manufacture of tires accounts for approximately half of all benzene used, according to Epstein's study. Another major usage is as an octane booster in gasoline. Nylons, pesticides, adhesives, laminates, coatings, inks, paints, varnishes and moldings all contain benzene.

Besides steelworkers, employees in petroleum and petrochemical refineries, and in chemical plants (especially those manufacturing rubber products and solvents) are at high risk from benzene exposure. Other types of workers exposed to benzene are printing pressmen and lithographers, shoemakers, gasoline pump attendants and professional artists and craftsmen.

For nearly 100 years, exposure to benzene has been known to cause blood diseases. But since 1960 evidence has shown that the chemical also causes aplastic anemia, leukemia and chromosomal danger. Aplastic anemia, benzene's best recognized effect, is chacterized by pallor and fatigue. It can exist with another condition known as pancytopenia. With pancytopenia, bleeding can occur in the skin and elsewhere in the body and susceptibility to infection is increased.

Sometimes even complete recovery from aplastic anemia is followed by the development of acute leukemia 20 years later. Cases of these two diseases have been reported in several types of workers, including printers in rotogravure plants, rubber workers, aircraft construction workers and leather and shoe workers.

An important benzene worker study was based on Turkish shoe workers who, between 1955 and 1960, began using adhesives containing high levels of benzene. They were exposed to levels in the 150 to 650 ppm range. Epstein said that individual cases of aplastic anemia among the shoe workers were detected in 1961. By 1977, 46 of them had developed the disease and 14 died from it. Five survivors later developed leukemia, from which they subsequently died.

In 1978 Dow Chemical Co. released a study confirming the occurrence of chromosome damage in workers with average benzene exposure levels of 2 to 3 ppm.

Textiles: 'Brown Lung'

Three hundred years ago an Italian physician first publicized the "continual coughs" that plagued those "who hackle in the flax and hemp." The cause, wrote Bernardino Ramazzini, was a "foul mischievous powder" — cotton dust.

Inhaling cotton dust over a period of time can cause a variety of health problems and, in many cases, can lead to a severe chronic respiratory disease called byssinosis or "brown lung." The disease results from a gradual narrowing of the victim's airways to a fraction of their original diameter.

According to OSHA, as many as 600,000 workers in the cotton industry are "at risk" and more than 35,000 cotton workers already have been crippled from cotton dust exposure. Thousands of others show some signs of brown lung.

While earlier breathing difficulties are thought to be reversible, a worker cannot recover from an advanced stage of brown-lung disease. Exposure to cotton dust also leads to increased risk of chronic bronchitis and emphysema.

Cotton dust comes from the stem and leaf material that sticks to the cotton plant when it arrives at textile mills. As the plant is processed into yarn by high-speed machinery, the dust flies into the lungs of textile workers. It is present wherever raw cotton is used. Raw cotton comes not only in bales but also as floor sweepings and other waste from cotton processing operations. In addition to cotton fiber or lint, cotton dust can contain substances such as fungi, soil, pesticides and ground-up plant matter. The dangerous particles small enough to enter workers' lungs are invisible.

Mining: 'Black Lung'

Mining, the subject of the earliest writings on occupational health, has long been viewed as a particularly hazardous occupation because of the danger of underground accidents. Mining disasters make a particularly strong call on public sympathy and usually are followed by controversy over responsibility for the accident.

Mine legislation has had a long history, but one of limited protection. After a series of mining accidents, the U. S. Bureau of Mines was established in 1910 in the Department of the Interior. But the bureau did not acquire authority to inspect mines until 1941 or to set and enforce safety-health standards until 1952. A mine explosion in December 1951 that took 119 lives near West Frankfort, Ill., spurred enactment of the federal Coal Mine Safety Act of 1952. Under this law, the bureau could close a mine if conditions presented an immediate danger. But its authority extended only to mines that employed at least 15 persons, a restriction that was not lifted until 1966. In the same year, Congress passed the Metal and Non-metallic Mine Safety Act extending protection to other miners.

Another coal-mine accident, claiming 78 lives at Farmington, W. Va., on Nov. 20, 1968, spurred enactment of the most stringent of all mine safety laws, the Coal Mine Health and Safety Act. It became law on Dec. 30, 1969, establishing mandatory health and safety standards for underground mining — in contrast to surface, or strip-mining. The standards applied to fire protection, roof supports, escape ways, communications systems and permissible levels of dust.

In the case of day-to-day mining accidents, the effect is instantaneous, the immediate cause not too hard to determine and the extent of injury readily assessed. In the case of disability or death from chronic lung diseases caused by mineral dusts, it is difficult to determine the degree to which environmental pollutants contribute.

According to OSHA, three out of four coal miners who live to retire on pension have pneumoconiosis or "black lung," an incurable, fatal disease caused by coal dust in their lungs. An estimated 4,000 miners die annually from black-lung disease.

Silicosis, another lung disease caused by dusts in mines and quarries, is even more prevalent than black lung. According to the World Health Organization, "of all occupational diseases, silicosis is the major cause of permanent disability and mortality and is the most costly in terms of compensation payment."

According to Eric Eckholm, the effect of coal dust on the lungs has been well known to doctors at least since 1813, when the "black lungs" of autopsied coal miners were described in medical literature. In 1974 an editorial in the respected British medical journal *The Lancet* charged that "between the wars, when the introduction of mechanization without dust control created gross disease on a mass scale, the complacency of experts . . . delayed effective dust suppression for a whole generation." *The Lancet* said that "there is overwhelming evidence that coal mining still uses up men and discards them to an exceptional extent."

In the early 1970s a committee of the U. S. National Academy of Sciences wrote that "the underground control of coal dust must be improved. Proper ventilation technology is available and has been for some time; the high incidence of pneumoconiosis is inexcusable."

The 1969 Coal Mine Health and Safety Act required that miners be given chest X-rays when their employment began and periodically thereafter. If a miner was found to be developing black lung, he was given an opportunity to transfer to a job in a less dusty part of the mine. The act also provided monthly cash payments to coal miners disabled by the disease or to their widows.

Under the Coal Mine Health and Safety Act of 1969, the air in a mine must be swept clean by forced ventilation of all but 2 milligrams per cubic meter of respirable coal dust — a "safe" standard that British studies indicated would result in 1 to 3 cases of black lung per 100 miners after 35 years of work.

After enactment of the black-lung program in 1969, Congress became impatient with the slow speed of claims processing and the high rate of claim denial. So amendments were passed in 1972 that eased eligibility requirements to include all dependents in an afflicted miner's household as beneficiaries, extended coverage to surface as well as underground miners and broadened the definition of black-lung disability. More than 118,000 of the 165,000 miners and miners' dependents whose claims had been previously denied wanted their claims reviewed under the new standard. The new rules diminished the importance of X-ray evidence and presumed that miners who had worked for many years in the mines had black lung disease.

In 1970 the tax-free black-lung payments were set at $136 a month and geared to raise automatically with the pay of civil service workers. By 1981 the payments were $279.80 a month for a claimant with no dependents, $419.60 with one dependent, $489.60 with two dependents and a maximum of $559.50 with three or more dependents.

From 1970 to 1977 the federal government paid the entire $5.6 billion cost of the black-lung program. Benefits for claims filed after July 1973 were paid by the mine operator who last employed the claimant for a one-year period. However, the government had difficulty identifying these "responsible" employers, partly because mine operators challenged many claims. Thus, the government itself had to pay the benefits. There were unsuccessful efforts to have the states adopt the program as part of their existing workers' compensaton systems, financed by employer premium payments.

A series of amendments, pushed through Congress in 1976 and 1977 by representatives of coal-producing states, ordered that all previously denied claims be reviewed under the new, more lenient rules. The changes increased the approval rate for claims from as low as 7.4 percent in the early 1970s to 50 percent in 1979. By 1979 more than 480,000 miners or their survivors — a number equal to the

Many video-display computer terminal (VDT) users experience illnesses — ranging from eyestrain to neck pain, muscular strain, back aches, skin rash and irritability.

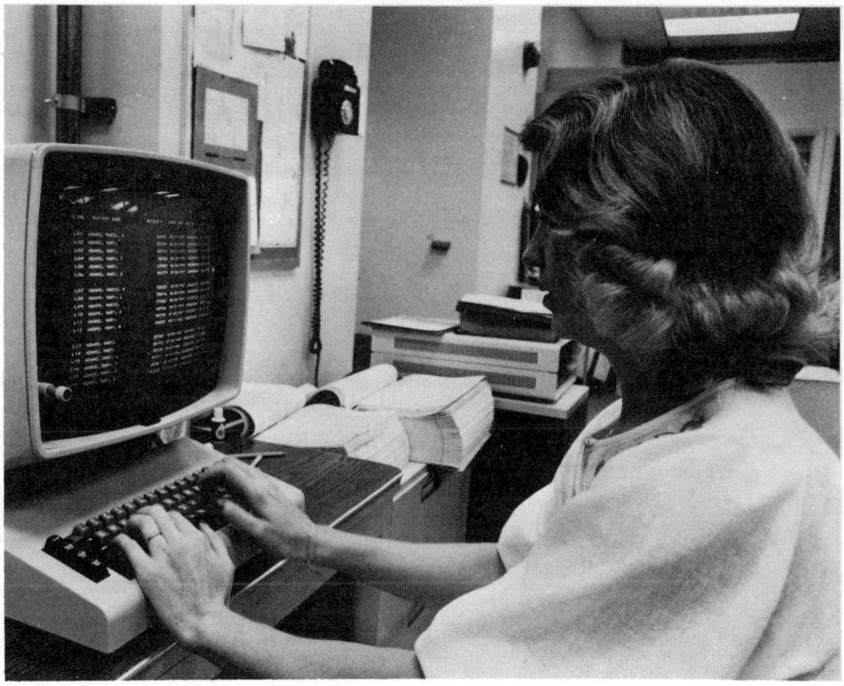

entire mining workforce in 1950 — had been awarded black-lung benefits.

By 1979 the benefits totaled approximately $8.3 billion. When the black-lung plan originally was adopted in 1969 its sponsors had estimated it would cost $90 million a year. But the cost passed $300 million a year in 1971, even with the low approval rate for applications.

In 1977 Congress created a government-run trust fund to cover the costs of the majority of black-lung cases for which "no responsible mine operator" could be determined. It was financed by a tonnage tax paid by the mine operators — 50 cents a ton on underground coal and 25 cents a ton on strip-mined coal. In effect, it was a federal workers' compensation program specialized for black lung.

But the uniform tax offered no incentive for coal-mine operators to exercise diligent dust-control practices. And the companies were allowed to deduct their trust fund payments from their federal tax liability.

In the mid-1970s it was found that miners and environmental technicians assigned to sample sections of mines were cheating on OSHA regulations. OSHA was getting "controlled samples" — fakes intended to deceive them into believing that coal-dust levels were being held within legal limits.

By August 1980 the General Accounting Office (GAO) estimated that coal miners and their families had received more than $31 million in black-lung disability or death payments that, in more than 88 percent of the cases, were not supported by adequate medical evidence. In addition to retroactive benefits that had been paid to the miners or their dependents since 1977, the same recipients were still receiving some $79 million a year, according to the GAO study. Although the payments were legal under 1977 amendments to the Federal Coal Mine Health and Safety Act, GAO argued that to prevent possible abuse "medical evidence should be restored as the basis for establishing eligibility."

In February 1981 the Reagan administration proposed to cut the $956 million deficit in the black-lung benefits program. The United Mine Workers union threatened to strike, arguing that the current deficit resulted not from recipients' abuse but from other factors, including $324.6 million in 1979 payments to miners who previously had been denied claims. Reagan proposed cutting the general tax revenue contribution to the fund by $1.96 billion through 1986, including $378 million in the next budget year. Although coal operators contribute to the fund the government makes up the deficit.

Reagan argued for tighter "proof of disability" standards and a "reasonable increase" in the current tax on coal production, which would end the need for federal subsidies by 1983. Because most of the program costs arise from cases already approved, the only choices left to the Reagan administration were to slash benefits to miners and their survivors, levy the burden on the operators, or force the taxpayer to pay the cost of past negligence. It was estimated that over the next 15 years the program would exceed revenues from the coal tax by more than $9 billion.

The black-lung benefits program has been administered by the Coal Mine Workers' Compensation division of the Labor Department since 1973.

Hazards of Office Work

An area of occupational safety and health that has been getting increased attention is office work. With the Labor Department predicting that more than half of all new jobs in the 1980s will be white-collar jobs, office hazards are becoming a major issue. Office-worker groups have formed in more than 30 states to demand a safe work environment.

Joel Makower, in a 1981 study, *Office Hazards: How Your Job Can Make You Sick*, said that office air pollution can be dangerous. Well-insulated, energy-efficient buildings trap toxic substances such as asbestos, benzene, carbon monoxide, formaldehyde and vinyl choloride. Other office pollutants include benzene and toluene, both contained in rubber cement and cleaning fluids. Both substances have been associated with various blood diseases. Methanol and ammonia, used in many duplicating-machine fluids, can irritate the eyes, nose and throat.

"There's probably more damage to human health from indoor air pollution than from outdoor pollution," said an epidemiologist at the World Health Organization. David Berg of the Environmental Protection Agency (EPA) estimated that as much as 10 percent of the lung cancer in the United States is caused by radon, a radioactive gas emitted from concrete and brick. Modern buildings often have windows that cannot be opened and inadequate heating and cooling systems.

In 1980 a Louis Harris poll taken for the Steelcase Co., a major manufacturer of office equipment, found that nearly 60 percent of those polled were dissatisfied with their office temperature. Many complained of distracting noise, poor lighting and chairs. Office photocopiers also produce potentially harmful pollutants, according to Makower. The EPA found that trinitrofluorenone (TNF), a chemical that coats the printing drums of some IBM copiers, causes gene mutations in bacterial and mammalian cells and may affect workers. Photocopier repair technicians are at the greatest risk from TNF. Ozone is another hazard in photocopiers, according to Makower. It inflames lung tissues and membranes, breaks down red blood cells, contributes to breathing difficulties and is suspected of producing changes in blood enzyme levels.
enzyme levels.

Typing Paper. Skin specialists have known for years that some individuals are allergic to the substances in typing paper, carbon paper, the paper used in duplicating machines. The newest problem is an allergy to some brands of carbonless copypayer.

In the June 12 *Journal of the American Medical Association*, Dr. James G. Marks Jr., dermatologist with the Hershey Medical Center of Pennsylvania State University College of Medicine, told of a college clerk who suffered skin rashes for more than a year before the cause was traced to the carbonless copy paper used for student registration. Avoiding the paper cured the rash.

Marks also cited earlier reports of paper allergy, including a female office worker who developed a rash on her hands from typing paper. One of the most severe cases involved a woman with such acute sensitivity to formaldehyde — a substance widely used in papermaking — that she could not handle most newspapers, books or magazines. She even reported developing a rash from lying on the paper cover spread over the doctor's examining table.

Video-Display Computer Terminals. Between 7 million and 10 million Americans spend their working hours in front of video-display computer terminals (VDTs), sometimes called CRTs. The screens display words on a cathode-ray tube. These keyboard/TV screen combinations have a broad and rapidly expanding range of applications in the workplace. They are used by private industry and government (the federal government is the world's largest buyer of computers and VDTs); in publishing, communications, banking and insurance; by computer operators and airline reservations clerks; and in offices of all kinds, large and small. They are even being used in grade school education programs, and experimental use of VDTs for information access in the home has begun. According to Makower, there will be 28 million VDTs in the United States by the end of the 1980s.

The VDT enables many companies to provide better services at lower costs. It saves time and has changed the nature of work for millions of workers. But an alarming number of VDT users are experiencing illnesses — ranging from eyestrain to neck pain, muscular strain, back aches, skin rash and irritability. Since their introduction into the workplace about 10 years ago, video-display terminals have been linked to a wide variety of disorders including cataracts, birth defects, altered behavior and heart disease.

"The problems associated with video display terminals are being studied at an increasingly frantic pace by government agencies, unions and universities around the world," wrote Makower. He pointed to a 1979 study by NIOSH on four newspaper offices and an insurance company. The study found more complaints of physical and psychological problems among VDT users than among people who did similar work without VDTS.

In 1980 the Canadian Press, Canada's leading wire service agency, quoted an airline organizer as predicting that VDT operators were going to be "the asbestos workers of the future."

Whether exposure to VDT radiation is harmful is a matter of scientific dispute. In 1981 the Food and Drug Administration (FDA) said VDTs emitted "insignificant" amounts of radiation. But Makower said in his study that an FDA representative conceded the agency had not performed a radiation test.

By the 1980s researchers were focusing attention on possible VDT hazards not related to radiation emission. The National Research Council's Committee on Vision, with support from NIOSH, conducted a symposium in August 1981 to explore eyesight disorders possibly caused by VDTs. The root of the problem, according to some of the symposium participants, may not be the VDT itself but poor "task structure" and workplace design. For example,

Government-Mandated Permissible Noise Levels in the Workplace

Hours Per Day	Decibel Sound Level
8	90
6	92
4	95
3	97
2	100
1-1/2	102
1	105
1/2	110
1/4 or less	115

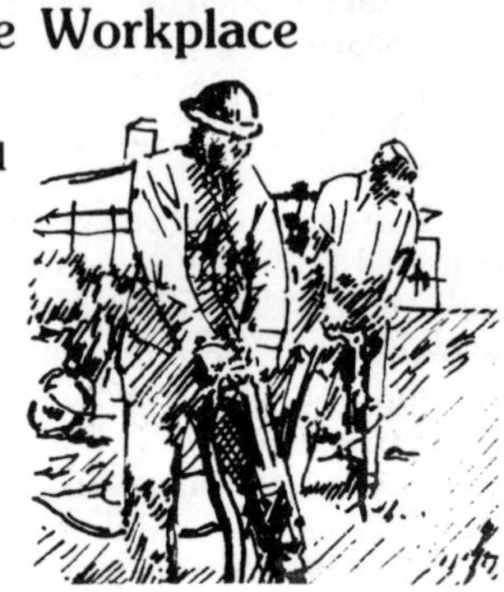

Steven Sauter of the University of Wisconsin said that VDTs up against windows, exposed to glare or located in hot, noisy, crowded environments could contribute to users' discomfort. Researchers have suggested that VDT users take regular breaks. NIOSH recommended that "there should be mandatory work-breaks of at least fifteen minutes every two hours for VDT operators under moderate visual demands and ten minutes every hour for operators under high visual demands, high work load, and . . . repetitive work tasks."

Stress in the Workplace

Some occupational illnesses seem to stem from psychological stresses. According to Dr. Hans Selye, originator of the concept of stress and the body's reaction to it, stress is the body's response to any demand made on it. Everyone has a different level of stress tolerance and is capable of handling different amounts and kinds of stress.

Job features that can bring about physical, psychological or psychosocial stress range from physical working conditions to the type of social interaction on the job. Some critical job stressors include workload, long work hours, fast work pace, time pressure, meaningless work tasks, the organizational climate, fear of job loss and lack of job satisfaction or career development. Recent OSHA emphasis on work-induced diseases, especially cancer, has made workers more aware of workplace hazards and adds to their anxiety. When a worker is excessively stressed, symptoms may be anxiety, fear, anger, tension, depression, difficulty in concentrating, loss of appetite, insomnia, fatigue and withdrawal. Functionally, stress symptoms may be headaches, muscle aches, nausea, constipation or diarrhea, irregular heart beat and frequent urination. Disorders such as migraine, coronary heart disease, high blood pressure, bronchial asthma, peptic ulcer, colitis, neurosis, some skin diseases and possibly arthritis frequently are associated with chronic stressful exposures. Aside from these well-known stress-related disorders, others that stress affects either directly or indirectly include diabetes, gout, migraine, glaucoma, hemorrhoids, asthma, allergies, acne, arthritis, back pain and cancer.

Physical working conditions also have an impact on worker stress. Noisy, smoky, crowded, poorly lighted and hot or cold workplace environments all play a role in a worker's attitude and motivation.

According to Makower's study, there is increasing evidence that spending long hours under fluorescent lights can increase stress and reduce resistance to colds and disease. Makower also noted that the layout of offices and the design of furniture contribute to both physical and psychological stress. For example, he contends that "open offices — with floor-to-ceiling walls replaced by space dividers — contribute to noise, crowding, and poor air circulation."

Except for noise, more workers complain about temperatures than any other stress-related working condition, according to one study. Extremes in cold or hot temperature have been demonstrated to contribute to stress. Illumination of proper intensity and direction with glare avoidance is needed to avoid eyestrain. Extremes in lighting, specifically glare, interfere with effective human behavior due to a decrease in visual contrast and legibility. Headaches, fatigue, and irritability are the common complaints associated with eyestrain.

Consequences of Stress

Early stress reactions are seen by changes in work performance or behavior. Unusual delays in completing work, increased frequency of mistakes, increased accidents, and acceptance of lower performance standards are also evidenced. Behavioral changes can be seen in attendance problems, poor personal hygiene, tremors, sudden weight change, argumentativeness, frequent requests for more information, suspiciousness, increased use of alcohol and drugs and increased smoking.

While occupational safety professionals may not agree on the actual percentage of fatal industrial incidents that are due to human factors, some studies have found that approximately 75 percent are due to human error. And safety professionals are becoming increasingly aware that stress can contribute to human error.

There is increasing evidence, according to Makower, that secretarial and routine clerical jobs are becoming associated with stress-related illnesses such as heart disease, hypertension, ulcers and nervous disorders. The National Heart, Lung, and Blood Institute, a branch of the National Institutes of Health, released a study in 1980 concluding that women clerical workers were much more likely to develop heart disease than professional women, housewives or male clerical workers. The study also found that women clerical workers were almost twice as likely to develop coronary disease as women in other jobs.

Air traffic controllers claim to suffer an unusually high risk of stress and hypertension as one consequence of their job. Yet a 1978 report by the Boston University School of Medicine cautioned against the conclusion that air traffic control work by itself causes hypertension.

"Our interpretation of the findings is that for individuals who are predisposed to developing hypertension by reason of a host of possible genetic and biological factors, exposure to air traffic control work increases the risk or perhaps hastens the rate of their developing hypertension," the report stated. The report also found that the context in which the controllers were performing their job, and the attitudes and feelings they had about their situation, influenced their risk for health changes.

Psychological principles are increasingly being applied to occupational stress. According to the 1979 Surgeon General's Report, some companies provide training in meditation and other relaxation techniques, and seminars on how to cope with stress at home and at work. Many companies employ psychologists or psychiatrists, or pay for such services outside the firm. Some companies redesign jobs to make them more meaningful. For example, instead of assembly lines requiring each worker to deal with small elements of a whole, some employers are now allowing workers to assemble entire products.

Noise Hazards

The problems of noise go beyond their contribution to stress. Each year thousands of Americans lose their hearing because of the loud noise in many factories and construction sites. Those who work in the construction, lumber, mining, steel and textile industries are especially exposed to deafening sound. OSHA currently sets the standard of noise for any workplace at 90 decibels. This means that if the noise level exceeds 90 decibels for eight hours a day or rises even higher for a shorter time, the company must install feasible engineering or administrative controls to reduce the noise level.

"By 'feasible' engineering controls we mean design changes," explained Richard J. Peppin, senior scientist at OSHA's Health Standards Office. "This could mean changing the gears of a machine or putting enclosures around it. Administrative controls essentially mean to rotate employees so that if they're exposed to say 95 decibels for eight hours, you get them so that they are there for only four hours.... Sometimes that works out but sometimes people are skilled at a certain job and they can't do that [be rotated]." If the company cannot make the needed engineering or administrative changes, OSHA recommends that they outfit the exposed workers with protective devices such as earcuffs (the headphone-like devices worn by airport workers) or earplugs.

Since 1974 OSHA has considered a proposal to lower the permissible eight-hour noise level from 90 to 85 decibels. The proposal, predictably, drew the support of labor groups and the opposition of business groups. Much of the opposition centered on a 1976 study by the agency which estimated that businesses would have to pay about $18.5 billion in engineering controls to reach the 85 decibel level.

Nicholas Ashford of MIT wrote in *Crisis in the Workplace* that excessive noise not only can impair hearing but "triggers changes in cardiovascular, endocrine, and neurological function." OSHA says that noise appears to cause quickened pulse rate, increased blood pressure and a narrowing of the blood vessels. Over a period of time, these may place an added burden on the heart. Noise may also put stress on other parts of the body by causing the abnormal secretion of hormones and tensing of muscles. Workers exposed to noise sometimes complain of nervousness, sleeplessness and fatigue. Noise exposure can reduce job performance and cause high rates of absenteeism.

According to OSHA, an estimated 14 million workers in the United States are exposed to hazardous noise. The OSHA regulations apply to workers mostly in the lumber, petroleum, coal, textile, electrical, gas, sanitary services and primary metals industries. "The primary benefit [of the regulations]," said Eula Bingham, then administrator of OSHA, "will be a substantial reduction in the incidence of occupational hearing impairment." In January 1981, during the waning days of the Carter administration, OSHA ordered industry to provide hearing protectors to all workers exposed to noise levels exceeding certain decibel rates. The ruling was scheduled to go into effect in April 1981 but OSHA deferred action after the change of administrations; in September the agency was still making changes in the ruling.

Health Care Work

Hospital and dental workers exposed to leaking anesthetic gases risk liver disease and miscarriages. Dentists using mercury experience higher rates of nervous and emotional disorders. One of the most serious problems is faced by X-ray technicians who suffer from radiation exposure.

Almost since its discovery in 1895 by the German physicist Wilhelm Roentgen, the X-ray has been recognized as an extraordinarily valuable medical tool — but one with clear risks for both the operator and the exposed individual. The premature deaths of more than 100 physicians and other investigators in the early years of radiological research have been attributed to excessive exposure to the invisible, painless rays.

The human health risks of excess radiation include blisters, skin burns and cancers of various types. Many experts believe excessive radiation also can impair the health of future generations by making subtle changes in human genes.

Researchers disagree on how to calculate precisely the dangers of relatively low doses of ionizing radiation, such as those emitted by X-ray machines. Some researchers predict 100 times more deaths from low doses of ionizing radiation than others, depending on their methods for estimating risk. (Ionizing radiation is radiation capable of producing cell damage which, if not repaired by the organism, can cause illness or death.)

In July 1980 the National Academy of Sciences revised its low-level radiation risk estimates, greatly reducing its predictions of deaths from low-level exposures. However, the revised estimates are controversial and are still being studied.

In the 1968 Radiation Safety Act, Congress mandated federal performance standards for electronic products that emit radiation, including X-ray machines. Under that law, the Bureau of Radiological Health (BRH) sets standards applying to all machines manufactured after 1974 and for replacement parts for older machinery.

Federal regulation of radiation is split among a number of agencies; the Environmental Protection Agency establishes general levels for radiation exposure, while the Nuclear Regulatory Commission shares responsibility with BRH for regulating current medical uses of radiologic procedures.

THE CHALLENGE: PROGRESS WITH SAFETY

During the 1960s, the accident rate in American industry began to climb dramatically and it continued to rise in the 1980s. New occupational diseases were discovered in alarming numbers.

OSHA gives several reasons for this deterioration of job safety and health conditions. One is increased mechanization. Another is the rapid increase in the production and use of industrial chemicals.

New materials such as petroleum-based chemicals and synthetic fabrics have been invented since the 1930s. Between 1958 and 1970 the number of industrial chemicals catalogued by one industry magazine jumped from 17,000 to 41,000 and, according to OSHA, only a few hundred had been tested for their long-term effects on workers' health.

As studies show, hazardous substances are not confined to the workplace. Members of families of asbestos workers have developed asbestos-related diseases, apparently resulting from exposure to fibers on the workers' clothing. Chemicals that threaten workers also may pollute the air and water in the general environment. In Hopewell, Va., for example, the pesticide Kepone not only caused sterility, tremors and liver damage among chemical workers but also hurt the fishing industry in the James River and polluted water as far away as New York and New Jersey. *(See box p. 52)*

Controlling Hazards

Since the early 1970s OSHA has recommended several ways to control workplace hazards. Many toxic chemicals can be replaced with other, less toxic ones; flexible wire and pipes often conduct less noise than rigid machine parts; and large-diameter centrifugal fans operating at slower speeds are quieter than small-diameter propeller fans operating at high speeds.

The agency further suggests that some welding operations that create dangerous gases and metal fumes can be replaced with "crimping" of metals to form a joint. Also, water can be used in processes that create a lot of dust.

If a hazard cannot be eliminated, OSHA suggests the following ways to contain its effect:

- Segregating the hazard in a room or building.
- Covering bins, conveyors and vats containing toxic substances.
- Installing "local exhaust" systems that have fans to draw workplace pollutants away from workers and into hoods or ducts to be captured by a filter or collector.
- Moving fresh air into an area and polluted air out ("dilution" ventilation) when local exhaust is not possible.
- Rotating workers in and out of the most dangerous jobs will limit the exposure until a permanent engineering solution is found.

Occupational health and safety has become a significant issue to many scientists, workers and government officials. Passage of the Occupational Safety and Health Act of 1970 provided an institutional approach to the increasing problem. Scientists began to understand the origin of some cancers. Workers became more involved in health and safety decisionmaking. As Eric Eckholm pointed out in his study, workers are "challenging the historic managerial monopoly on job related information."

Yet critical areas of occupational health need further study. As the 1979 Surgeon General's Report concluded, these areas include: the role of occupational exposures in producing birth defects and the special problems of women exposed to hazardous substances, occupational causes of respiratory disease alone or in combination with smoking, the role of job stress and exposure to physical and chemical agents in cardiovascular disease, the behavioral changes induced by chronic exposure to low levels of chemicals, the health effects of occupational exposure to heat and radiation, the interaction between these and chemical agents, and methods for analyzing thresholds of exposures to hazardous workplace conditions. Finally, there is still much to learn about what combinations of regulations and incentives work best to bring about changes in both employer and employee attitudes and practices to reduce occupational risks.

There are significant problems that have hindered occupational safety and health research, according to the 1979 Surgeon General's Report. Inadequate data and the long latency periods before disease develops prevents knowledge about the risks of approximately 1,000 new chemicals introduced each year. The worker's first symptoms may be so vague as to be dismissed — a pervasive or recurrent spell of fatigue, dizziness, shortness of breath, loss of appetite, difficulty in sleeping, or visual or hearing irregularities. Since many of those afflicted are young, healthy and with little history of prior illness, there may be a tendency to postpone medical examinations until the affliction is well-established. In some cases the damage is not revealed until some time after the individual has left the contaminated workplace. The damage may then be irreversible.

The variety of ways which people come in contact with hazardous agents, the lack of recorded information about the intensity, duration and combinations of exposures, the confidentiality of employers over trade secrets, and of workers and occupational physicians over personal health records and the fact that workers are often not told the names of the chemicals they work with all obstruct the research in this field.

Samuel Epstein, in his study, asserted that in general workers are denied knowledge of the types and concentrations of chemicals they are exposed to. He also argued that often workers are not informed whether chemicals have been adequately tested, whether they are toxic under conditions in the plant, or whether they are carcinogenic.

Companies and regulators have been accused of keeping secret the research findings that could save workers. Eckholm wrote that many decades ago studies in central Europe showed that uranium miners were dying of lung cancer with unusual frequency, and that the risk could be reduced by installing adequate ventilation. But in the United States, Ashford wrote, the "failure of public and private decisionmakers to utilize this widely disseminated information has exacted a terrible toll" among uranium miners. As recently as 1971 thousands of American uranium miners still worked under conditions that tripled their chances of getting lung cancer.

Similarly, Dr. Joseph K. Wagonner of NIOSH observed that decades after Japan and several European countries banned the use of certain carcinogenic chemicals in the dye industry, "thousands of American workers are still literally sloshing in them."

In August 1981 *The Washington Post* said federal agencies knew the names of hundreds of thousands of people who had been exposed to cancer-causing chemicals on their jobs, but had made no effort to tell them about the risk to their health. No apparent effort had been made to name or notify 21 million workers — one in every four — who were known to have been exposed to hazardous materials regulated by OSHA.

NIOSH, "a primary holder of this information," the Post said, "has used the lists of names only for research purposes waiting for the people on them to die. Then the names are followed up, and if the causes of death can be learned, they become part of the tally the government uses to set up control standards for dangerous substances."

Two joint notification pilot projects of NIOSH and the Workers' Institute for Safety and Health (WISH), an arm of the AFL-CIO, were scheduled to begin in August 1981. One of the pilot projects was for 1,100 chemical plant workers in Augusta, Ga. NIOSH had learned of their exposure to a known carcinogen in 1972.

The agency maintained that it would cost too much for the government to find everyone, notify them and then provide follow-up services. NIOSH saw its role as a research agency, not a public health agency, according to executive officer Dr. Ken Coene.

The agency estimated at a 1977 Senate hearing that it would cost up to $40 million to find and notify all of the estimated 21 million workers who have been exposed to a hazardous substance. Giving them all medical surveillance — not treatment — just to spot a developing illness, would cost $54 billion.

And, judging from the Reagan administration's emphasis on lowering the costs of occupational safety and health, it was unlikely that all of those workers would be treated. *Business Week* magazine said it was "increasingly clear" that OSHA's direction under Thorne Auchter "will be significantly different in both style and substance from that of his predecessor [Eula Bingham]. . . ."

OSHA was expected to work more closely with industry and to try to implement safety regulations that would keep industry costs at a minimum. Auchter told an interviewer that "the question of the least costly approach has an awful lot of merit." He said he wanted to lower the lost-workday rates of hazardous companies and "get out of the safer worksites." OSHA estimated that about 82,000 manufacturing companies (one-fourth of the total) exceeded the national average for lost workdays.

In one of the most heated arguments since OSHA's beginning, union leaders argued in 1981 that the agency under Reagan and Auchter might backtrack on the emotional issues of cotton dust standards, lead standards and the labeling of toxic chemicals. Labor leaders and Reagan also clashed over safety devices in the workplace. Instead of costly insulation and ventilation systems, the administration favored protective equipment such as earplugs and respirators.

Business Week in September 1981 predicted that industry would see "dramatic reversals" in OSHA's inspection, citation and penalty practices. Among the significant changes under discussion, according to the magazine, were:

- A new targeting system to exempt some employers from inspections at general manufacturing operations.
- Fewer inspections as a response to worker complaints.
- Labor-management committees that would exempt qualifying employers from most inspections.

Whatever changes were eventually made, it was widely predicted that OSHA could become one of the first government agencies chosen by the Reagan administration for a major overhaul.

8

Regulation: Worth the Cost?

Vietnam veterans exposed to a herbicide so powerful it could strip the leaves from every tree in a forest in 24 hours... farmers who pastured their sheep downwind from the U.S. nuclear test site in Nevada... soldiers who were marched into the radioactive fallout for "stress tests"... families living above the buried chemicals at New York's Love Canal... farm workers sprayed with agricultural chemicals ... uranium miners, chemical workers...

The number of groups was growing rapidly in 1981 — people who claimed they were victims of harmful health effects from radiation, toxic chemicals or other environmental factors, and were seeking help. They wanted the federal government, or someone, to pay their medical bills and compensate them for disabilities they said they had suffered, or might suffer, through no fault of their own — cancer, miscarriages, sterility, birth defects in their children.

In 1980 they put new pressures on Congress and the courts for that help. The Vietnam veterans claimed that the potent herbicide Agent Orange sickened them and caused defects in the children they later fathered. Western ranchers and soldiers exposed to radioactive fallout from the Nevada nuclear tests claimed a heightened incidence of cancer. These two groups, apparently the most organized, filed sizable lawsuits and persuaded members of Congress to introduce bills on their behalf.

Uncharted Territory

In trying to push environmental law beyond disease prevention efforts into the area of compensation, the veterans and other self-identified victim groups were venturing into a legal/scientific quagmire that environmental groups and their congressional allies had generally avoided, for several reasons.

One problem was that illnesses blamed on environmental agents might actually be developed from multiple causes, acting over a long period of time. Victims might never be able to prove the strict cause-and-effect relationship required by most existing legal systems — tort law, state workers' compensation programs, the Veterans Administration (VA) disability program. Another major problem was cost. Compensating an unknown number of victims for illness, long-term disability, and possibly even the lifetime earning losses of their children born with defects, could run into billions of dollars. The federal government had been no more anxious to assume such a burden than had private industry.

But the increasingly militant "victim" groups argued that they should have special help because:

- They had been involuntarily exposed.
- They had not been informed about possible hazards.
- They could not get aid through existing legal systems because of evidence standards and time limits.

What they wanted was either direct compensation payments or changes in certain legal "presumptions" so that they could more easily collect damages in lawsuits or from existing programs such as those of the Veterans Administration. That would mean major changes in the systems themselves, to accommodate the new concept of environment-related disease.

An Ongoing Problem

Science has always lagged behind public perception that "something causes cancer" and other environmental diseases. To illustrate, Dr. Irving J. Selikoff, chief of the environmental sciences laboratory at Mount Sinai School of Medicine in New York and an expert in industrial diseases, cites a classic, if extreme, example: In 1507 it was reported that women in a German-Czech mining region were remarrying with startling frequency — as many as nine times apiece. The reason: Their husbands, who worked in the mines, died very young. More than four centuries passed before scientists discovered that the miners' premature deaths were caused by radioactive pitchblende in the mines.

In 1969 Congress established a program to compensate coal miners afflicted with "black lung," a disease caused by prolonged exposure to coal dust. It also compensated a miner's dependents, if he was totally disabled and had survivors when he died. Originally, the federal government paid the claims, at a cost of more than $1 billion a year, but in 1978 the law was revised and the responsibility for compensating black-lung victims was shifted to the mining industry. A tax was imposed on all coal mined, to finance trust funds to pay disability and survivors' claims.

Progress in the 1970s

During the 1970s Congress passed numerous landmark environmental laws — clean air, clean water, toxic substances, pesticide and occupational health statutes — all mandating the elimination or control of pollutants believed to cause illness. But while a basic assumption of the legislation was that pollutants harm human health, in only a few cases did Congress go further, to decide that environmental agents already had caused abnormal, compensable conditions.

A program enacted in 1977 compensated Marshall Islanders who were exposed in 1954 to radioactive fallout from a nuclear weapons test and who later developed thyroid cancer and related diseases. In another instance, the Senate in 1976 approved a bill to compensate Michigan residents who were exposed to polybrominated biphenyls (PBBs) in their food after a 1973 mixup in which livestock feed was contaminated with the toxic chemical. But the House never approved the bill.

In 1978, amid rising concern about the costs of environmental pollution controls, Congress directed the National Center for Health Statistics to begin putting together a national data base on environmental illness so that its cost could be estimated.

Since 1978 an ominous succession of new hazards has come to light, many of them more difficult to deal with than the pollutants addressed in the environmental legislation already on the books. These hazards, such as toxic wastes, may affect the worker in the workplace and also menace the health of the public at large.

COMPENSATION: A CHANGING CONCEPT

Existing systems of victim compensation are varied and under review. Some systems require that a connection be established between the source of exposure to an agent and the resulting disease, and others do not. Some require that a party must be shown to be legally responsible for causing a disease before he is forced to pay compensation. Under tort liability law, a party can be compensated only when a sufficient relationship is shown between harm and particular activities. The damaged individual must prove that the party causing the injury was negligent. In the case of diseases caused by chemical agents, it is often impossible to prove direct negligence because the effects of many of the agents are not known. Other obstacles to successful suits include the high cost of health-effect studies, statutes of limitation that require a lawsuit to be brought within one to four years of exposure, and the absence of data on exposure levels.

The law has been slow to recognize the concept of environmentally caused disease — for both political and scientific reasons. Chemical manufacturers and other businesses that could be hurt financially have resisted the idea, while lawmakers, judges and administrators have sought stronger proof than researchers could give them.

Numerous lawsuits have been issued against private companies and the federal government to gain compensation through government programs. Shipyard workers who have contracted asbestosis, lung cancers and mesothelioma have sued asbestos manufacturers and the federal government. Residents near Love Canal in Niagara Falls, N.Y., have sued the Hooker Chemical Co. for property damage, miscarriages, cancer, birth defects and other serious illnesses caused by chemical contamination, and residents of Jackson Township, N.J., have sued the SCM Corp. for allegedly operating a dumpsite that contaminated drinking water supplies and caused cancer and kidney ailments.

The chief scientific/legal problem of compensation has been that so little has been known about many illnesses such as cancer and birth defects. And the fact that many of these disorders were common makes it difficult to prove that a specific case was "an act of God, and not Dow Chemical," as a congressional aide put it.

For example, some 30 percent of pregnancies ended in miscarriages and up to 8 percent of babies were born with defects in 1980. Pinpointing the cause in every case was beyond science. Scientists had the most trouble with low-level exposures to radiation because it was harder to rule out other "competing" potential causes of cancer. In addition, many of the complaints of Agent Orange veterans and individuals living near toxic waste sites and spills — fatigue, neurological sensations, psychological problems — could also be explained by other factors.

Against this background, the "victims" have had trouble developing clear proof that their cases were uniquely deserving of special treatment. Many workers' compensation plans have not covered what have been called "ordinary diseases of life." In general, workers' compensation, public assistance, private insurance plans, the VA compensation program and tort law have been far more responsive to acute illnesses and accidents than to chronic, environment-related disease. Consequently, for liability to be determined, most systems required very specific evidence, both of the exposure itself and of the connection between the substance and medical symptoms.

The contamination of milk supplies in Michigan in 1973 was an example of the difficulties of tort litigation on toxic substance pollution. Farmers contaminated with PBB sued the Michigan Chemical Co. (the producer of the PBBs) and others. After a 14-month trial — the longest in Michigan history — the court's decision went against the farmers. Although they had suffered damages, they could not prove that PBB had caused adverse health effects in their animals.

Two major questions that arise from instances like the Michigan PBB incident are 1) Does the legal system enable people with environmentally caused disease to obtain compensation for their injuries? 2) Do our government and legal systems provide enough deterrents to pollution?

Superfund Debate

Legislation enacted by Congress in December 1980 to help clean up toxic waste accidents and dumps did not include provisions to ensure victim compensation in cases of environmental disasters. A compensation proposal contained in the Senate's original version of the superfund bill would have made companies liable for any toxic releases from their factories, non-consumer products, workplaces and waste sites, in addition to emissions already regulated by clean air and water laws. The chemical industry strongly opposed the measure.

A Chemical Manufacturers Association (CMA) position paper maintained that the chemical industry had spent $6.7 billion — more than any other industry — to comply with pollution control laws. The companies did not want to be held liable for toxic emissions that were not

The Supreme Court and Regulation

Hopeful of a receptive hearing, business took several actions of federal regulators to the Supreme Court in early 1981 — arguing that they infringed on property rights or unduly limited state powers.

The court heard arguments in a major challenge of this type on Jan. 21. In the cases — *American Textile Manufacturers' Institute* v. *Marshall, National Cotton Council* v. *Marshall* — the textile industry opposed cotton dust exposure standards adopted by the Occupational Safety and Health Administration (OSHA). For the industry, former Solicitor General Robert Bork argued that OSHA adopted these standards without due consideration for the costs they would impose upon textile manufacturers.

The cotton dust cases were one of a series of challenges to OSHA standards. The business community pressed for a ruling requiring OSHA to show a balance between the costs to the employer and the benefits to employees.

Despite such challenges, the court handed the regulatory agencies a string of victories between December 1980 and March 1981.

On Dec. 2 the court unanimously held that the Environmental Protection Agency (EPA) need not concern itself with the economic impact of compliance with water pollution laws, thereby rebuffing arguments that some crushed stone, sand and gravel plants might have to close unless they received variances from 1977 clean water standards *(EPA* v. *National Crushed Stone Association).*

Also in December the court ruled that businesses finding themselves under investigation by the Federal Trade Commission must await the completion of those proceedings before they could challenge them in federal court *(FTC* v. *Standard Oil of California).*

During February and March the court upheld the power and practices of the Federal Communications Commission (FCC) and the Interstate Commerce Commission (ICC).

A long-running battle between the FCC and the Court of Appeals for the District of Columbia Circuit ended March 24, 1981, when the Supreme Court upheld the FCC's refusal to consider changes in the entertainment format of a radio station when reviewing an application for license renewal or transfer *(FCC* v. *WNCN Listeners Guild).*

Also in March, the court held unanimously that an ICC decision to approve abandonment of certain railroad service could not be challenged in state courts *(Chicago and North Western Transportation Co. v. Kalo Brick & Tile Co.)*

regulated by existing air and water pollution laws.

Also debated was the basic question of whether the fund should compensate victims or merely provide emergency cleanup. Concerned with inflation fighting and budget austerity, the Carter administration felt that victim compensation should be handled by private lawsuits against the responsible company. If the fund were to compensate victims, one Environmental Protection Agency (EPA) spokesman said, it would quickly go bankrupt. But environmentalists and senators argued that holding companies liable for victim compensation would be a powerful incentive for proper waste handling.

The Senate bill would have set aside one-third of the superfund to compensate victims for out-of-pocket medical expenses and lost wages. But mindful of the huge costs of compensating victims with long-term diseases such as cancer, senators limited reimbursements for out-of-pocket medical expenses to those incurred within six years after the person was first exposed to the toxic substance. Thus the fund would not cover diseases that took 20 or 30 years to show up.

An argument for victim compensation was the inadequacy of many state laws, which require that suits be filed within one or two years from the time the exposure first occurred. Often victims were not aware that they had been exposed to a dangerous substance until they became ill many years later.

Under the House bill proposed by Bob Eckhardt, D-Texas (1967-81), then chairman of the House Commerce Oversight Subcommittee, taxpayers would pay all the costs of cleaning up old dumpsites. He opposed requiring current producers to pay for earlier shoddy disposal practices.

CMA argued that society should pay for the cleanup because it benefited from inadequate disposal in the form of cheaper products. Chemical companies also objected to across-the-board fees on the entire industry because they would make companies that disposed of wastes properly share the cost of cleanup for careless firms. Others argued that the polluter should pay for cleanup because he benefited most from cheap disposal.

Industry representatives said their liability should end as soon as the wastes leave their factories. They maintained that they should not be held liable for the negligence of transporters or disposal-site operators.

But Justice Department attorneys argued that the easiest way to improve waste handling was to make waste generators and handlers police themselves. If a company knew it would be held liable for the actions of its haulers, it would make sure they acted properly.

In the end, the combination of forces arguing against inclusion of the Senate provision proved stronger than those in favor. The victims' compensation provision was dropped from the final version of the bill, which authorized $1.6 billion for the superfund. *(Details, p. 38)*

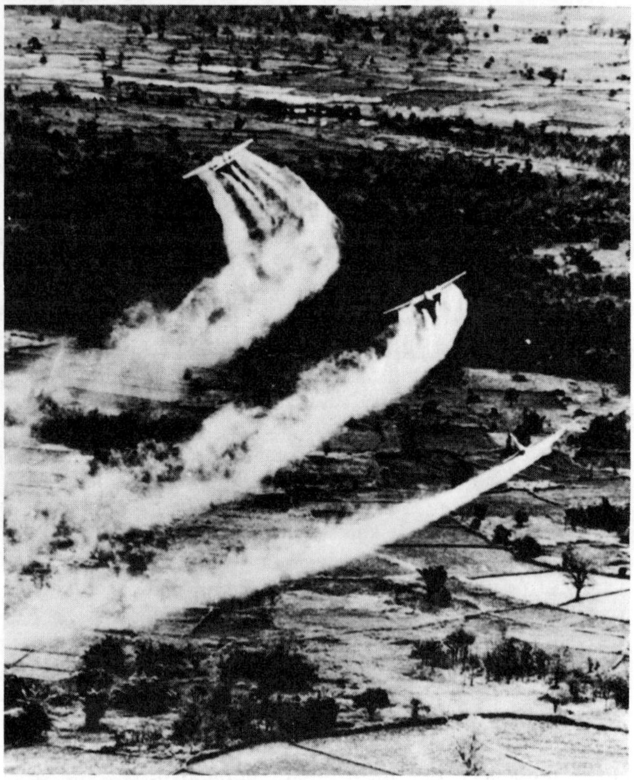

U.S. Air Force planes sprayed the defoliant Agent Orange over dense vegetation in South Vietnam in 1966.

Lack of Support

The growth of interest in protecting consumers from unsafe products has been accompanied by a growth of product liability lawsuits. Writing in the September/October 1977 issue of *Regulation,* Richard Epstein, law professor at the University of Chicago, noted that "the law of products liability has undergone numerous changes that have, taken together, profoundly increased the probability that a successful suit for damages will be brought against the maker or seller of a product. A speeding motorist may recover full damages from an automobile manufacturer for injuries that he himself could have avoided by reasonable care. A plaintiff who is burned by throwing perfume upon a lighted candle can recover from the manufacturer or retailer of the perfume because they did not warn that perfume is flammable."

In many cases, the consequences of this change have been reflected in rising insurance rates and business failures. "Before we make the obligations of manufacturers too onerous, we should bear in mind the perils of such expansion," Epstein concluded. "There is the risk of standardless litigation. There is the risk of making manufacturers and sellers bear the risk of loss when others in the chain of distribution, including the injured party, are better able to prevent the harm in question."

Agreeing with Epstein, Walter Guzzardi Jr. wrote in *Fortune,* April 9, 1979, "What is made safe for the village idiot will cost the man of common sense more. Many people would choose to be careful, or to buy their insurance in some other form. Nonsmokers don't want to pay extra for fireproof bedsheets; people who fasten seat belts don't need the costly air bag. Buyers and sellers should share more equitably the total costs of accidents — the costs to the consumer of property damage, medical expenses and forgone income, and the costs to the manufacturer of making a safer product."

In the past, environmental groups had not pushed strongly for victim compensation because their resources were limited and because they regarded prevention and cleanup as more urgent priorities — much as medical researchers have argued that funds spent on discovering a polio vaccine did more good for more people than dollars invested in iron lungs for those who already had the disease. The EPA shared that basic assumption. So did key members of Congress such as James J. Florio, D-N.J., chairman of the House Commerce Transportation Subcommittee, one of several panels with jurisdiction over the superfund legislation.

Another factor adding to inaction in the past was that, until the superfund legislation came along, compensation showed up in Congress as a parochial issue. Members limited their bills to a specific problem in their state or district, or to a special group such as the veterans. "Narrowing the group" to limit the potential cost of a bill had been a respected legislative tactic for softening opposition. But a narrow bill might not attract broad enough support to pass. Such bills have had a high failure rate in the past.

Not only was support for environmental disease compensation weak, but there was strong industry opposition to the idea. The chemical industry continued to raise serious questions about the concept of environmental illness, per se, as well as about the validity of charges against specific substances. Chemical and other companies resisted incorporating the concepts of "environmental" or "occupational" disease into law.

The Dow Chemical Co., which successfully blocked past federal actions to remove the suspect component of Agent Orange from the domestic market, in 1980 was actively contesting veterans' claims in a major federal court suit in New York. It was not that the product contributed significantly to Dow's profits. "This stuff is .000 percent of a nine-and-a-quarter billion-dollar-a-year business," said Dow spokesman Phillip Schneider. The real issue was the quality of scientific findings on which legal decisions were made, said Dow attorney Don Freyer. After 30 years of manufacturing the herbicide, Dow had "a large data base that just eloquently demonstrates that this isn't harmful. If we can't demonstrate it in this case, then no one can make any chemicals," Freyer warned.

In 1981 both the House and Senate approved a bill directing Veterans Administration hospitals to give "priority medical treatment" to veterans who had been exposed to Agent Orange. The bill also directed the VA to extend the scope of its Agent Orange study to include the effects of other toxic chemicals that had been used in Vietnam. As of September 1981 the bill had not received final passage.

CURRENT ISSUE: COST-BENEFIT ANALYSIS

"Regulations cost American business an estimated $102 billion a year, about $30 billion of it in mountains of paperwork. All this adds to the crushing burden of inflation."

That comment, made by Sen. Thomas F. Eagleton, D-Mo., in early 1979, echoed the sentiments of many in Congress and in the business community concerned about the pervasiveness and rising costs of regulation. (Eagleton in 1981 was chairman of a Senate Democratic task force on regulatory reform.)

Among examples of reported regulatory costs:

- The Small Business Administration (SBA) reported in December 1979 that paperwork requirements of small business by regulatory agencies cost each firm an average of $1,270 a year.
- Data Resources Inc. estimated that the cost of meeting environmental regulations during 1979 was $12.3 billion, up from $9.6 billion in 1978.
- Louis Lasagna, a professor at the University of Rochester Medical Center, reported in the November/December 1979 *Regulation* that pre-market testing of new drugs required by the Food and Drug Administration cost up to $50 million.
- In January 1978 Dow Chemical Co. released a study showing that the impact of federal regulations cost the company $186 million, a 27 percent increase over 1975. The study classified $69 million of the cost as "excessive."
- The University of Pennsylvania found that the cost of complying with 12 federal programs jumped from $350,000 in 1972 to $3.2 million in 1977.
- In March 1979 R. J. Reynolds Industries Inc. reported that the costs of meeting regulations of nearly 40 federal agencies as well as regulations of various foreign, state and local regulatory bodies was $29 million in 1977.
- Fifty cents of the cost of an average prescription made by Eli Lilly & Co., the pharmaceutical concern, goes for compliance with federal regulations.
- According to estimates by Richard Posner of the University of Chicago, federal regulation of milk prices under the Agricultural Act of 1937 cost consumers an estimated 10 percent of their milk bills, or nearly $1 billion, in 1977.

While few persons advocate a return to *laissez-faire* capitalism, in which government had little or no role in regulating corporate behavior, many by 1981 were arguing for a large-scale cutback in complex and sometimes conflicting federal rules affecting health, the environment and other areas. Business people said that their desire to ease government restraints was not selfish. The entire nation would benefit from the higher productivity and lower prices that deregulation would bring, they said.

Federal requirements imposed on factories and manufactured products have resulted in substantial price hikes for consumer goods, according to Murray L. Weidenbaum, chairman of President Reagan's Council of Economic Advisers. "Virtually every study of regulatory experience indicates both needless expense and ineffective operations," he said.

Measuring the Costs

In addition to the direct costs, as measured by the federal budgets for regulatory agencies (almost $8 billion for 16 major agencies in fiscal 1981), there are the costs incurred by the private sector in meeting regulatory reporting and other requirements.

A study by the Council on Environmental Quality put the estimated cost of incremental expenditures for pollution control by the EPA at $9 billion for air pollution, $4.7 billion for water pollution and $0.7 billion for solid waste in 1975. The council estimated that by 1984 annual incremental costs would rise to $18.6 billion for air, $19.5 billion for water, $1.3 billion for solid waste and $0.6 billion for land reclamation. Although it is difficult to measure the benefits derived from such expenditures in terms of an enhanced and more healthy environment, the Senate Government Operations Committee cited a number of studies indicating that air pollution programs were more likely than water pollution programs to offset their costs with savings in damage prevention.

McKean Study

Writing in the Summer 1980 issue of *Policy Analysis*, University of Virginia economist Roland McKean noted the high costs of enforcing environmental and safety regulations. He divided the related costs into three categories: 1) avoidance costs on the part of the regulated parties (lobbying against a rule, concealing noncompliance, going to court to protest a rule); 2) costs borne or imposed by the regulatory agency (inspections, recordkeeping, prosecuting violators); and 3) costs incurred in the form of a reduction in benefits due to imperfect or incomplete enforcement. It was the third category that he believed was the most costly.

McKean pointed to a number of factors that made a regulation difficult or expensive to enforce. There may be problems in identifying or measuring the regulated behavior and determining its source; regulations may be ambiguous; there may be no consensus regarding the goals of regulation; and more than one agency may be involved.

Weidenbaum Study

One of the most widely cited analyses of the costs of regulation was a study prepared for Congress' Joint Economic Subcommittee on Growth and Stabilization by Murray Weidenbaum, then a professor at the Center for the Study of American Business, Washington University, St. Louis, Mo. Weidenbaum estimated that the total cost of regulation was $102.7 billion in fiscal 1979 ($4.8 billion for administration and $97.9 billion for compliance). The study, released April 8, 1978, was generally critical of the existing regulatory system. Among the areas cited by Weidenbaum as being adversely affected by regulation:

- *Automobiles* — Compulsory catalytic converters to reduce air pollution and seat belts added $666 to the price tag of a 1978 model. The converter increased national fuel consumption by approximately $3 billion a year.
- *Consumers* — "The costs of complying with government regulations are inevitably passed on by business to the consumer in the form of higher prices," noted Weidenbaum.
- *Workers* — "Government regulation, albeit unintentionally, can have strongly adverse effects on employment. . . . Many industry facilities and entire factories have been closed down — with substantial but unmeasurable effects on employment — because of the high costs of meeting environmental, safety and other regulatory requirements."

Weidenbaum argued that one hidden cost of government regulation was its adverse effect on innovation. "The longer it takes for a new product to be approved by a government agency — or the more costly the approval process — the less likely that the new product will be created," he wrote. "In any event, innovation will be delayed."

For example, he cited a 1973 study by Sam Peltzman of the University of Chicago, who estimated that the 1962 amendments to the Food and Drug Act had delayed the introduction of effective drugs by about four years and had also led to higher prices for pharmaceutical products. Professor Lasagna made a similar point in his *Regulation* article, pointing out that some highly effective but marginally profitable drugs were never marketed because the required testing would have made them prohibitively expensive.

Weidenbaum contended that regulation impeded economic growth by claiming a rising share of new capital formation. He noted that Edward Denison of the Brookings Institution (writing in the January 1978 *Survey of Current Business*) had conducted a study to estimate the loss of productivity caused by meeting government pollution and job safety standards. According to Denison, by 1975 output per unit of input in the non-residential business sector of the economy was 1.4 percent smaller than it would have been if business had operated under the regulatory conditions of 1967. Of that amount, 1 percent was due to pollution abatement and 0.4 percent to employee safety and health programs.

Business Roundtable Study

On March 14, 1979, the Business Roundtable — chief executive officers of approximately 190 major companies —

Estimated Pollution Expenditures, 1979-88

Program	Total Annual Costs* 1979	1988	Cumulative ('79-'88)
Air Pollution			
Public	2.1	3.5	27.8
Private			
Mobile	8.1	14.7	115.8
Industrial	5.4	9.0	74.0
Electric Utilities	9.8	15.0	121.2
Subtotal	25.4	42.2	338.8
Water Pollution			
Public	11.9	19.6	145.1
Private			
Industrial	7.6	11.5	93.5
Electric Utilities	.9	1.5	11.4
Subtotal	20.4	32.6	250.0
Solid Waste			
Public	2.0	3.1	27.1
Private	5.2	9.1	73.8
Subtotal	7.2	12.2	100.9
Toxic Substances	.3	1.1	8.2
Drinking Water	.7	1.3	10.5
Noise	.1	1.6	6.9
Pesticides	.1	.1	1.7
Land Reclamation	1.7	1.8	18.0
Total	55.9	92.9	735.0

**billions of 1979 dollars*

Source: Council on Environmental Quality

The figures listed here reflect anticipated costs of compliance with environmental regulations as of mid-1980. According to the Council on Environmental Quality, these figures are estimated and show ranges of cost rather than exact figures.

released a study showing that the regulatory policies of six federal agencies cost 48 major corporations operating in more than 20 industries a total of $2.6 billion in directly measurable effects in 1977. This compared with capital expenditures by the companies of $25.8 billion, research and development costs of $6 billion and net income after taxes of $16.6 billion.

The study, managed by the accounting firm of Arthur Andersen & Co., was distinguished from other regulatory cost studies by its specificity. It not only identified incremental costs by general classification, such as operating and administrative costs, but also provided a breakdown of costs of specific regulations. For example, 29 percent of incremental costs attributed to the EPA were related to water treatment regulations.

The Roundtable stressed that its study did not measure the cost of the regulations of all agencies (the only agencies studied were EPA, the Equal Employment Opportunity Commission, OSHA, the Department of Energy, the FTC and the Labor Department's administration of the Employee Retirement Income Security Act); costs incurred by many industries; or the costs of state regulations. It also omitted secondary costs of regulation, which are difficult to quantify. Examples of secondary costs were described as delays in construction of new plants and equipment, the misallocation of resources and the loss of productivity that is caused by regulation.

Overall, the study indicated that manufacturing companies bore the highest costs of regulation — $2.3 billion of incremental costs. EPA regulations imposed incremental costs of $2 billion, 77 percent of the $2.6 billion total for all six agencies combined, while OSHA regulations imposed incremental costs of $184 million, a small portion of the participating companies' total expenditures for worker safety and health in 1977.

The impact of regulation showed a wide variation among industries. As an illustration, the incremental cost of OSHA rules averaged $6 a year for each worker in the banking industry, but $220 a year for a worker in the chemical industry.

In addition, certain regulations were found to be especially burdensome while others imposed relatively small costs. To illustrate the former, two regulations by the EPA accounted for $900 million of incremental costs in 1977 — Control of Air Pollution from New Motor Vehicles, and the National Ambient Air Quality Standard for Particulates.

Support for Regulation

To many environmentalists and consumer advocates, much of the talk about the inflationary impact of regulation has been as a ploy by business to trim its costs at the expense of human health. Most of the information about the cost of regulation has been generated by business and, therefore, has been greatly exaggerated, they have argued. Mark Green, then director of Nader's Congress Watch, told the Senate Commerce Committee in November 1978 hearings:

> There is a powerful fad being marketed by much of the business community and others ... that government action is invariably wrong and pernicious. Business critics of regulation often list regulations that seem to be bizarre and foolish, but it would be unfortunate if trivial and picayune examples distorted the seriousness of this debate. For what is at stake here is not so much where to locate outhouses as what to do about the 1,000 people a day who die of a cancer in this country, or the 20 million Americans injured in product-related defects annually.

Green also contested the argument of Weidenbaum and others that regulation impedes technological change. Writing in the Jan. 21, 1979, *Washington Post,* he noted:

> Before the Food and Drug Administration banned spray cans using fluorocarbons, the industry said there was no alternative. The day after the ban went into effect, the country had a new pump spray that didn't use fluorocarbons, and that was *cheaper* than aerosol cans. After Washington imposed strict safety standards for car bumpers, auto engineers developed bumpers that are far stronger and lighter — and that save consumers an average $100 in repair costs over the life of the car.

The Cost of Life and Health

Green and other supporters of regulation — particularly in the health, safety and environmental areas — have rejected industry's cost-benefit approach to regulation in these fields. "Given the current state of economic art," Green wrote, "mathematical cost-benefit analyses are about as neutral as voter literacy tests in the Old South. They are often ideological documents designed to prove preconceived notions."

Robert Stulberg, staff attorney for Public Citizen Inc. Health Research Group, asked, "How can you possibly put a dollar figure on the cost of a human life? Why don't they carry out their computations to when a worker falls from a scaffold or dies in a grain shaft explosion? To attribute the inflation rate to few and meager health standards is fallacious. Take a look at what the inflation has been in companies' net profits."

Sen. Gary Hart, D-Colo., agreed with Stulberg that business' inflation argument was fallacious because the benefits of regulation are not part of the equation. "Assume the cost to society of pollution damage such as respiratory disease is $1,000," he wrote in the January 1979 *EPA Journal.* "The $4,400 car with pollution control equipment is actually a new commodity which produces more net benefits to society than the lower-priced $4,000 car."

"You have to look at all the costs," said Rafe Pomerance, legislative director of Friends of the Earth. "The costs of health, visibility, nuisance, irritation. Everybody knows that property values are affected by air pollution."

"What is the price tag for lives saved by avoiding future diseases, since asbestos and other substances in our lives today cause cancer in 30 years?" queried Green. "How much will you pay for a 6-year-old who is not disfigured from flammable sleepwear? How do we calculate the exact benefits of being able to see across the Grand Canyon, of avoiding needless destruction of our recreation areas?"

Attempts at Measurement

Despite Green's contention that many benefits of regulation "involve immeasurable or moral considerations," efforts have been made to quantify the benefits resulting from regulation and the costs that would be incurred without it.

The EPA, for example, estimated that the cost of repainting surfaces damaged by polluted air was almost $650 million in 1970. OSHA calculated that its cotton dust standards would prevent 1,749 cases of brown lung a year, thus saving more than $500 million in medical costs. A study for the EPA and the Council on Environmental Quality by Data Resources Inc. of Cambridge, Mass., concluded that environmental controls actually would decrease unemployment slightly (by 0.2 to 0.3 percent annually) and would result in only a tiny increase in the inflation rate (from 0.1 to 0.2 percent a year) over the next eight years. That study, while conceding that pollution controls would bring about job losses among production workers in industries such as steel and paper, concluded that overall unemployment would be more than offset by hiring workers to construct, install and service mandated anti-pollution devices and sewers.

In October 1979 the Corporate Accountability Research Group released a study showing $36 billion in benefits from health and safety regulations, compared to costs of $31.2 billion. The study found that federal auto and highway regulations had saved 100,000 lives between 1966 and 1979, that product safety standards reduced accidental crib deaths by 50 percent and that cleaner air mandated by EPA would reduce the mortality rate by 7 percent.

The study also pointed out that the extra $500 required to meet bumper restraint and fuel economy standards that were slated to become effective by 1984 would be offset within two years by added savings, through lower bumper repair bills and reduced gasoline costs.

One problem of the cost-benefit approach is that the analyses are frequently "in the eye of the beholder," according to Delaware Republican William Roth Jr., chairman of the Senate Governmental Affairs Committee. "You don't have to be in [Washington] too long to know you can get figures to prove or justify almost anything you want to do," he said.

Democratic Rep. George Danielson of California said, "I'm not against cost-benefit [analysis] if it is one of a group of criteria. But you cannot reduce everything on Earth down to dollars and cents."

Another criticism of the approach is that the figures generally come from industry and "the costs are in the hands of the companies who have every incentive to exaggerate," said Nancy Drabble of Congress Watch. A report by the House Commerce Oversight and Investigations Subcommittee accused industries of predicting "large compliance costs and major impacts ... knowing that such projections are likely to induce regulators or the courts to water down or delay ... a proposed regulation." Moreover, some economists say it is difficult to predict with much accuracy the costs of new technology needed to comply with regulations.

Reagan Push for Cost-Benefit Approach

After President Reagan early in his presidency issued an executive order requiring cost-benefit analyses, Sen. Eagleton wrote to his Democratic colleagues March 20, 1981, saying that Reagan's order could slow the regulatory process dramatically and could insulate administration decisionmaking from public and congressional oversight. "At a minimum, these [cost-benefit] approaches could add needless delay and expense to the administrative process," he said. "Worse still, necessary regulations in such areas as nuclear safety and toxic waste protection could remain unissued merely because the value of avoiding atomic catastrophe or future genetic damage could not be precisely toted up in an accountant's ledger."

Eagleton said there was consensus among his seven-member Senate task force "that regulations are too often foisted on the public without an adequate analysis of their costs and benefits," but that members of the task force were "seriously concerned about mathematically strict cost-benefit analysis proposals which fail to recognize the imprecision inherent in the technique."

Defense of the regulatory process also came from an unlikely source — Reagan's budget-cutting budget director, David A. Stockman. "There's a major residual role for government in regulating workplace safety and the environment," Stockman said.

R. David Pittle, a member of the Consumer Product Safety Commission, said that "Although there have been instances where government regulations have gone awry, many of the attacks against agencies are inaccurate and unfair. Many thoughtful Americans do understand that a certain amount of government involvement in the market is necessary to make it function properly, especially in areas such as product safety, where the individual consumers often cannot exercise much influence over the safety of the products available to them."

The administration's reform efforts "do not constitute a Neanderthal plea to ignore the real problems of pollution, discrimination, and so on," said CEA Chairman Weidenbaum. "Precisely to the contrary: they are offered in the belief that every task government undertakes should be performed ably and that the existing regulatory process simply is not working well.... In view of the magnitude of the resources devoted to regulatory purposes, the public deserves better than it has been getting."

REGULATORY REFORM: OUTLOOK FOR THE FUTURE

"American society experienced a virtual explosion in government regulation during the past decade," President Reagan told a joint session of Congress Feb. 18, 1981. "The result has been higher prices, higher unemployment and lower productivity growth.... We have no intention of dismantling the regulatory agencies — especially those necessary to protect [the] environment and to ensure the public health and safety. However, we must come to grips with inefficient and burdensome regulations — eliminate those we can and reform the others."

The deregulation efforts of Reagan and other presidents focused on cutting the plethora of rules issued by old-line agencies such as the Interstate Commerce Commission (ICC), as well as by the newer regulators such as the Occupational Safety and Health Administration (OSHA).

Outside the government, many business people, unhappy with what they considered unnecessary and costly aspects of the regulatory maze, lobbied for more flexibility in health and safety standards and argued that the process should be streamlined overall. Spokesmen for groups such as the Chamber of Commerce of the United States, the Business Roundtable and the National Federation of Independent Business said the labyrinth of federal rules and costly, time-consuming procedures for approving them dampened productivity, fueled inflation and blunted America's competitive edge abroad.

They also argued that federal regulations penalized consumers in many cases. "The Truth in Lending law is so broad as to enable regulators to write regulations so complex [that] no business can afford to comply with the law," said M. Kendall Fleeharty, director of the Chamber of Commerce's Regulatory Action Center. "The ... regulations cost far more than the marketplace advantages [of regulation] to the consumer."

In addition, business complained that agencies frequently chose the more expensive alternative when issuing a rule, thereby driving up the costs of production. OSHA "doesn't want to talk about ear plugs" for workers in noisy factories, Fleeharty said. "They only want to talk about noise abatement equipment, which costs millions of dollars."

Reliance on Competition

In contrast to the general business view, consumer and environmental activists and labor groups warned that deregulatory "overkill" could negate the progress made in cleaning up the environment, providing safer and more healthy working conditions and protecting consumers from hazardous products. At the same time, many of them advocated reducing or abolishing federal controls that protected some economic sectors from marketplace competition. Sen. Edward M. Kennedy, D-Mass., summarized this view in a speech before a conference on regulatory reform in May 1979. "If Americans are to believe in their government, regulation must be — and be seen to be — fair, reasonable and effective. In the area of social regulation — traffic safety, food purity, drug efficacy, environmental protection, job safety and health — deregulation is unlikely to be the answer; here, the choice will be how to regulate, not between regulation or none." But, Kennedy continued, "where health and safety are not paramount, and industry consists of several firms in a reasonably competitive market, the most likely answer is not to regulate."

Reagan and Deregulation

Armed with what he viewed as an election mandate, Reagan upon taking office immediately began to attack the regulatory maze through a series of administration actions that could be implemented more quickly than legislation. White House aides and congressional Republicans also went to work on bills to revamp basic agency laws, to streamline the bureaucracy and to make the executive actions part of permanent legislation.

All of Reagan's top economic advisers were on record as favoring deregulation. They included Vice President George Bush; CEA Chairman Weidenbaum; Office of Management and Budget Director Stockman; James C. Miller III, director of the Office of Information and Regulatory Affairs at OMB; and Martin Anderson, Reagan's chief domestic policy adviser.

"A dramatic substantial rescission of the regulatory burden is needed both for the short term cash flow relief it will provide to business firms and the long term signals it will provide to corporate investment planners," said Stockman in a report to the president. "All told, there are easily in excess of $100 billion in new environmental, safety and energy compliance costs scheduled for the early 1980s."

"The Reagan administration is thinking big about regulatory reform," said OMB's Miller. OMB published a report early in 1981 that maintained EPA was beginning to expand at an alarming rate and that its influence was going far beyond its budget. The most significant indication of EPA's regulation costs was what OMB called "incremental cost." These costs included those for pollution control that went beyond what would have been incurred had there been no regulation.

Reagan Strategy

Two days after he was sworn in on Jan. 20, Reagan announced the creation of his Presidential Task Force on Regulatory Relief, chaired by Vice President Bush. The other members were Treasury Secretary Donald T. Regan, Attorney General William French Smith, Commerce Secretary Malcolm Baldrige, Labor Secretary Raymond J. Donovan, OMB Director Stockman, CEA Chairman Weidenbaum and domestic policy adviser Anderson. OMB's Miller was the executive director. The panel was authorized to review major regulatory proposals by executive branch agencies, assess executive branch regulations already on the books, oversee the development of legislative proposals, and make recommendations on regulatory personnel and how to reform regulation through executive orders, agency actions and legislative changes.

According to Weidenbaum, a key element in the group's anticipated effectiveness was that "the task force at the top of the structure doesn't have any interest group constituency to protect and defend. Its only constituency is the president and the president's program for rationalizing regulation."

Establishment of the task force was followed by Executive Order 12288, issued Jan. 29. The order terminated the Council on Wage and Price Stability's (COWPS) major function — monitoring price and wage increases and setting voluntary guidelines for them. The agency, set up in 1974, had been a failure at fighting inflation, Reagan said.

Another early move to assert greater White House control over regulation came on Feb. 17, 1981. On that day, Reagan issued a second executive order (12291), which gave OMB's Stockman and Miller wide powers over the regulatory apparatus. It required executive agencies to prepare a regulatory impact analysis for all new and existing major regulations. Subject to direction from the presidential task force, Miller's office was given authority to issue criteria for deciding when a regulation was "major" (there was no set dollar figure) and to tell an agency to perform an economic analysis for any rule. Regulatory analyses would have to be performed for "major" rules and would have to be approved by OMB before being published. Agencies were required to apply cost-benefit analyses to all rulemaking and adopt the least costly alternative. Twice a year, they would have to publish a regulatory agenda of rules under consideration.

The new authority for the OMB was much broader than that vested in Carter's Regulatory Analysis Review

The Regulatory Maze: Agencies Involved...

Increased public attention to environmental problems and work-related health hazards helped the number of federal agencies involved in those areas to proliferate during the 1970s. The two major agencies in those fields are the Environmental Protection Agency (EPA) and the Occupational Safety and Health Administration (OSHA). *(Background, p. 4)* Other agencies active in those fields include:

Agricultural Stabilization and Conservation Service (ASCS). Administers various voluntary land-use programs to protect, expand and conserve farmlands, wetlands and forests. *(Agriculture Department)*

Army Corps of Engineers. Regulates all construction projects in the navigable waterways of the United States; promulgates regulations governing the transportation and dumping of dredged materials in navigable waters; develops, plans and builds various structures — dams, reservoirs, levees, harbors, waterways and locks — to protect areas from floods, supply water for municipal and industrial use, create recreational areas, improve water and wildlife quality, and protect the shorelines of oceans and lakes. *(Defense Department)*

Bureau of Land Management (BLM). Administers public lands located mainly in the western United States and Alaska. Resources managed include timber, minerals, oil and gas, geothermal energy, wildlife habitats, endangered plant and animal species, rangeland vegetation, recreation areas, wild and scenic rivers, wild horses and burros, designated conservation and wilderness areas and open space lands. *(Interior Department)*

Consumer Product Safety Commission (CPSC). Establishes mandatory safety standards governing the design, construction, contents, performance and labeling of consumer products; develops rules and regulations to enforce standards. Hazard-related programs include acute chemical and environmental hazards.

Federal Aviation Administration (FAA). Establishes and enforces rules and regulations for safety standards covering all aspects of civil aviation, including noise and exhaust emissions from aircraft (in cooperation with the EPA). *(Transportation Department)*

Federal Energy Regulatory Commission (FERC). Issues licenses for hydroelectric power projects that contain conditions for protection of fish and wildlife and water quality and provide for recreational opportunities, flood control and the efficient and safe operation of project dams. *(Energy Department)*

Federal Highway Administration (FHWA). Sets functional safety standards for the design, construction and maintenance of the nation's highways and establishes safety standards for commercial motor carriers in interstate or foreign commerce; regulates the movement of dangerous cargoes on highways and administers programs to reduce motor carrier noise. *(Transportation Department)*

Federal Maritime Commission (FMC). Certifies the financial responsibility of vessels that carry oil or other hazardous material to cover cost of cleaning up spills in navigable waters of the United States and adjoining shorelines.

Federal Trade Commission (FTC). Protects the public from false and deceptive advertising, particularly that involving food, drugs, cosmetics and therapeutic devices. Issues report on "tar" and nicotine contents of cigarettes.

Food and Drug Administration (FDA). Administers laws to ensure the purity and safety of foods, drugs and cosmetics. Develops programs to reduce human exposure to radiation; conducts research on the effects of radiation exposure. Conducts research on the biological effects of potentially toxic chemical substances found in the environment. *(Health and Human Services Department)*

Materials Transportation Bureau. Develops and enforces equipment and operating safety regulations for the transportation of all materials by pipeline; carries out inspection, compliance and enforcement actions for transport of all hazardous materials (including radioactive materials) by air, water, highway and rail. *(Transportation Department)*

Mine Safety and Health Administration (MSHA). Develops and promulgates mandatory mine safety and health standards and ensures compliance with such standards. Aims to prevent and reduce mine accidents and occupational diseases. *(Labor Department)*

Group (RARG), which Reagan disbanded. The RARG studied only about 10 regulations a year and issued reports only *after* the proposals had been published in the *Federal Register.* Under the new procedures, OMB, under the direction of the presidential task force, would review regulations *before* they were published. The agency would have to delay action until the review was completed. However, OMB was not given absolute veto power over all agency decisions, according to C. Boyden Gray, counsel to Vice President George Bush. Gray conceded that OMB "could tell agencies to redo the anlaysis," causing quite a few frequent delays. "But they couldn't hold something off to displace the agency's decisionmaking authority," Gray added.

... In Environment and Occupational Health

National Bureau of Standards (NBS). Conducts research and provides technical information on the protection of public health and safety, environmental quality, the improvement of industrial productivity and the promotion of better materials use. *(Commerce Department)*

National Institute for Occupational Safety and Health (NIOSH). Researches and develops occupational safety and health standards. *(Department of Health and Human Services)*

National Oceanic and Atmospheric Administration (NOAA). Describes, monitors and predicts conditions in the atmosphere, ocean, sun and space environment; disseminates environmental data through a system of meteorological, oceanographic, geophysical and solar-terrestrial data centers; manages and conserves living marine resources and their habitats, including certain endangered species and marine mammals. *(Commerce Department)*

National Park Service. Administers programs to conserve the scenery, natural and historic objects and wildlife in the nation's parks. *(Interior Department)*

National Transportation Safety Board (NTSB). Investigates and reports on the transportation of hazardous materials. *(Transportation Department)*

Nuclear Regulatory Commission (NRC). Licenses the construction and operation of nuclear reactors and other facilities; licenses the possession, use, transportation, handling and disposal of nuclear materials.

Office of Conservation and Renewable Energy. Directs energy conservation programs; expands use of biomass, alcohol fuels and urban waste; studies the problems involved in acid rain and carbon dioxide associated with coal burning. *(Energy Department)*

Office of Surface Mining Reclamation and Enforcement. Protects society and the environment from the adverse effects of coal mining operations; establishes minimum national standards for regulating surface effects of coal mining; promotes reclamation of previously mined lands. *(Interior Department)*

Office of Water Research and Technology. Supervises the nation's water quality and quantity; research support includes controlling the quality and quantity of ground water and surface water; conservation techniques and technologies; protection of fragile water ecosystems and other natural resources; and water management planning. *(Interior Department)*

Soil Conservation Service (SCS). Administers national program to develop and conserve soil and water resources; offers technical assistance on agricultural pollution control and environmental improvement projects. *(Agriculture Department)*

U.S. Coast Guard. In the area of water pollution works with Materials Transportation Bureau to ensure that shipowners clean up oil or hazardous materials discharged into navigable waters. *(Transportation Department)*

U.S. Fish and Wildlife Service. Regulates the development, protection, rearing and stocking of wildlife resources and their habitats; protects migratory and game birds, fish and wildlife, endangered and threatened species, enforces regulations for hunters of migratory waterfowl; preserves wetlands as natural habitats. *(Interior Department)*

U.S. Forest Service. Manages the national forests and grasslands and regulates the use of forest resources; regulates activities of commercial foresters working in national forests to ensure that the methods employed do not substantially damage the environment. *(Interior Department)*

U.S. Geological Survey (USGS). Classifies and manages mineral and water resources on federal lands, including the Outer Continental Shelf. Maintains the Earth Resources Observation System (EROS) Data Center that conducts and sponsors research to apply data findings in areas including mapping, geography, mineral and land resources, water resources, rangeland, wildlife and environmental monitoring. *(Interior Department)*

Water and Power Resources Service. Develops and manages water and power resources in the western states. Projects include flood control, river regulation, outdoor recreational opportunities, fish and wildlife enhancement and water quality improvement. *(Interior Department)*

Later Decisions

Meanwhile, a number of Cabinet secretaries issued their own regulatory directives. On Feb. 12, 1981, Labor Secretary Donovan withdrew a major rule requiring the labeling of hazardous chemicals in the workplace. The rule had been a major source of confrontation between labor and business. The administration also indicated its intention to change some environmental and health rules such as the Interior Department's surface mining regulations and the Labor Department's general rules governing chemical carcinogens. Under review were federal programs for the handicapped and OSHA noise control policies. Under consideration as well were proposals to reduce and streamline regulations for approval of new drugs.

On March 25 Bush announced that 63 health, energy, environmental and other rules would be modified or canceled, including 36 Carter administration "midnight" regulations frozen in January. The other 27 were existing regulations that eventually could be modified. Then, on April 6, Bush announced the administration planned to ease, drop or postpone an additional 34 environmental and safety rules for automobiles and trucks.

A prime target for review was the Department of Health and Human Services (HHS), which issues about 500 rules a year (most of them related to actions of the Food and Drug Administration and the Health Care Financing Administration). "Overzealous interpretation of statute and legislative intent by government regulators was a major frustration for me and many of my Senate colleagues," said HHS Secretary Richard S. Schweiker, former ranking Republican on the Labor and Human Resources Committee. "In my new role [as secretary], I can now zero in on those programs which have been tinkered and tampered with to the point they exceed the law itself."

Another target for reform was the Consumer Product Safety Commission, which was up for reauthorization in 1981. The administration wanted to shift the agency's focus from setting rules and standards to providing education and information.

One major test of the administration's commitment to, and congressional support for, cost-benefit analysis would come with revision of the Clean Air Act, due to expire Sept. 30, 1981. The act would be reviewed against the backdrop of a troubled economy and amidst arguments that the law causes unemployment, industrial stagnation and hampers the development of domestic energy. A November 1980 report by the Business Roundtable, which contended that the law cost industry $400 billion since 1970, recommended applying cost-benefit analysis in developing future clean air standards. Existing law required health standards to be set without regard to costs.

"As I look at our agenda for the rest of the year [1981], I see the hearings on Clean Air Act revision looming very large," said Weidenbaum. "Substantively that is going to be an important event for the future direction of all safety, health and environmental regulation, because many of the major questions that are common to all regulation in those areas will be met in developing proposals for the Clean Air Act."

Legislating Reform

While a great deal of reform can be accomplished administratively through executive orders and the appointment of sympathetic individuals to important positions, it takes legislation to make orders permanent and to institute government-wide reforms.

A Reagan administration budget fact sheet said: "Not all of our regulatory problems can be solved satisfactorily through more effective regulatory management and decisionmaking. Statutory constraints often preclude effective regulatory decisions." The administration pointed out that many laws were conflicting, overlapping or inconsistent.

According to Gray, the vice president's counsel, the administration could live with a reform proposal introduced by Sen. Paul Laxalt, R-Nev., a close Reagan adviser and chairman of the Judiciary Regulatory Reform Subcommittee. But Gray and other administration spokesmen said they were worried that Congress would place new demands on regulators that could interfere with the White House's efforts to reform the system through executive orders. The administration was concerned that the cost-benefit restrictions in the Laxalt bill might end up being stricter than those Reagan had imposed. Executive branch officials indicated they might want to waive cost-benefit analyses in some cases to speed up deregulation. They also feared that there would be amendments to allow one chamber of Congress to veto the actions and regulations of executive agencies. OMB's Miller said he was concerned that Congress might pay too much attention to a regulatory reform bill and not enough to revising basic statutes, such as the Clean Air Act.

A draft version of the Laxalt bill would force agencies to measure the costs and benefits of each proposed major rule, but it would not require them to choose the least costly option if they could justify the need for a more expensive approach. Outside parties would not be able to challenge a rule in court simply because they did not like the way the cost-benefit tests were performed. The entire rule would have to be found arbitrary or capricious before it could be overturned. In addition, agencies would have to review their rules every 10 years, subjecting those they wanted to amend or drop to new cost-benefit tests.

The Laxalt bill also contained the so-called Bumpers provision, named after Sen. Dale Bumpers, D-Ark., who unsuccessfully offered it as an amendment to other regulatory reform legislation in 1980. It would strengthen court review of agency decisionmaking.

In the House, Rep. Danielson introduced a bill similar to one reported by the Judiciary Committee in 1980. It differed from the Senate draft in that it lacked a strict cost-benefit provision. Instead, it would require regulators to perform a two-step economic review of proposed regulations. Regulators would have to state why a rule was needed, provide an analysis of its benefits and its "adverse economic effects" and explain why a rule with a less adverse effect was not chosen.

The bill would require agencies to review rules every 10 years and measure their economic impact, but it would not require them to kill burdensome rules. The measure also contained a two-house legislative veto requiring the president's signature. Like the Senate bill, Danielson's measure contained a Bumpers provision.

Prospects for Change

As of late 1981 the outlook for congressional action on comprehensive regulatory reform was uncertain. The administration had misgivings about some of the features of the various bills under consideration, and it was joined by labor, consumer and environmental groups, who opposed in particular the legislative veto, expanded court powers and strict cost-benefit analyses. The groups parted company with the administration on other issues, however, and were fighting its efforts to weaken or roll back health, safety and environment regulations.

A number of scholars also were questioning some of the proposals being aired on Capitol Hill. Among them was Antonin Scalia, co-editor of *Regulation,* who warned that "the imposition of new procedural impediments [by Congress] can only succeed, during the Reagan administration, in preserving the administrative decisions of the past."

In particular, Scalia was critical of legislative veto proposals and a statutory cost-benefit analysis requirement. Such "executive enfeebling measures," he wrote, "do not specifically deter regulation. What they deter is change. Imposed upon a regulation-prone executive, they will on balance slow the increase of regulation; but imposed upon an executive that is seeking to dissolve the encrusted regulation of past decades, they will impede the dissolution."

But administration officials were confident that their approach would cut miles of red tape and benefit business and the public alike. "What the president is attempting to do in this area," said Vice President Bush, "is find a balance between safety in the workplace and environmental protection and, at the same time, eliminate from our economy unneeded regulations so that we can grow and increase our nation's productive capacity."

Environment and Health

Chronology of Legislation, 1970-1980

1970

The first year of what has been called the environmental decade witnessed several important federal actions related to environmental health. In a symbolic gesture emphasizing the importance of the environment, President Richard Nixon signed the National Environmental Policy Act Jan. 1 as his first official act of 1970. The act, which Congress had cleared the preceding December, made environmental protection a matter of national policy.

In February Nixon sent Congress a major environmental message outlining a 37-point program of legislative and administrative actions. What was needed, he said, was "total mobilization" to clean up the environment. And in July Nixon sent Congress a reorganization plan establishing an independent Environmental Protection Agency. The new agency, which came into being Dec. 2, consolidated major anti-pollution programs that previously were scattered throughout the government.

Congress also was busy, passing three bills that formed much of the modern foundation of the federal government's effort to protect the health of the environment and its inhabitants. The Clean Air Amendments of 1970 established specific deadlines for a 90 percent reduction of certain pollutants from new automobiles and established controls on emission of pollutants by new factories and other stationary sources of air pollution. Passage of that bill came even though the auto industry claimed it could not meet the deadlines in the bill. Those deadlines were also opposed by the Nixon administration.

The federal government was also authorized to enter most American workplaces to assure their health and safety. The Occupational Safety and Health Act, which was to become one of the most controversial laws enacted during the decade, authorized the secretary of labor to set and enforce safety and health standards for some 55 million workers.

The Water Quality Improvement Act set liability for cleanup costs of oil spills. Related legislation to help communities build water sewage treatment plants did not get out of committee in either chamber.

The Resources Recovery Act of 1970 contained a three-year, $463 million authorization for solid waste disposal. The measure gave greater emphasis than existing federal programs to the recycling and recovery of materials from solid wastes.

Other environmental health laws passed by Congress in 1970 banned advertisement of cigarettes on radio and television and sought to eliminate the causes of lead-based paint poisoning.

Clean Air Act

Responding to growing public concern about the declining quality of the nation's air, Congress Dec. 18, 1970, completed action on a landmark air pollution control bill. The $1.1 billion, three-year program (HR 17255 — PL 91-604) set specific deadlines for the reduction of certain hazardous automobile emissions, established air quality standards for other air pollutants and gave the Environmental Protection Agency (EPA) and the states tools to enforce compliance with those standards. The goal was to clean up the nation's air in the 1970s.

President Nixon signed the bill Dec. 31 despite his opposition to one set of its provisions. The administration and the automobile industry had both exerted pressure on Congress to allow the EPA to set deadlines for cleaning up harmful exhaust fumes emitted by new model cars. Instead, Congress decided to write those deadlines into the law.

PL 91-604 required that model-year 1975 cars emit 90 percent less carbon monoxide and hydrocarbons than did model-year 1970 cars. It also specified that nitrogen oxide emissions from 1976 model cars be reduced by 90 percent compared with model-year 1971 levels. The law permitted the EPA administrator to grant a one-year extension, which he did in 1973. *(Box, p. 137)*

Other provisions of the bill as cleared included establishment of new research programs and assistance to the states to set up pollution control programs. The legislation put controls on emissions by new stationary sources of pollution and established new anti-pollution regulations for auto fuels and for aircraft engines and fuels.

The final version of the bill was much closer to the original Senate bill than it was to the far weaker House version.

The House bill contained no deadline by which automobile manufacturers had to reduce auto emissions, had weaker requirements for testing new cars and controlling vehicle fuels, and authorized lower funding for research and other activities.

'Earth Day'

Observance of "Earth Day" in 1970 by millions of Americans marked the peak of national harmony on environmental issues. Celebrated April 22, the day was devoted to study and protest of environmental problems, including several large rallies in New York City and Washington, D.C., environmental "teach-ins" and various community cleanup projects.

Congress adjourned for the day as at least 23 senators and 15 representatives spoke on environmental issues at gatherings across the nation.

President Nixon took no formal role in the proceedings, but a White House spokesman released a statement saying the president "feels the activities show the concern of people of all walks of life over the dangers to our environment."

The effort, originally suggested by Sen. Gaylord Nelson, D-Wis., was designed to focus national attention on environmental problems, just as the 1969 demonstrations against the Vietnam War sharpened public opinion on that issue. Nelson and Rep. Paul N. McCloskey Jr., R-Calif., sponsored a group, the Environmental Teach-In, formed early in 1970 to organize Earth Day activities. The group estimated that at least 2,000 colleges, 10,000 primary and secondary schools and 2,000 communities undertook Earth Day observances.

Earth Day was lengthened to Earth Week by presidential proclamation in 1971 and again in 1972. But enthusiasm for "save the earth" activities dwindled each year as the public began to question the economic costs of cleaning up the environment.

Background

Most air is contained in the first 2,000 feet of the troposphere. Since man discovered fire — and began polluting the air — this shallow layer of air surrounding the earth had become a giant wastebasket for the byproducts of massive combustion. With the coming of the industrial age, the problem was compounded by factories spewing hazardous substances into the air.

According to scientists, the atmosphere had a natural self-cleansing process that operated as long as there was enough time and space allowed. But scientists warned that humans had not been permitting nature sufficient time to catch its breath between assaults on the purity of the air. It would be a mistake, they claimed, not to take the air pollution problem seriously. Some said it would be fatal.

Pollution Sources. Air polluters were divided into two categories — stationary (factories) and mobile (automobiles and other vehicles). Each year the stationary polluters were discharging two million tons of carbon monoxide, nine million tons of sulfur oxides, two million tons of nitrogen oxides, four million tons of hydrocarbons and six million tons of particulate matter into the air.

The big three industrial polluters were petroleum refineries (4.2 million tons of pollutants), smelters (4.15 million tons) and iron foundries (3.7 million tons). Power plants and the heating systems used in homes were also high on the list of stationary polluters.

Mobile polluters composed the largest single contributor to pollution in the atmosphere. Exhaust from cars, trucks and buses spewed about 90 million tons of contaminants into the atmosphere every year — about 60 percent of the total air pollution.

Previous Legislation. The federal government became involved in the problems of air pollution just after the Korean War. The first congressional action came in 1955 with the passage of a bill (PL 84-159) that authorized the Public Health Service to conduct air pollution research. The $5 million authorized by the act was to cover expenses for fiscal years 1956-60.

The Clean Air Act of 1963 (PL 88-206) increased air pollution authorizations to $95 million for fiscal years 1964-67 and provided for a series of steps — culminating in legal action — that states, municipalities and the federal government could take to end interstate and intrastate air pollution (although for intrastate pollution the federal government could act only at the request of the state's governor).

A second title (PL 89-272) was added to the Clean Air Act in 1965 directing the secretary of Health, Education and Welfare (HEW) to establish emission standards for new motor vehicles. The first standards for hydrocarbon and carbon monoxide exhaust emissions were published in 1966 and were applicable to most new gas-powered motor vehicles beginning with the model-year 1968.

Legislation enacted in 1967 (PL 90-148) substantially strengthened the powers of local, state and federal authorities. It authorized the HEW secretary to designate air quality regions throughout the country; provided full federal financing for regional control commissions to be established by state governors; and empowered the HEW secretary to enforce air quality standards in the control regions if the states failed to adopt such standards and an acceptable pollution abatement plan within 15 months after receiving federal guidelines on air purity. The act also empowered the HEW secretary to go to court to prosecute violations of standards in an air quality region after 180 days' notice of violation. By the end of 1970 no state had full-scale standards and implementation plans in effect for any pollutants.

Provisions

As signed by the president Dec. 31, the Clean Air Act Amendments of 1970 (HR 17255 — PL 91-604) contained the following major provisions:

Air Quality Standards

- Required the EPA administrator to publish a list of air pollution agents for which air quality criteria would be issued; the first such list had to be published within 30 days of enactment of the bill. Specific criteria had to be issued within 12 months after the pollutants were designated.
- Required the administration to publish national primary and secondary ambient (average) air quality standards for each agent already cited as a pollutant when the

bill went into effect. For other pollution agents, the administrator had to publish national standards at the same time pollutants were designated. (Primary standards specified the minimum air quality needed to protect public health and secondary standards promoted public welfare.) The administrator had to promulgate primary air quality standards; states had to devise plans for secondary standards.

• Authorized the administrator to specify and set emission standards for hazardous air pollutants — those having a proven relationship to increased human death rates or serious illness. The administrator could grant waivers of up to two years for compliance with the standards. The president also was authorized to grant such waivers if he found technology did not exist or if national security required such action. States had the primary responsibility for enforcing the regulations.

• Required the administrator to publish periodically, starting within 90 days of enactment of the bill, lists of the categories of new stationary pollution sources and set emission standards. The administrator could formulate or enforce plans where states failed to act.

• Required the administrator to emphasize research on the effects of air pollution agents, singly and in combinations, on public health and welfare.

State Implementation Plans

• Required each state, after public hearings, to adopt plans for implementing, maintaining and enforcing the standards and goals promulgated for each air control region, or portion of a region, within that state. Such plans had to be submitted to the federal government within nine months after the standards and goals were promulgated and were to be approved or disapproved within four months. The administrator could approve the plan if it provided for attainment of primary air quality standards in three years; included emission requirements and schedules of compliance; included provisions for monitoring devices; included effective procedures to control new pollution sources; provided for inter-governmental cooperation; provided that each state would have adequate personnel, funding and authority to enforce the plan; and provided for periodic inspection and testing of motor vehicles. The administrator could grant extensions of up to 18 months for submission of plans, and up to three years for implementation of plans.

• Authorized the administrator to formulate plans for states that did not submit plans or that submitted plans which were not approved; the administrator could also provide for hearings if the states made no such provisions and he could require the revision of already approved plans if he later found them to be inadequate.

• Required each state to be responsible for air quality within its boundaries. Existing interstate and intrastate air quality control regions were maintained; the administrator was directed to designate other control regions within 90 days.

• Authorized the EPA to provide up to two-thirds of the planning costs and up to half of the operating costs of establishing or improving air quality control programs serving a single municipality, or up to 75 percent of planning costs and 60 percent of operating costs for programs serving two or more municipalities. Part of these grants could be in the form of technical aid provided by federal personnel.

• Authorized the EPA to provide 100 percent of costs for two years, and 75 percent of costs thereafter, for implementation plans for interstate air quality control regions.

Automobile and Fuel Regulations

• Authorized the administrator to set emission standards for all potentially dangerous pollutants from new motor vehicles and engines.

• Required that engines of automobiles and other light duty vehicles, beginning with model-year 1975, had to comply with standards lowering emissions of carbon monoxide and hydrocarbons by 90 percent compared with the model-year 1970 levels; and by model-year 1976 with standards lowering emissions of nitrogen oxide by 90 percent compared with the model-year 1971 level. The administrator had to report annually to Congress on matters relevant to control systems.

• Permitted manufacturers to apply for one-year extensions of the carbon monoxide and hydrocarbon deadlines after Jan. 1, 1972, and for the nitrogen oxide deadline after Jan. 1, 1973. The administrator had to act on the requests within 60 days; if he granted the requests, he was required to establish interim standards at the same time. The National Academy of Sciences was authorized to study the technological feasibility of meeting the standards.

• Required passenger car pollution control standards to be effective for five years or 50,000 miles, whichever was less, according to regulations set by the administrator. He could also set standards for other types of vehicles and engines.

• Prohibited the sale of new cars or engines not in compliance with standards; prohibited the removal of pollution

Auto Deadline Extended

In April 1973 Environmental Protection Agency Administrator William D. Ruckelshaus used his authority under the 1970 Clean Air Act Amendments to grant the auto industry's request for a one-year extension of the 1975 deadline for compliance with strict emission standards for carbon monoxide and hydrocarbons. Several weeks later on July 30 he announced a one-year extension of the 1976 deadline for a third auto pollutant, nitrogen oxide.

Interim standards stricter than the industry wanted were imposed in every state but California, where tougher standards were permitted. California suffered from a severe auto pollution problem.

Ruckelshaus, who had turned down several earlier industry requests for delays in the 1975 deadline, finally relented after the auto companies warned that they could not install pollution control devices in time to meet the deadlines imposed by the 1970 law and thus would be forced to shut down.

control devices. Violations would be subject to a civil penalty of up to $10,000.

• Required the administrator to conduct tests on new vehicles or engines submitted by manufacturers or new pollution abatement devices and to issue one-year certifications of conformity. The administrator also could perform assembly line tests and suspend or revoke certification of non-conforming vehicles manufactured after that date or produced prior to that date and still in the manufacturer's possession. The suspension would continue until conformity was again achieved. EPA employees could inspect plants and records.

• Required warranties for pollution abatement equipment, under standards set by the administrator, that would cover all purchasers and would require the manufacturer to bear costs of repairs to achieve compliance. After a vehicle had been sold, an inspection of its pollution abatement devices could be made only with the owner's permission.

• Authorized the administrator to control or prohibit sale of any fuel or fuel additive if the emissions from it would endanger public health or interfere with passenger cars' pollution control devices. The administrator had to take into account technical and cost factors. No state could implement regulations regarding fuels that were stricter than federal levels unless such regulations were part of its air quality plan. Civil penalties were set at $10,000 per day.

• Authorized the administrator to grant states up to two-thirds of the cost of developing and maintaining effective vehicle inspection programs and emission testing and control programs.

• Established a federal low-emission vehicle procurement program in the federal government. The government was authorized to purchase any vehicles certified to be low-polluting at a premium price of up to 150 percent of the lowest cost of conventional car models that they were replacing. The premium could be raised to 200 percent for especially innovative cars. The bill authorized $5 million for fiscal 1971 and $25 million annually for fiscal 1972 and 1973.

• Authorized the administrator to encourage research on air pollution in relation to fuels and low-emission alternatives to the existing internal combustion engine with authorizations of $75 million for 1971; $125 million for fiscal 1972 and $150 million for fiscal 1973.

• Authorized the administrator to seek injunctions to stop pollution sources that endangered public health if local or state authorities had not acted to seek abatement.

• Authorized citizens or groups to bring suits in federal courts against either the administrator — for failure to perform specified duties — or alleged violators, including government agencies.

• Authorized the attorney general to go to court to require that the owner of any patent relating to emission limitations make the information available to any person who needed it in order to comply with standards set by the bill. The court would determine payments to the patent owners.

• Set punishments for violations of implementation plans. The administrator was required to give prior notification to both the person violating the plans and the state in which the violation occurred. If corrective action was not taken, he could issue an order requiring compliance or bring civil suits against the violator. A person who knowingly violated an implementation plan or an abatement order could be punished by a fine of up to $25,000 for each day of violation and a year in prison, or up to $50,000 per day and two years in prison for persons with previous violations. Anyone convicted of falsifying information or tampering with monitoring devices was subject to a fine of up to $10,000 and six months in prison.

Aircraft

• Required the administrator, following a study and hearings, to formulate standards for aircraft emissions. The secretary of transportation was to help formulate the standards and enforce them. States could not implement standards more stringent than those set by the federal government. The administrator of the Federal Aviation Administration had to set aviation fuel standards, following consultation with the EPA administrator.

Noise Pollution

• Established within the EPA a new Office of Noise Abatement and Control to study noise pollution and its effect on the public health and welfare. The office would be authorized to look into problems associated with all types of noise, including sonic booms. One year after enactment of the bill, the administrator would be required to report on the study to the president and Congress and to request new legislation. The bill authorized $30 million for the noise program.

Funds

• Authorized for carrying out provisions of the act other than those specified above: fiscal 1971, $125 million; fiscal 1972, $225 million; and fiscal 1973, $300 million.

Solid Waste Management

Increased concern for environmental protection prompted Congress in 1970 to shift the focus of federal solid waste programs to the recovery and reuse of resources and energy from the materials discarded by society. Most earlier federal efforts had concentrated on the disposal of solid wastes.

Congress Oct. 13 sent to the president a three-year $462.75 million extension (HR 11833 — PL 91-512) of federal solid waste disposal programs. The new legislation, the Resources Recovery Act of 1970, set up a program of demonstration and construction grants for innovative solid waste management systems, provided technical and financial assistance to state and local agencies in planning and developing resource recovery and waste disposal systems and established major research programs to develop methods of dealing with solid wastes.

HR 11833 also established a two-year, $2 million study by a new National Commission on Materials Policy.

HR 11833 provided that all solid waste programs administered by the Department of Health, Education and Welfare (HEW) would be transferred to the Environmental Protection Agency after it was set up Dec. 2, 1970.

Background

Congress in 1965 passed the Solid Waste Disposal Act (PL 89-272) to begin a national research and development program for improved methods of solid waste disposal and to provide technical and financial aid to state and local governments in developing, establishing and conducting solid waste disposal programs.

The 1965 law authorized up to 50 percent of the cost of state or interstate surveys of disposal practices and grants for demonstration projects, including up to two-thirds of a project's construction costs. Responsibility for the program was split between HEW and the Interior Department. Interior had responsibility for solid waste resulting from mineral or fossil fuels; HEW had jurisdiction over all other aspects.

In 1968 Congress extended the act through fiscal 1970 (PL 90-574).

On April 10, 1970, President Nixon sent a message to Congress urging legislators to redirect federal solid waste efforts toward reducing the amount of waste created and recycling waste materials.

Nixon signed HR 11833 Oct. 26, although he expressed some concern about the spending levels in the bill. The measure authorized substantially more federal spending for solid waste programs than Nixon had requested in his fiscal 1971 budget.

Provisions

Major provisions of HR 11833, the Resource Recovery Act of 1970:

- Directed the secretary of HEW to promote research on health and welfare effects of waste, operation and financing of solid waste disposal programs, reduction of the amount of waste, and development and application of better methods of collecting and disposing of solid waste and of processing and recovering materials and energy from solid wastes and components of solid waste.
- Directed the secretary of HEW to conduct studies on economic means of recovering useful materials from solid waste; uses of such materials and the market impact of such recovery; appropriate incentive programs, including tax incentives, to aid in solid waste disposal; reasonable changes in existing production and packaging methods to reduce the amount of solid waste; waste collection and containerization; and proposals for imposing disposal charges.

The secretary was to report annually on such studies to the president and Congress.

- Authorized the HEW Department to establish demonstration projects or techniques developed through its special studies.
- Authorized planning grants of up to two-thirds of the cost for single municipalities and three-quarters of the cost for other areas, for making surveys of solid waste problems, preparing solid waste disposal plans (with emphasis on recycling wastes), developing proposals for pilot projects and planning programs for collecting and processing abandoned vehicle hulks.
- Authorized grants to public agencies for demonstration of resource recovery systems or construction of innovative solid waste disposal facilities. The federal share of demonstration grants would be 75 percent; the federal share of construction grants would be 50 percent if the project served only a single municipality and 75 percent in other cases. Federal funds would be used only for design and construction, plus first-year operation and maintenance costs in the case of demonstration grants. Funds could not be used for land acquisition. No more than 15 percent of the annual authorization could be used in any one state.
- Authorized the secretary of HEW, as soon as practicable, to formulate guidelines for solid waste recovery, collection, separation and disposal systems, as well as model codes and ordinances.
- Authorized $41.5 million for all HEW solid waste programs for fiscal 1971.
- Authorized for HEW demonstration and construction grants: fiscal 1972, $80 million; fiscal 1973, $140 million. For other HEW programs (including research): fiscal 1972, $72 million; fiscal 1973; $76 million.
- Authorized for Interior Department solid waste programs: fiscal 1971, $8.75 million; fiscal 1972, $20 million; fiscal 1973, $22.5 million.
- Created a seven-member National Commission on Materials Policy to develop by June 30, 1973, a national waste materials policy.

The commission would study national and international materials requirements, the relationship of materials policy to population and environmental quality, means of using more materials that could be recycled or reused or that would self-destruct and means of improving and coordinating information on materials usage. The bill authorized $2 million for the study.

NEPA Signing Begins Environmental Decade

As his first official act of the new decade, President Nixon Jan. 1, 1970, signed into law the National Environmental Policy Act of 1969 (NEPA).

Approved by Congress Dec. 22, 1969, the landmark legislation declared that it was the federal government's continuing policy "to use all practicable means and measures, including financial and technical assistance, in a manner calculated to foster and promote the general welfare, to create and maintain conditions under which man and nature can exist in productive harmony, and fulfill the social, economic, and other requirements of present and future generations of America."

In what was to become the most far-reaching — and controversial — provision of the new law, the bill directed federal agencies to consider the impact on the environment of all major activities and to include in every recommendation an analysis of that effect and alternatives to the proposal.

The bill also set up a three-man Council on Environmental Quality to advise the president and Congress on environmental matters. The first three members appointed to that council were: Under Secretary of the Interior Russell E. Train, former head of the Conservation Foundation, chairman; Robert Cahn, an environmental reporter for the *Christian Science Monitor*; and Gordon J. F. MacDonald, vice chancellor of the University of California at Santa Barbara.

Water Quality Improvement

After a five-month deadlock between House and Senate conferees, Congress March 25 approved a major water pollution control bill (HR 4148 — PL 91-224) to help clean up the nation's waterways. The Water Quality Improvement Act of 1970, aimed primarily at oil spills, was signed into law April 3 by President Nixon.

In addition to making petroleum companies liable for up to $14 million in cleanup costs for oil spills. HR 4148 also outlawed the flushing of raw sewage from boat toilets, strengthened restrictions on thermal pollution from nuclear power plants and ordered development of criteria covering the effects of pesticides in streams, rivers and other waters.

The bill also created an Office of Environmental Quality to act as a staff for the president's Council on Environmental Quality. The council had been established in 1970 to advise the president and Congress on environmental issues.

Provisions

As signed into law April 3, HR 4148:

- Declared it to be U.S. policy that there should be no oil discharges into navigable waters of the United States or adjoining shorelines.
- Authorized the president to act to remove an oil spill unless properly done by the owner or operator responsible for the spill.
- Established a liability to the United States for an oil spill of up to $100 per gross ton of oil or $14 million, whichever was lower, for a vessel and $8 million for an onshore or offshore facility unless the spill resulted from an act of God, war, U.S. government negligence or an act or omission of a third party.
- Established unlimited liability if an oil spill resulted from willful negligence or misconduct.
- Authorized the president to designate those discharges, other than oil, that constituted dangerous substances and to clean up such substances, unless accomplished immediately by an owner or operator of a vessel or onshore or offshore facility.
- Provided means for the establishment of federal standards for marine sanitation devices to prevent discharge of untreated sewage into navigable waters of the United States.
- Authorized the federal government to enter into agreements with states or other political subdivisions or agencies to carry out demonstration projects on new methods and techniques for the elimination or control of pollution within the watersheds of the Great Lakes.
- Required compliance with water quality standards and the purposes of the act by all federal agencies and departments engaged in public works activities of any kind.
- Required any applicant for a federal license or permit involving the construction or operation of facilities that could result in the discharge of substances into navigable waters to obtain a certification from the state in which the discharge would originate stating that there was reasonable assurance that such activity would not violate water quality standards.
- Established in the Executive Office of the President an Office of Environmental Quality, to be directed by the chairman of the Council on Environmental Quality.

EPA Created

Heightened concern for the safety of the environment resulted in the creation of the independent Environmental Protection Agency (EPA) in 1970.

Under the reorganization plan to create the agency, which President Nixon submitted to Congress in July, all major federal programs to combat pollution would be consolidated under the jurisdiction of the new agency. Offices and programs transferred to EPA included the Federal Water Quality Administration and certain other pesticide research programs formerly in the Interior Department; the National Air Pollution Control Administration, and divisions of the Environmental Control Administration and Food and Drug Administration, formerly in the Department of Health, Education and Welfare; the pesticides registration authority of the Department of Agriculture; the environmental standard-setting function of the Atomic Energy Commission; the functions of the Federal Radiation Council and certain research authority of the Council on Environmental Quality.

The reorganization plan took effect when Congress failed to pass a resolution vetoing it. The House defeated a veto resolution by voice vote. A veto resolution was not even considered in the Senate.

The first EPA administrator was William D. Ruckelshaus, an assistant attorney general in the Justice Department's civil division at the time of his appointment. The Senate confirmed Ruckelshaus Dec. 2, 1970.

Water Pollution

Neither the House nor the Senate Public Works committees completed action in 1970 on water pollution legislation intended to aid communities building water sewage treatment plants. Bills under consideration — including an administration proposal — would have increased aid to communities for construction of facilities, streamlined existing programs and strengthened enforcement. The existing authorizations for water pollution programs were to expire June 30, 1971. A comprehensive water pollution control bill was approved in 1972. *(Story, p. 145)*

In related action, President Nixon Aug. 11 vetoed the first fiscal 1971 appropriations bill (HR 17548) for the Department of Housing and Urban Development (HUD), in part because it contained $500 million — $350 million more than his budget request — for HUD's basic water and sewer facilities grants. Nixon signed a second bill (HR 19830 — PL 91-556) that appropriated $350 million for the program.

Nuclear Licensing

Congress in December 1970 cleared a bill (HR 18679 — PL 91-560) requiring the Atomic Energy Commission (AEC) to regard nuclear power plants as profit-making commercial ventures subject to licensing in accordance with the competitive criteria of federal antitrust laws. A controversial provision that effectively would have stripped from the Environmental Protection Agency its newly acquired authority to set radiation standards was deleted prior to final passage of the bill.

As cleared by Congress, PL 91-560 eliminated from the Atomic Energy Act of 1954 the provision that required the AEC to find a "practical value" before licensing a plant for commercial or industrial purposes.

Lead Paint Poisoning

Congress Dec. 31, 1970, cleared a bill (HR 19172 — PL 91-695) authorizing $30 million over fiscal years 1971-73 to eliminate the causes and incidence of lead-based paint poisoning.

The bill authorized: $5.01 million for the secretary of Housing and Urban Development (HUD) to determine the extent of lead paint poisoning and methods by which the paint could be removed from residential housing; $15 million for grants to local governments to eliminate lead-based paint hazards and $9.99 million to assist local governments to detect and treat lead paint poisoning.

Cigarette Advertising Ban

Congress March 19, 1970, ended six years of controversy over federal government efforts to regulate or prohibit cigarette advertising by clearing legislation (HR 6543 — PL 91-222) banning all cigarette commercials on radio and television or on any other medium of electronic communication subject to the jurisdiction of the Federal Communications Commission. The ban was effective Jan. 2, 1971.

The bill was passed 13 months after HR 6543 was introduced in 1969 with the intention of extending a provision of the Cigarette Labeling and Advertising Act of 1965 (PL 89-92) that prohibited any federal, state or local government from requiring health warnings in cigarette advertising.

The Senate and House had passed differing versions of HR 6543 in 1969. The Senate measure banned cigarette advertising on radio and television and strengthened the warning on cigarette packages. The House version contained no reference to advertising on radio and television and provided a weaker label warning. The final version differed only slightly from the Senate version of the bill.

As signed into law, HR 6543 (PL 91-222):

- Made it unlawful to advertise cigarettes on radio or television beginning Jan. 2, 1971.
- Changed the mandatory wording on cigarette packages from: "Caution: Cigarette Smoking May Be Hazardous to Your Health" to: "Warning: The Surgeon General Has Determined That Cigarette Smoking Is Dangerous To Your Health."
- Prohibited any affirmative action by the Federal Trade Commission (FTC) on printed cigarette advertising until July 1, 1971, and outlined the steps for congressional approval that would have to occur before the FTC could issue any health-related regulation of such advertising.
- Prohibited all state and local health-related regulation or prohibition of cigarette advertising.

Occupational Safety

Congress in 1970 completed action on the Occupational Safety and Health Act (S 2193 — PL 91-596) to establish a comprehensive on-the-job safety program for about 55 million industrial, farm and construction workers employed by firms engaged in interstate commerce.

Labor had sought the legislation because most workers complained that state safety and health agencies were failing to cope adequately with the problem of occupational deaths, injuries and illnesses. The law allowed random inspections of work places to be made without warning and required immediate penalties for violations of the federal regulations. These "first-instance sanctions" were intended to prod employers into complying before they were inspected.

Background

PL 91-596 was the first comprehensive safety and health act Congress ever enacted. Prior to that legislation, laws in the job-safety field were a specialized few: the Walsh-Healey Act of 1936, which established certain safety criteria for workers on federal contracts; the Longshoremen's and Harbor Workers' Act amendment of 1958, which required employers to maintain safe conditions; mine safety laws enacted in 1941, 1947, 1952 and 1969; and a construction safety law enacted in 1969.

In 1968 President Lyndon B. Johnson proposed an occupational safety and health bill that would have given the secretary of labor power to set and enforce federal standards. Johnson said the federal government offered the worker only a "patchwork of obsolete and ineffective laws."

The Johnson proposal met strong resistance from business groups, Republicans and conservative Democrats, and it was never enacted.

In 1969 President Richard Nixon asked Congress to establish a National Occupational Safety and Health Board with the power to set standards for the protection of most of the nation's workers. To encourage the states to submit plans for expanding and improving their own occupational safety and health programs, the president said that federal standards would not take effect in states where a plan was at least as strong as a federal standard.

The Nixon plan was supported by most employers and the House, but labor and liberal Democrats were able to convince the Senate to enact a far stronger bill. The Senate version prevailed in conference.

Provisions

To guarantee workers' safety and health, PL 91-596 set up three separate agencies:

- The Occupational Safety and Health Administration (OSHA) within the Department of Labor to promulgate health and safety standards and to enforce those regulations.

- An independent, three-member board, the Occupational Safety and Health Review Commission (OSHRC), to rule on penalties issued by OSHA inspectors and challenged by employers.
- The National Institute of Occupational Safety and Health (NIOSH) within the Department of Health, Education and Welfare to prepare the research for establishing safety standards.

Enforcement

To enforce the standards, the act authorized OSHA inspectors to visit work places without prior notice. Inspections would be made in the event of an accident, if an employee filed a valid complaint or by random selection.

For each violation of a safety or health regulation found, the inspector was required to issue a citation and propose a penalty. The citation was to be posted at the site of the violation until the violation was corrected or for three days, whichever was longer. The act specified that an employee representative, as well as the employer, could accompany the OSHA inspector during his tour.

Citations could be issued for four categories of safety or health hazards:

- *De minimus* violations were those that had no direct bearing on the health or safety of the worker.
- Non-serious violations, defined as conditions that related to job safety but probably would not cause serious injury or death, carried discretionary penalties of up to $1,000.
- A serious violation, one in which there was a substantial probability that death or serious injury could result, carried a mandatory penalty of up to $1,000.
- A violation posing an imminent danger to employees was to be abated immediately. If it was not, the inspector could seek compliance through the courts. Willful or repeated violations carried a penalty of up to $10,000 or six months in prison.

Employers also could be cited for other violations of the OSHA regulations, including failure to post a citation, failure to maintain certain records required by OSHA and failure to report an accident or fatality.

Employers could apply to OSHA for a variance from a specific health or safety regulation if they could prove that the facility or procedure was at least as effective as that covered by the standard. Small businesses could apply for long-term loans from the Small Business Administration to offset any financial difficulty resulting from compliance with OSHA standards.

Businesses could consult with OSHA personnel to ascertain measures necessary to come into compliance with the standards but the consulting could not be done at the place of business.

Review Commission

If a business wanted to challenge a citation or contest a penalty, it had 15 days from the time it received the citation to appeal to OSHRC. An administrative law judge would conduct an investigation and then issue his opinion, which could be appealed to the review commission itself. If a citation was not contested within 15 days, it was considered final.

An employer also could petition the review commission if he believed that the time stipulated for abatement of a hazard was unreasonable. Such petitions had to be filed before the abatement time expired.

State Standards

The law authorized the secretary of labor to approve state plans to develop and enforce safety and health standards if the secretary found the plans complied with the federal law. The legislation authorized federal grants for up to 90 percent of costs to states to identify needs, develop plans and improve administration and enforcement of standards; and it provided federal grants for up to 50 percent of costs to assist states in carrying out occupational safety and health standards.

1971

Congress in 1971 began work on several bills affecting environmental health but did not complete action on any of them. The bills encompassed water pollution control, pesticide regulation, ocean dumping and marine safety. Charges that the supersonic transport aircraft (SST) was potentially environmentally harmful also persuaded Congress to stop funding for federal participation in development of the SST.

Meanwhile there were signs that an ecological backlash was setting in, as the public began to weigh the costs of cleaning up the environment. President Nixon's public statements reflected that shift. In his "clean energy" message in June, Nixon stressed the importance of developing a safe fast-breeder nuclear reactor by 1980 and maintained that it was possible to "balance environmental and energy needs." On Aug. 6 he warned against seeking "ecological perfection at the cost of bankrupting the very taxpaying enterprises which pay for the social advance the nation seeks." And in another address a month later, Nixon declared that "we are not going to allow the environment issue . . . to destroy the industrial system that made this the great country it is."

Water Pollution

Legislation aimed at making the nation's waterways virtually pollution-free by 1985 and authorizing $16.8 billion to do the job passed the Senate unanimously in 1971.

The Senate bill (S 2770) increased dramatically the federal investment in construction of sewer treatment plants and required local governments to charge industrial users fees to pay for the treatment of their pollutants. It also required federal permits for discharging any wastes into navigable waters; industrial polluters would be required to install the most up-to-date abatement equipment available.

Shortly after Senate approval, the Nixon administration announced its opposition to the bill on the grounds it gave too much authority to the federal government and not enough to the states. The White House called upon the House Public Works Committee to reopen hearings on the measure. Those hearings were held shortly before Congress adjourned for the year and the committee did not file its report until 1972. Congress completed action on the measure in 1972. *(Story, p. 145)*

Existing federal water pollution control programs had expired June 30, but Congress passed two temporary extensions. A third extension was not enacted in 1971 and existing legislation technically expired Oct. 31.

Ocean Dumping

A bill (HR 9727) to control the dumping of waste material in the oceans passed both houses but was lodged in conference at the end of 1971. Congress completed action on the measure in the final week of the 1972 session. *(Story, p. 146)*

The major differences between the two versions concerned the definition of waters covered, the dumping of dredge material and designation of marine sanctuaries to be preserved for recreational, ecological and esthetic values.

Supersonic Transport

Environmental considerations were a key to Congress' refusal in 1971 to continue the federal government's participation in the construction of a supersonic transport plane (SST). The funding cutoff was a serious rebuff to the Nixon administration and the U.S. aviation industry.

Congressional termination of federal funds for the project had the effect of ending the U.S. SST operation for the foreseeable future because private financing of the aircraft seemed improbable.

The administration and aviation industry, supported by labor and regional interests, contended that continued federal support was necessary to maintain U.S. superiority in aerospace technology and marketing, to sustain a sound U.S. balance of payments and to avoid massive unemployment and deterioration in the aerospace industry.

But charges were levied that the fleet of SSTs could contaminate the atmosphere, generate harmful noise and even trigger a cancer-producing fallout. It was also argued that no market existed for the aircraft, that its only beneficiaries would be wealthy travelers and that federal funds should be directed instead toward more generally beneficial activities.

The House rejected the funding March 18 by a 217-204 vote. The Senate rejected it March 24 by a 51-46 vote.

By halting federal participation in the project, the congressional action resulted in the layoff of an estimated 7,000 employees at the Seattle plant of the Boeing Company, the main contractor. By 1971 the U.S. government had contributed about $840 million to the project and Boeing $125 million. The firm was working on two prototype aircraft to compete with the Anglo-French Concorde and the Soviet TU-144.

Marine Safety

Congress did not complete action on legislation to promote marine safety and protect the environment in harbors and navigable waters.

The House approved a bill (HR 8140) to establish federal controls in marine areas to reduce the increasing frequency of vessel accidents and to avoid pollution of ports, waterways and adjoining shorelines. The Senate took no action on the bill in 1971, but the measure cleared Congress in revised form in 1972.

Pesticide Regulation

Legislation regulating the manufacture, distribution and use of pesticides was approved by the House in 1971. But the Senate did not act until 1972, when Congress cleared the measure (HR 10792). *(1972 action, p. 148)*

Growing concern since the early 1960s over the effect of pesticides on humans, wildlife and the environment in general had produced pressure for stricter federal control over certification and the use of pesticides. Existing legislation, enacted in 1947, was primarily a labeling law.

1972

Passage of several major environment bills in 1972 gave the 92nd Congress an impressive record for acting to protect environmental health.

Major bills enacted set federal controls over water pollution, ocean dumping, coastal zones, noise and pesticides. Another bill significantly liberalized black lung benefits. The water pollution control measure was enacted over President Nixon's veto.

In other action, both chambers passed toxic chemicals control legislation, but the measure died when the House refused to accept a few late Senate changes. The Senate also passed a ban on the synthetic hormone diethylstilbestrol (DES), but the House did not take any action.

Noise Control

On the last day of the session, Congress set up the first comprehensive federal program aimed at curbing noise harmful to the human environment.

The Noise Control Act of 1972 (HR 11021 — PL 92-574) gave the federal government authority to set standards limiting certain commercial sources of noise, such as construction and transportation equipment, motors, engines and electric or electronic devices. It also directed the Environmental Protection Agency (EPA) to propose noise standards for aircraft but gave the Federal Aviation Commission (FAA) final authority to reject standards that it found unsafe or impractical.

Noise: Annoying and Dangerous

Research amassed by 1972 indicated that noise, which had increased markedly in previous years, was not only annoying but also harmful. Researchers were unanimous on one fact: noise caused hearing loss. Permanent damage occurred when a person was exposed to a sound level of 85 decibels (a decibel is a measure of sound) over a period of years, although that person was unlikely to notice the hearing impairment until it was too late to do anything about it.

While normal conversation occurred at about 60 decibels, heavy traffic operated at about 90 decibels, a riveting machine blasted away at 110 decibels and the noise level at a discotheque could reach 120 decibels. The threshold of pain was put variously at between 130 and 150 decibels.

Other research related noise to a variety of other ailments besides hearing loss, ranging from nervous tension headaches to neurosis. Doctors at the December 1969 meeting of the American Association for the Advancement of Science reported on experiments that indicated that noise:

- Caused blood vessels to constrict, cutting the flow of blood to key parts of the body.
- Affected the whole autonomous nervous system, which controlled the involuntary functions of the heart, blood vessels, muscles and glands.
- Could cause seizures in epileptics.
- Disturbed unborn children and might harm them.

An EPA report estimated that noise subjected about 40 million Americans to hearing damage or other mental or physical hazards and that up to 64 million people lived in homes that were affected by aircraft, traffic or construction noise.

Despite widespread discussion of the detrimental effects of noise, the only measures enacted by Congress prior to 1972 were a 1968 bill providing for aircraft noise abatement (PL 90-411) and a section of the Clean Air Amendments of 1970 (PL 91-604) that required EPA to conduct a study of noise.

Provisions

As signed into law, the Noise Control Act of 1972:

- Declared it national policy to protect the public health and welfare from detrimental noise, to coordinate federal research and activities in noise control, to set federal noise emission standards for commercial products and to provide information to the public.
- Exempted military combat weapons, rockets or experimental federal equipment from the act's requirements.
- Required the EPA administrator to issue within nine months of enactment noise criteria based on scientific knowledge; to publish within 12 months noise levels to protect public health, welfare and safety; and to identify within 18 months products that were major sources of noise and to give techniques for controlling their emissions.
- Required the administrator to set noise emission standards within 18 months for products distributed in interstate commerce designated as major noise sources, including construction and transportation equipment, motors, engines and electrical and electronic equipment.
- Required EPA standards to be based on the reduction in noise emissions achievable with the best available control technology, taking into account the cost of compliance.
- Required product manufacturers to warrant new products to conform to the federal regulations.
- Pre-empted state and local authority to set noise emission standards that would be enforceable against manufactured products; but allowed states to set and enforce limits on environmental noise through licensing, regulation or restriction on use.
- Directed the EPA administrator to report within nine months of enactment on the adequacy of FAA flight and operational noise controls, the adequacy of emission standards on new and existing aircraft (including recommendations for retrofitting engines and phasing out existing aircraft), cumulative airport noise exposure levels and other airport noise control measures.
- Required the FAA, after consultation with the EPA and the Transportation Department, to set or amend standards for measurement, control and abatement of aircraft noise and sonic booms.
- Required the EPA to submit to the FAA proposed regulations to control and reduce aircraft noise and sonic booms; required the FAA to begin proposed rule-making procedures within 30 days and to hold hearings within 60 days. Required FAA to approve, modify or reject EPA's proposed rules; however, if any EPA rules were rejected FAA would have to explain its reasons publicly and in detail; including information on safety, public interest, economics and technology; required all inter-agency communications to be printed in the *Federal Register.*
- Directed the EPA administrator to issue labeling requirements for products that emitted excessive noise or were intended to reduce noise.
- Required the secretary of the Treasury to regulate imported products for noise emissions.
- Required the administrator to issue, within nine months of enactment, noise emission standards for railroads and motor carriers (trucks and buses) in interstate commerce; gave the secretary of transportation authority to enforce these standards; allowed states to set higher standards or restrict movement if made necessary by special local conditions.
- Directed the EPA administrator to identify low-noise-emission products with the help of an advisory committee and to certify them for preferential use by federal agencies if the General Services Administration determined that their costs were not more than 125 percent of the retail price of the least expensive alternate product; authorized $1 million for fiscal year 1973 and $2 million per year for 1974 and 1975 to help purchase such products.
- Authorized citizen suits in federal courts against violators or against the EPA or FAA for failure to carry out mandatory provisions of the act.
- Authorized $3 million for fiscal 1973, $6 million for 1974 and $12 million for 1975 to carry out the act.

Toxic Substances Control

A bill (S 1478) to establish a federal regulatory system for potentially hazardous chemicals died in the final days of the 92nd Congress when the House failed to agree to changes made by the Senate in the original House-passed version.

Among the potentially harmful materials to be regulated under the legislation were the elements asbestos, lead and mercury; organic chemicals such as polychlorinated biphenyls (PCBs); and phosphate detergents.

The major difference between the House and Senate versions involved pre-market testing requirements for new chemical substances. Unlike the original Senate bill, the less protective House bill would have exempted from pre-market testing those new chemicals with no known potential hazards.

Congress was unable to reach agreement on the issue until 1976. *(1976 action, p. 158)*

Water Pollution

On the last day of the 1972 session, Congress overrode President Nixon's veto of the Federal Water Pollution Control Act Amendments of 1972 (S 2770 — PL 92-500), the most comprehensive and expensive environmental legislation enacted up to that time.

The amendments initiated a major change in the basic federal approach to water pollution by adding strict limits on what could be discharged into waterways to existing standards to maintain and improve water quality.

The bill set a national goal of eliminating all pollutant discharges into U.S. waters by 1985 and an interim goal of making the waters safe for fish, shellfish, wildlife and people by July 1, 1983. S 2770 contained authorizations of $24.7 billion over three years, through fiscal 1975, including more than $18 billion in federal grants to the states for construction of waste treatment plants.

S 2770 set up a new pollutant discharge permit program under stiff guidelines administered by the Environmental Protection Agency (EPA), replacing an old program established under the Refuse Act of 1899. States could operate their own permit program if EPA approved, but the agency could take over state programs that failed to meet federal standards and could veto individual permits under certain circumstances.

Citizens were allowed to sue polluters, the federal government or the EPA if they had interests — economic or recreational — that were adversely affected.

Industry — the nation's largest user of water — was particularly affected by the legislation. Industries were required by mid-1977 to use the "best practicable" technology for treatment of any discharges into U.S. waters. By mid-1983, they were directed to install the "best available" equipment. The bill established a 15-member national commission to study the costs and benefits of achieving the 1983 deadline and to report to Congress.

In a major departure from the language of both the House and Senate versions of the bill, the final version exempted most EPA actions under S 2770 from provisions of the National Environmental Policy Act of 1969 (PL 91-190), which required the filing of detailed environmental impact statements for federal projects significantly affecting the environment.

Senate approval of a tough water cleanup bill in 1971 had prompted concerted lobby efforts on the part of the administration and industry to soften the abatement deadlines and grant more power to state authorities. But the final version of the bill paralleled Senate language in many respects and was far stiffer than the administration-backed measure approved by the House in 1972.

Nixon had withheld approval of the controversial measure while he awaited the outcome of a bill setting a federal spending ceiling and giving the president authority to decide where spending cuts should be made. When the Senate Oct. 17 refused to grant him such broad authority, Nixon vetoed the water bill. In his veto message, Nixon, who had proposed a $6 billion federal program, called S 2770 "staggering, budget-wrecking."

The Senate promptly voted to override the veto in the pre-dawn hours of Oct. 18. The House rejected the veto later the same day. The votes in both houses were well over the two-thirds majority necessary to override a veto.

Provisions

As cleared by Congress over the president's veto, S 2770 contained major provisions that:

Title I — Research

- Declared it the act's objective to restore and maintain the chemical, physical and biological integrity of the nation's waters.
- Established as a national goal elimination of pollutant discharges into U.S. waters by 1985 and as an interim goal achievement of water quality safe for fish, shellfish, wildlife and recreation by July 1, 1983.
- Established as a national goal elimination of discharges of toxic pollutants in toxic amounts, providing federal financial aid to build public waste treatment works, developing area-wide waste treatment management plans and making a major research effort to develop technology to eliminate pollutant discharges.
- Directed the administrator of the Environmental Protection Agency to administer the act and provide for public participation in development of regulations.
- Authorized the administrator to make a maximum of 50 percent federal grants to states for administrative expenses of planning agencies (for a maximum of three years) developing comprehensive water quality control plans for river basins, bays or lakes.
- Directed the administrator to study the special water pollution problems caused by oil spills, marine sewage equipment (especially on small boats), pesticides, waste oil, estuary pollution, total sewage, agricultural and other rural pollution, fresh water aquatic ecosystems, river systems and thermal discharges.
- Authorized the administrator to make a maximum of 75 percent research and development grants (for demonstration purposes only) for storm sewers, joint municipal-industrial treatment systems, water recycling methods and agricultural pollution.
- Directed the administrator to set up special demonstration projects (with a maximum of 75 percent federal participation) to eliminate pollution of the Great Lakes, with particular attention to the rehabilitation and environmental repair of Lake Erie.
- Directed the administrator to identify and eliminate stationary toxic pollution sources in ports and harbors.

Title II — Construction Grants

- Declared the purpose of the title to require waste treatment management plans and practices that applied the best practicable technology, were on an area-wide basis, encouraged recycling and reclamation and integrated facilities.
- Authorized the administrator to make grants to state or local agencies for the construction of publicly owned treatment works, up to 75 percent of the costs.
- Authorized grants to be allotted to the states on the basis of need, as determined by the EPA.
- Authorized some reimbursement of states and municipalities for treatment work construction begun between 1966 and 1972 (not more than 80 percent) and between 1956 and 1966 (not more than 30 percent).

• Directed the president to prepare a water resources plan for all U.S. basins; plans had to be completed by Jan. 1, 1980, with annual progress reports to Congress required.

Title III — Standards and Enforcement

• Made the discharge of any pollutant by any person unlawful except as authorized by a discharge permit *(Title IV).*

• Provided that existing interstate and intrastate water quality standards remain in effect subject to EPA approval and revision.

• Directed the administrator to develop and publish detailed water quality information and guidelines for effluent limitations.

• Required industrial dischargers by July 1, 1977, to meet effluent limitations based on use of the "best practicable control technology currently available" as defined by the EPA administrator. Required publicly owned treatment works to meet effluent limitations based on secondary treatment (the second step in waste treatment in which bacteria consume the organic parts of the wastes) by the same date.

• Required industrial discharges by July 1, 1983, to meet effluent limitations based on use of the "best available technology economically achievable" as determined by the administrator. Limits would be based on categories or classes of industries and would be aimed at elimination of discharges if technologically and economically achievable. Industries could seek relief based on economic capability. Public treatment works had to use best practicable technology over the life of the works by the same date.

• Directed the administrator to list categories of industrial pollution sources and set national performance standards — including zero-discharge, if practicable — for each new source. States could take over enforcement if laws were as strict as federal standards. If new factories complied with provisions of the bill, they would not be subject to more stringent standards for at least 10 years.

• Directed the administrator to submit a water quality inventory report to Congress by Jan. 1, 1974, and required states to submit such reports by Jan. 1, 1975.

• Directed the administrator to list toxic (seriously harmful to human or other life) pollutants and to set effluent limitations — including prohibition of discharge, if needed — to provide "an ample margin of safety."

• Prohibited discharge of radiological, chemical or biological warfare agents or high-level radioactive waste.

• Required the administrator to set effluent limitations for thermal discharges (discharge of water at different temperature from receiving waters) that would ensure a balanced population of fish, shellfish and wildlife.

• Provided criminal penalties of between $2,500 and $25,000 per day or one year in prison or both; $50,000 per day or two years or both for second offenses; and civil penalties of up to $10,000 per day.

• Declared it to be U.S. policy that there should be no discharges of oil or hazardous substances into U.S. waters, adjoining shorelines or contiguous zone waters.

• Set civil penalties for oil or hazardous substance discharges of up to $50,000 (per discharge), with no limit for willful discharges.

• Directed the states to prepare plans to restore fresh water lakes and authorized federal grants for clean lakes projects.

• Established a 15-member national commission to investigate the technological aspects of achieving the 1983 economic, social and environmental goals in the act.

Title IV — Permits and Licenses

• Required applicants for federal discharge licenses or permits to first obtain state, interstate agency or EPA certification that the discharge would comply with effluent limits set under the act.

• Authorized the EPA administrator, after opportunity for public hearings, to issue permits for pollutant discharges, including previously exempt municipal discharges, under certain conditions and if they met other requirements of the act.

• Authorized states to conduct their own discharge permit programs if approved by the EPA.

• Declared existing permits issued under the 1899 Refuse Act to be valid, but provided that no new permits could be issued after enactment of S 2770.

• Authorized the administrator to suspend state programs that did not meet federal guidelines; but the administrator could veto individual state permits only during the interim period before the guidelines were issued.

Title V — General Provisions

• Gave the administrator emergency powers to bring suit in district court to stop pollution presenting an imminent health or welfare hazard.

• Authorized citizen suits against the U.S. government, other federal agencies or the EPA administrator. Defined citizens as persons having an interest adversely affected.

• Provided for judicial review of the administrator's actions in circuit courts of appeals.

• Provided that nothing in the act would deny the right of states or interstate agencies to set pollution control standards at least as stringent as federal standards.

• Established an Environmental Financing Authority to help finance the non-federal share of the costs of any waste treatment construction project.

• Exempted EPA actions under the act from the requirements for filing a statement detailing the impact on the environment of major federal projects as mandated by the National Environmental Policy Act of 1969 (PL 91-190), except for federal grants for construction of publicly owned sewage treatment plants and permits issued for pollutant discharges from new sources.

Ocean Dumping

After being tied up in conference for nearly a year, a bill (HR 9727 — PL 95-532) banning the unregulated dumping of waste materials into the oceans and coastal waters cleared Congress in the last week of the 1972 session.

The bill declared a national policy of regulating ocean dumping to protect human health and welfare, the marine environment and the economic potential of ocean resources. It banned the transportation out to sea or dumping under any circumstances of radiological, chemical or biological warfare agents or high-level radioactive wastes. And it set tough civil and criminal penalties of up to $50,000, with each day of violation to be considered a separate offense.

Provisions

As signed into law Oct. 23, HR 9727:

- Prohibited the transportation out to sea or dumping into the territorial waters or contiguous zones (the area outside the coastal zone but within the 12-mile territorial limit) of any radiological, chemical or biological warfare agent or any high-level radioactive waste.
- Authorized the Environmental Protection Agency (EPA) to issue permits, after opportunity for public hearings, for the transportation out to sea and dumping of waste materials if they would not unreasonably endanger human health and welfare or the marine environment.
- Authorized the secretary of the Army, through the Corps of Engineers, to issue permits for the transportation out to sea and dumping of dredged or fill material under similar restrictions contained in EPA permits; gave the EPA administrator veto power over Corps of Engineers permits.
- Required permits to designate the type and amount of material to be dumped, dumping location, permit expiration date and other information; authorized issuance of general permits; required all permits to be reviewed periodically and all information to be made public.
- Set civil penalties of up to $50,000; set criminal penalties of up to $50,000 or a year in prison or both; provided that each day of violation would be considered a separate offense; exempted from penalties emergency dumping to safeguard life at sea.
- Pre-empted state authority to regulate ocean dumping but allowed states to adopt dumping criteria and issue regulations if approved by the EPA administrator.
- Authorized appropriations of $3.6 million for fiscal year 1973 and $5.5 million for fiscal 1974 to conduct the anti-dumping program.
- Authorized $6 million annually for three years for research programs on ocean dumping and the long-range effects of pollution and other man-induced changes of ocean systems.
- Provided for designation of marine sanctuaries to be preserved for recreational, ecological or esthetic values.

Related Action

An international convention prohibiting the dumping of poisonous materials into the oceans was signed by the United States Dec. 29, 1972. Negotiated by representatives of 91 countries, including all of the world's major maritime nations, the Convention on the Prevention of Marine Pollution by Dumping of Wastes and Other Matter forbade the unloading at sea of high-level radioactive wastes, biological and chemical warfare agents, crude oil, some pesticides and durable plastics; it also required a permit for the discharge of less harmful materials such as cyanides and flourides. The convention was more comprehensive in the number of types of substances whose discharge was prohibited than PL 92-532.

Coastal Zone Management

Congress established a national program for the management and protection of U.S. coastal waters and adjacent shorelines in the Coastal Zone Management Act of 1972 (S 3507 — PL 92-583).

The $186 million measure authorized federal grants to the states to help them develop coastal management programs under federal guidelines. The grants would pay up to two-thirds of the cost of state programs each year.

The bill was designed to protect the resources of coastal waters against increasing population and other pressures on the areas. Areas covered under the bill included coastal waters, bays, sounds, lagoons and estuaries, the Great Lakes, and adjacent shorelands such as tidal areas, salt marshes, wetlands and beaches. The measure declared a national policy of preserving, protecting, restoring and developing the coastal zones in the national interest.

A House committee report called the U.S. coast "the nation's most valuable geographic asset" and said it probably was the area "most threatened with deterioration and irreparable damage." There are about 100,000 miles of U.S. coastline and 75 percent of the population lives in coastal states, the report said.

A Senate committee report said that according to some projections, more than 80 percent of the population would live within 50 miles of a coast by the year 2000.

Provisions

As signed into law Oct. 27, S 3507 contained major provisions that:

- Declared it the national policy to preserve, protect, develop and, wherever possible, restore the nation's coastal zone resources.
- Defined coastal zones as coastal waters and adjacent shorelands, including tidal areas, salt marshes, wetlands and beaches; defined coastal waters to include the Great Lakes and their connecting waters or sounds, bays, lagoons and estuaries.
- Authorized the secretary of commerce to make annual grants to coastal states to help them develop and administer coastal-zone management programs under federal guidelines but provided that individual grants could not exceed two-thirds of the cost of a program.
- Required the secretary to review state management programs and performance, and authorized termination of financial assistance in cases of poor performance.
- Authorized the secretary to make grants of up to 50 percent of the costs (not to exceed $2 million) for acquisition, development and operation of estuarine sanctuaries for research purposes.
- Authorized appropriations of $9 million annually for fiscal years 1973-77 for program planning grants, $30 million annually for 1974-77 for administrative grants, up to $6 million for fiscal 1974 for estuarine sanctuary grants and $3 million annually for 1973-77 for general administrative expenses.

Marine Safety

Congress in 1972 moved to prevent oil spills and other accidents in the nation's ports and waterways when it approved legislation (HR 8140 — PL 92-340) authorizing the Coast Guard to supervise marine traffic in congested areas. The law also called for federal design and construction standards for vessels carrying hazardous bulk liquid materials.

Provisions

As signed into law (PL 92-340) July 10, HR 8140, the Ports and Waterways Safety Act:

- Authorized the secretary of transportation to establish comprehensive regulations for the design, construction, maintenance and operation of vessels carrying bulk cargoes for the purpose of protecting the marine environment. (Bulk cargoes were defined as materials such as inflammable or combustible liquids, oil of any kind, hazardous polluting liquids; bulk dry cargoes were excluded from provisions of the act.)
- Set Jan. 1, 1976, as the latest day by which initial design and construction standards would have to be applied to vessels in foreign trade or foreign registry.
- Authorized the secretary of transportation to establish and operate marine traffic systems and controls for congested waterways and to prescribe safety equipment and procedures for docks and other structures.
- Provided a maximum civil penalty of $10,000 and criminal penalties of not less than $5,000 nor more than $50,000 or five years imprisonment, or both, for violations of the act.

Nuclear Licensing

Responding to warnings of future blackouts and brownouts, Congress May 17, 1972, cleared a bill (HR 14655 — PL 92-307) authorizing the Atomic Energy Commission (AEC) to issue temporary operating licenses for certain nuclear power plants whose operation was necessary to ensure an adequate power supply. About 13 power plants were affected by the bill.

A provision for public hearings with "expedited procedures" on applications for temporary licenses was included in the bill. The AEC and the power industry opposed the provision, contending that speedy licensing could not be achieved unless the hearing requirement was waived.

PL 92-307 amended the Atomic Energy Act of 1954 by adding a new section authorizing the issuance of interim operating license until Oct. 30, 1973, for reactors whose applications for a full operating license had been contested. The bill specified that all applications filed before Sept. 1, 1971, had to meet the requirements of the National Environmental Policy Act of 1969 (PL 91-190).

Related Development. In related action, the Senate failed to act on a House-passed measure that would have freed nuclear power licensing procedures from the environmental considerations imposed by the National Environmental Policy Act of 1969 (PL 91-190). HR 13752 would have permitted temporary licensing of nuclear power plants prior to completion of environmental impact statements by the Atomic Energy Commission.

Cyclamate Compensation

The House July 24, 1972, by a 177-170 vote, passed a bill (HR 13366) permitting domestic food growers, processors, packers and distributors to sue for payment by the federal government to recover losses sustained as a result of the 1969 ban on cyclamates.

Cyclamates were used as sweeteners in a wide variety of diet foods and drinks, as a cheaper substitute for sugar in processed foods and as a coating or sweetener for numerous drug products. Testing performed in the 1960s found that the sweeteners caused cancer in laboratory animals; federal law required substances producing cancer in test animals to be banned from human consumption. The Department of Health, Education and Welfare began to phase out the use of cyclamates in foods and other substances on Oct. 18, 1969. A total ban on use of the sweetener took effect on Aug. 14, 1970.

A Senate Judiciary subcommittee held hearings on the bill in September but took no further action and the indemnity measure died.

Pesticides Regulation

Congress in 1972 replaced existing laws regulating the use of pesticides with new legislation (HR 10729 — PL 92-516) giving the government broader authority to control the vast array of pesticides and other pest killers.

In the first major change in federal regulation of pesticides in 25 years, Congress required that all pesticides be registered with the Environmental Protection Agency (EPA), which would control the manufacture, distribution and use of pesticides. Only those involved in interstate commerce had been regulated by existing law, the Insecticide, Fungicide and Rodenticide Act of 1947, which was primarily a labeling law.

The new legislation, the Federal Environmental Pesticide Control Act of 1972, made it easier to ban hazardous pesticides and imposed penalties for their improper use. Under existing law, the government had to complete a long and complicated procedure before banning a pesticide it found dangerous. And while it could require proper labeling, no penalties were prescribed for improper use.

As cleared by Congress, HR 10729 divided pesticides into two categories — general use and restricted use. Restricted pesticides would have to be clearly labeled and could be used only by certified applicators. The bill required pesticide manufacturers to submit detailed information to the EPA with their registration applications, including labels, claims to be made, directions for use, the chemical formula and test results.

Under a controversial provision originally added by the House Agriculture Committee, pesticide manufacturers or retailers could be compensated if their products were declared an imminent hazard by EPA and removed from the market. No payment would be made, however, if the pesticide owners knew in advance that their products were harmful and still continued to use or produce them. Original House action had been completed in 1971.

Provisions

As signed into law Oct. 21, major provisions of HR 10729:

- Required all pesticides in U.S. commerce to be registered with EPA.
- Required registration applicants to submit detailed information on the pesticide, including labeling, claims to be made, directions on use, chemical formula and test results.

• Allowed test data supporting one application to be used in support of another application if the original registrant agreed and was paid a reasonable amount for the information.

• Required all information in support of an application (except trade secrets) to be made public 30 days after the registration.

• Provided that the lack of a proven need for a pesticide could not be a criterion for denying registration.

• Authorized the EPA administrator to cancel the registration, change the classification or hold hearings on pesticides that, when used in accordance with commonly recognized practice, caused "unreasonable" adverse affects on the environment.

• Authorized the EPA administrator to suspend registrations of pesticides that presented an imminent hazard to health or the environment; provided an opportunity for hearings and judicial review.

• Authorized indemnity payments to pesticide manufacturers or owners whose product was declared to be an imminent hazard unless they knew in advance that the products were illegal under the act.

• Provided that exported pesticides had to meet the laws of the foreign purchaser only and that imported pesticides had to meet U.S. standards.

• Established two classifications of pesticides: 1) general use and 2) restricted use; restricted pesticides would have to be clearly labeled and could be used only by certified applicators.

• Required EPA to set standards for federal or state certification of private and commercial applicators and gave the EPA administrator the authority to reject state programs.

• Allowed states to impose stronger regulations on the sale or use of pesticides than those enforced by the federal government, but prohibited different state packaging or labeling requirements.

• Set civil penalties of up to $5,000 for each offense or up to $1,000 for pesticide applicators; set criminal penalties for manufacturers of up to $25,000 or a year in prison or both, or up to $1,000 or 30 days in prison for private applicators.

• Authorized appropriations of whatever sums were necessary to carry out provisions of the act.

DES Controversy

The Senate Sept. 20, 1972, passed a bill (S 2818) providing for an immediate ban on the use of the growth hormone DES (diethylstilbestrol) in animal feed but permitting use of DES animal ear implants at least until Jan. 1, 1973.

There was no House action on the bill, which died at the end of the 92nd Congress. In 1975, the Senate again approved a DES ban and the House again failed to act. The Food and Drug Administration (FDA) finally banned the controversial substance for use as a growth stimulant in 1979. *(1975 action, p. 155)*

DES, used in animal feed to stimulate rapid weight gain, had been found to cause cancer in laboratory mice. A growing body of evidence indicated a direct link between young women having a rare form of vaginal cancer and their mothers who were given DES, a synthetic hormone, during pregnancy to prevent spontaneous abortion.

DES residues had been detected with increasing frequency in beef and lamb livers despite FDA regulations designed to eliminate such residues. The Delaney clause, a provision of the Food Additive Amendments (to the Food, Drug and Cosmetic Act) of 1958 states that a food additive could not be approved if the substance caused cancer in laboratory animals — even if some presumably safe level for human food use could be established. The clause did not forbid the use of a cancer-causing substance in animal feed, but it did require that all such substances be eliminated from the animal before it was slaughtered.

The FDA issued a ban on DES in animal feed in 1972, but the order was overturned in 1974 by a federal court on grounds that the agency had not given manufacturers of the drug a full hearing. The FDA again proposed a ban in 1976, but it did not take effect until 1979.

Black Lung Benefits

A bill (HR 9212 — PL 92-303) liberalizing eligibility standards for benefits to coal miners stricken by pneumoconiosis (black lung disease) cleared Congress May 10.

HR 9212 amended Title IV of the landmark Coal Mine Health and Safety Act of 1969 (PL 91-173), which established federal safety standards at coal mines and authorized a compensation program for miners and widows of miners totally disabled or killed by pneumoconiosis.

The disease, which is caused by the inhalation of fine coal dust particles, leads in its advanced stages to severe breathing difficulty and premature death.

As cleared by Congress, HR 9212 enabled a miner to more easily establish his entitlement to black lung benefits by vastly broadening the definition of total disability and forbidding the denial of benefits solely on the basis of a negative chest X-ray.

The bill also delayed until 1974 the responsibility of industry to start paying new lifetime claims. And it made benefit payments available to orphans of miners, who were inadvertently excluded under the 1969 law.

Provisions

As signed into law May 19, HR 9212:

• Provided disability benefits to orphans of deceased miners and permitted dependent parents, brothers or sisters of a deceased miner to receive such benefits, where no widow or child survived him, if they had been totally dependent on the miner and had lived in his household for one year prior to his death.

• Extended for 18 months — to July 1, 1973, from Jan. 1, 1972 — the filing period for claiming disability benefits during which time the federal government would assume responsibility for the cost of such benefits for the remainder of a beneficiary's life; authorized federal payment of claims filed during the period July 1, 1973, to Dec. 31, 1973, for that period only. Beginning Jan. 1, 1974, claims were to be filed under state workers' compensation laws.

• Extended the program for five years to Dec. 30, 1981, and authorized the payment of disability benefits on all claims filed prior to that date for the remainder of a beneficiary's life.

• Prohibited the denial of a claim solely on the basis of a

negative chest X-ray, and provided that miners with 15 years' service prior to July 1, 1971, who were disabled by a respiratory disease would be presumed disabled by pneumoconiosis unless proven to the contrary.

- Broadened the definition of total disability to include any respiratory impairment that prevented a miner from engaging in his usual occupation.
- Authorized the payment of benefits to miners working on surface or strip mine operations.
- Prohibited discrimination by employers against any miner solely because he had contracted pneumoconiosis.
- Authorized the secretary of the Department of Health, Education and Welfare to issue grants for construction of pneumoconiosis treatment facilities and to initiate research on devices to test for the presence of black lung disease.

1973

Congress passed no significant environmental health legislation in 1973, although it voted to extend the lead-based paint poisoning prevention program and amended state sewage construction grant allocations authorized by the 1972 water pollution control act.

A measure to place federal regulations on the marketing of toxic substances died for the second year in a row and Congress was unable to override the president's veto of a bill to restore the rural water and sewer grant program.

Toxic Substances Control

As they had in 1972, the House and Senate failed to reconcile differing versions of legislation to control the marketing of toxic substances.

The Senate favored stiffer controls than the House, particularly on the issue of pre-market testing. Its version was preferred by environmentalists and by labor unions, whose member-workers risked exposure to dangerous chemicals during their manufacture. The more limited House bill came closer to the proposals backed by the Nixon administration and the chemical industry.

Congress finally reached a compromise on the controversial issue in 1976. *(1976 action, p. 158)*

Rural Sewer Grants

Supporters were unable to save the rural water and sewer grant program, which had been terminated by the Nixon administration Jan. 10, 1973. The House April 10 failed to override a veto by President Nixon on a bill (HR 3298) that would have restored the program. The vote was 225-189 — 51 votes short of the two-thirds majority needed to override a veto.

The program was established by Congress in 1965 to provide matching grants to soil and water associations and local public agencies for construction of water supply and sewage disposal systems in rural areas.

The administration cancelled the program in 1973 for budgetary reasons, claiming that rising farm incomes meant rural communities had more money to spend on water and sanitation systems and required little federal assistance. Of the $150 million appropriated for fiscal 1973 for the program, only $30 million had been spent prior to its cancellation.

Water Pollution

Congress cleared a bill (S 2812 — PL 93-243) adjusting the allocation formula for state sewage construction grants under the Federal Water Pollution Control Act of 1972 (PL 92-500).

The purpose of the bill was to ensure that all states received a minimum allocation even though President Nixon had impounded some of the funds authorized for the construction program. The bill assured states that they would receive at least as much in fiscal 1975 as they received in fiscal 1972.

The 1972 water pollution law authorized $18 billion for grants to states for construction and improvement of waste treatment plants with the federal government paying 75 percent of total costs. The law provided for obligation of the funds through contract authority, thus avoiding the necessity for separate appropriations legislation.

President Nixon announced in November 1972 that, as an anti-inflationary move, he would not allocate $6 billion of the $11 billion authorized for fiscal 1973-74. In January 1974, Nixon impounded $3 billion of the $7 billion authorized for fiscal 1975, bringing the total of funds impounded to $9 billion.

Pollution Control Extensions

Congress cleared two routine bills extending through fiscal 1974 funding authorizations for two environmental laws.

One bill (HR 5445 — PL 93-15) extended the 1970 Clean Air Amendments and the other (HR 5446 — PL 93-14) extended the 1970 Solid Waste Disposal Act (PL 91-512).

Lead Paint Poisoning

Congress in 1973 approved a two-year extension of the Lead-Based Paint Poisoning Prevention Act of 1970. A key feature of the extension legislation (S 607 — PL 93-151) set a limit on the allowable lead content of interior paints.

Authorities estimated that 400,000 children in the United States suffered from lead poisoning. Many were poisoned by eating paint chips peeling from the walls of older houses.

S 607 required the secretaries of the departments of Health, Education and Welfare, and Housing and Urban Development to prohibit the use of lead-based paint in residential buildings constructed or renovated with federal assistance or in any toy, drinking or eating utensil or piece of furniture distributed or manufactured after enactment of the bill. The bill defined lead-based paint as any paint containing more than 0.5 percent lead by weight. On Jan. 1, 1975, that limit would be lowered to 0.06 percent.

1974

It was a largely discouraging year for environmentalists. Congress established a new program to safeguard drinking water supplies in response to well-publicized reports of contamination. But it also relaxed air pollution standards to allow more coal burning and postponed auto emission standards for another year. In addition, President Ford vetoed a bill that extended the federal program insuring the public against a nuclear power accident.

In other action, Congress abolished the Atomic Energy Commission, giving its research and development functions to a new Energy Research and Development Administration and its regulatory and safety functions to a Nuclear Regulatory Commission. The Senate passed a bill to strengthen food safety laws, but the House did not act on it.

Clean Air Amendments

The national energy crisis and the government's decision to strive for reduced dependence on foreign energy sources prompted Congress in 1974 to postpone air pollution control deadlines for both auto manufacturers and industrial polluters. The legislation represented the first substantial change in the 1970 Clean Air Act Amendments. *(1970 law, p. 135)*

The 1974 Energy Supply and Environmental Coordination Act (HR 14368 — PL 93-319) delayed final auto emission standards a second time — from 1976 to 1977 model cars for hydrocarbons (HC) and carbon monoxide (CO), and from 1977 to 1978 for nitrogen oxides (NOx).

The auto industry argued that the first such one-year delay, granted by the EPA in 1973, had not given them enough time to perfect the technology needed to meet the final standards without severe economic repercussions.

The bill gave manufacturers a chance to apply to the EPA for yet another one-year postponement of the 1977 deadline for compliance with final HC and CO standards.

PL 93-319 also eased requirements for compliance with air quality standards by certain industrial polluters. The Clean Air Act required those polluters to meet state emission control standards by mid-1975 or mid-1977 at the latest. To comply, many electric utilities were forced to choose between converting their power plants from coal to cleaner burning fuels — such as oil, natural gas and low-sulfur coal — or installing emission-control equipment (usually stack gas "scrubbers"). Most plants chose to switch to clean-burning fuels and found themselves in a bind as such fuels became increasingly scarce and the pressure was on to use the plentiful domestic coal supplies.

To stimulate coal production and ease the impact of the "clean fuel deficit," the energy supply bill required electric power plants that could burn coal to do so through 1978, and authorized the Federal Energy Administration to order other fuel-burning plants to convert to coal. The Environmental Protection Agency (EPA) was to extend the final emission deadlines for converting plants through 1978, provided that primary air standards were not already being exceeded in the air control region in question.

In an effort to allocate clean-burning fuel to heavily polluted areas where it was needed most, the EPA was directed to encourage states to review emission control plans to eliminate unnecessarily strict requirements.

PL 93-319 also extended Clean Air Act authorizations for one year, through June 30, 1975. That enabled Congress to put off a complete review of the act and to sidestep a series of controversial clean air amendments proposed by the Nixon administration in March. *(1975 action, p. 153)*

Safe Drinking Water

Spurred by reports of drinking water contamination, Congress in 1974 cleared legislation (S 433 — PL 93-523) authorizing the Environmental Protection Agency (EPA) to set national standards for drinking water.

The 1974 Safe Drinking Water Act directed the EPA to set maximum allowable levels for certain chemical and bacteriological pollutants in some 240,000 water systems (those serving more than 25 customers). Previous federal drinking water programs were limited primarily to prevention of the spread of communicable diseases through drinking water involved in interstate commerce.

Congress had been debating national drinking water standards since 1972, when the Senate passed a bill similar to the 1974 measure but the House failed to act. The Senate passed S 433 in mid-1973. The House did not pass its version of the bill until late 1974, in the wake of two widely publicized reports that dramatized the problem.

The first report, released Nov. 7 by the Environmental Defense Fund (EDF), a public interest group, warned of a "significant relationship" between cancer deaths and drinking water taken from the lower Mississippi River near New Orleans, La.

The following day the EPA released its own survey of New Orleans drinking water, which had turned up 66 organic chemicals — some of them suspected carcinogens. In a nationally televised press conference, EPA administrator Russell E. Train announced that the agency was beginning a major project to review drinking water supplies in 80 cities.

Another EDF report released in early December suggested that the New Orleans problem was widespread.

President Ford signed the national standards bill Dec. 16 despite reservations about interfering with state authority to regulate water supplies and about the level of federal expenditures involved.

Provisions

As signed into law, major provisions of S 433 (PL 93-523):

- Required EPA, within 180 days of enactment, to issue interim primary standards to safeguard the quality of public drinking water supplies; required the regulations to take effect within 18 months of their issuance.

• Required EPA to contract with the National Academy of Sciences for a study of appropriate maximum contaminant levels in drinking water; required the academy to report to Congress within two years of enactment.

• Required EPA, within 100 days after the academy report, to establish maximum allowable levels for contaminants in drinking water under revised primary standards; authorized EPA to require specific treatment techniques for each contaminant.

• Required the revised primary standards to take effect within 27 months and 10 days after the report (within 51 months and 10 days of enactment).

• Required EPA to establish secondary standards governing the taste, appearance and odor of drinking water.

• Gave principal authority for enforcement of the standards to states that had adopted EPA primary standards and complied with other federal regulations for inspection and sampling of water supplies.

• Required EPA to notify states of violations of primary standards.

• Allowed EPA to bring civil suits to force correction of the violations if 1) the state failed to correct violations within 60 days and failed to file a required report with EPA, 2) EPA determined that a state that failed to correct violations within 60 days, but did file the report, "abused its discretion" in carrying out primary enforcement, or 3) the state had not adopted EPA primary standards and did not have principal enforcement power.

• Required operators of public water systems to notify their users of violations of EPA regulations.

• Allowed states with primary enforcement authority to grant variances to water systems unable to comply with maximum contaminant or treatment regulations because of the nature of raw water sources.

• Allowed states to grant seven- to nine-year exemptions from the regulations to existing water systems unable to comply because of economic or other compelling factors; required exempted systems to meet a partial compliance schedule during those years.

• Required EPA to establish regulations for state programs protecting underground water sources; required states complying with the regulations to ban underground injection of wastes without a permit within three years of enactment.

• Gave EPA backup authority to enforce the standards through court action.

• Gave EPA authority to deal immediately with drinking water emergencies; gave EPA emergency authority to allocate treatment chemicals including chlorine.

• Authorized $75 million for fiscal 1975-77 for research and training programs dealing with safe drinking water; authorized $52.5 million for fiscal 1976-77 for state grants and guaranteed each state 1 percent of grant funds appropriated; authorized $25 million for fiscal 1975-77 for special projects or demonstrations; authorized $4 million for fiscal 1975-77 for a survey of drinking water supplies in rural areas.

• Authorized EPA to guarantee private loans of up to $50,000 to small public water systems.

• Authorized judicial review of EPA regulations and state decisions to grant or not grant variances or exemptions from primary standards.

• Authorized citizens to bring civil actions against persons alleged to be in violation of the act and against EPA for alleged failure to carry out required duties after the bill had been enacted for 27 months.

Solid Waste Management

For the second year in a row, Congress cleared a one-year stopgap authorization for the Environmental Protection Agency's solid waste management program (HR 16045 — PL 93-611).

Congress enacted a major revision of the program in 1976. *(Story, p. 156)*

AEC Abolition

Congress in 1974 abolished the Atomic Energy Commission (AEC) and transferred most of its research and development functions to a new federal agency, the Energy Research and Development Administration (ERDA). Nuclear licensing, regulation and safety responsibilities were placed in a new Nuclear Regulatory Commission (NRC).

ERDA. In addition to the AEC programs, ERDA acquired fossil-fuel energy research programs from the Interior Department and geothermal and solar energy development programs from the National Science Foundation. ERDA's responsibilities also included nuclear weapons research and development for the Defense Department. The bulk of ERDA's $2.6 billion budget and 7,000-member staff, however, came from the former AEC.

Nuclear Regulatory Commission. The legislation (HR 11510 — PL 93-438) established a five-member Nuclear Regulatory Commission, appointed by the president, to take over the AEC's safety and regulatory functions. Other provisions pertaining to the new NRC:

• Created an Office of Nuclear Reaction Regulation and an Office of Nuclear Regulatory Research.

• Upgraded the AEC's regulatory division into an Office of Nuclear Material Safety and Safeguards.

• Made the safety office responsible for protecting commercial facilities against threats, sabotage or theft of nuclear materials.

• Required employees of firms regulated by the commission to report immediately to the NRC any violation of the Atomic Energy Act or any case of facilities having a safety defect that could create a substantial safety hazard.

• Directed the commission to report quarterly to Congress on any abnormal occurrences at licensed nuclear facilities; such incidents would have to be reported to the public within 15 days of an occurrence.

Nuclear Accident Insurance

President Ford in 1974 vetoed a bill (HR 15323) extending for five years the federal program insuring the public and the nuclear power industry against a nuclear power accident.

Ford favored the extension but vetoed the measure because of a provision that he claimed usurped his constitutional power to give the final stamp of approval to legislation. Concerned about the safety of expanding the use of nuclear power, Congress had inserted in HR 15323 language giving it the opportunity to disapprove the extension later in the year, if warranted by the results of a study on nuclear safety due to be completed in late 1974.

Congress extended the accident insurance program in

NRC Commissioners

Abolition of the Atomic Energy Commission at the end of 1974 gave President Gerald R. Ford the opportunity to name the entire membership of its successor, the Nuclear Regulatory Commission. As its chairman, Ford selected former astronaut William A. Anders, a Nixon-nominated member of the AEC. Dixy Lee Ray, who had been AEC chairman, became assistant secretary of state for oceans and international environmental and scientific affairs. As the other members of the Nuclear Regulatory Commission, Ford selected Victor Gilinsky from the Rand Corporation, Richard T. Kennedy from the National Security Council staff, Edward A. Mason from the Massachusetts Institute of Technology and Marcus A. Rowden, former general counsel to the AEC. They were all confirmed by the Senate in December.

To head the new Energy Research and Development Administration, Ford selected Robert C. Seamans Jr., former secretary of the Air Force (1969-73) and, at the time of his nomination, president of the National Academy of Engineering. The Senate confirmed Seamans in December.

1975 but omitted the provision to which Ford had objected because the study found little likelihood of a serious nuclear accident. *(Background, 1975 action, p. 154)*

Food Safety

The Senate July 11, 1974, passed without controversy a bill (S 2373) requiring increased government monitoring of food processing operations and comprehensive labeling of food products. However, the House did not act on the measure. A similar bill (S 641) passed by the Senate in 1976 also died without House action. *(Details, p. 159)*

S 2373 was described by its supporters as the most comprehensive revision of food safety law since enactment of the Federal Food, Drug and Cosmetic Act of 1938. That law gave the Food and Drug Administration (FDA) authority to inspect food processing plants and prohibited interstate commerce in adulterated or misbranded foods and drugs.

The 1974 measure was inspired by food scares such as the 1973 "mushroom crisis," which resulted in recalls of large quantities of contaminated canned mushrooms. In addition, a General Accounting Office study released in 1972 found that about 40 percent of the nation's 80,000 food processing plants operated under insanitary conditions.

As approved by the Senate, S 2373 required food processors to set their own standards for food wholesomeness, gave the FDA new tools to enforce those standards and required fuller labeling on food products. Processors of meat, poultry and eggs were not covered by the bill because they were regulated by the Agriculture Department.

OSHA Consultation Services

Although bills to repeal or even moderately amend the controversial Occupational Safety and Health Act of 1970 (PL 91-596) got nowhere during 1974, Congress decided to meet small businesses halfway on the issue of federal consultation services.

As an amendment to the Labor-Health, Education and Welfare appropriations bill for fiscal 1975 (HR 15580 — PL 93-517), Congress earmarked $5 million for a new program to advise small businesses on health and safety regulations. Businesses had complained that for a variety of reasons, they were unable to determine exactly which federal health and safety standards applied to their operations.

The bill also excused firms with 10 or fewer employees from OSHA's record-keeping and reporting requirements; previously such an exemption had applied only to firms with a maximum of seven employees.

1975

Farm and chemical interests attacked the federal pesticide control program as a drag on food production but failed to convince Congress that the program should be curtailed. Congress extended the pesticide regulation program through March 1977. It also extended for 10 years the program of federal insurance to compensate the public in the event of a major nuclear accident; a similar bill had been vetoed in 1974.

House and Senate committees worked on comprehensive amendments to the 1970 Clean Air Amendments, but no bills were reported in 1975. Nonetheless, it became obvious that Congress would relax the original requirements of the law to accommodate energy and economic demands.

The Supreme Court ruled against the Nixon administration's impoundment of billions of dollars intended for sewage treatment projects. But a national commission reported that the ambitious goal of the 1972 water pollution control law — cleaning up the nation's waters by 1985 — was not likely to be achieved.

Clean Air Amendments

Committees in both the House and Senate worked throughout 1975 on comprehensive amendments to the 1970 Clean Air Act (PL 91-604). But neither chamber debated the measure until 1976, when a Senate filibuster launched just before Congress was scheduled to adjourn killed the conference version. *(1970 law, p. 135; 1976 action, p. 156)*

The 1970 act was scheduled to expire midway through 1975. However, funding for its programs was continued for one year under a continuing appropriations resolution (H J Res 499 — PL 94-41).

Also in 1975, the Environmental Protection Agency granted auto manufacturers another year's extension of the auto emission control standards established by the 1970 law. That left interim standards in effect until model-year 1978 cars, when stricter limits on emissions of hydrocarbons, carbon monoxide and nitrogen oxide would be put in place.

Nuclear Accident Insurance

Congress in 1975 approved a 10-year extension (HR 8631 — PL 94-197) of the program of federal insurance against a nuclear power accident. PL 94-197 extended the program until Aug. 1, 1987, and provided for phasing out the government's role as insurer as the amount of available private insurance and the number of operating nuclear power plants increased.

The insurance program, created by the Price-Anderson Act of 1957 (PL 85-256), was designed to assure the public of compensation for any damages resulting from a nuclear power accident and to limit the liability of the industry for damages from a single accident. Such reassurance was needed to encourage the development of the infant nuclear power industry.

PL 85-256 required nuclear power plants to obtain the maximum private insurance coverage available — in 1957, about $60 million. It limited the industry's liability for any one accident to $560 million and the government assumed responsibility for paying the $500 million difference.

As the amount of insurance obtainable from private sources increased (to $110 million by 1974), the government's liability decreased, but the $560 million limit on the industry's liability remained in place.

Concerned by the growing reliance of government officials on nuclear power as the prime energy source of the future, environmentalists and others began in the early 1970s to question the safety of expanding nuclear power production. That concern was heightened after 115,000 gallons of liquid radioactive nuclear waste leaked from an Atomic Energy Commission facility at Hanford, Wash.

Some of this criticism spilled into the debate on extension of the federal insurance program. Critics argued that the liability limit was unnecessary if nuclear power was as safe as the industry claimed but that it was too low if a severe accident occurred.

In 1974 President Ford vetoed a five-year extension of the insurance program. He did not object to extension of the program but to a provision that allowed Congress to nullify the legislation later if it felt that such an action was warranted by a nuclear reactor safety study due for release late in 1974.

The study, headed by Norman C. Rasmussen of the Massachusetts Institute of Technology, was finally released in October 1975. It found that the likelihood of a serious nuclear accident with severe consequences for the public was quite small. The 1975 bill therefore did not contain the provisions to which President Ford had objected in 1974.

Provisions

As signed into law, PL 94-197 amended the Atomic Energy Act of 1954 to:

- Extend coverage of the insurance system set up by the Price-Anderson Act to nuclear plants licensed before Aug. 1, 1987. Existing law allowed coverage only for plants licensed before Aug. 1, 1977.
- Phase out the government's role as insurer by requiring all licensed nuclear power plants to pay, in the event of a nuclear accident resulting in damages exceeding the amount of available private insurance, a "deferred premium" between $2 million and $5 million per plant in order to provide funds to pay the damages up to $560 million. The government would continue to pay damages in excess of the combined total of private insurance and deferred premiums up to the $560 million limit.
- Allow the liability limit to increase once the private insurance/deferred premium total reached $560 million. The limit would increase as the total of private and industry commitments increased.
- Extend Price-Anderson insurance coverage to ocean shipment of fuel between licensed nuclear power plants outside the territorial limits of the United States and to nuclear facilities licensed by the government but located outside those territorial limits.
- Extend to 20 years from 10 years the statute of limitations applying to damage suits resulting from nuclear accidents.
- Require the Nuclear Regulatory Commission to report to the Joint Atomic Energy Committee, senators and representatives from affected states and districts on the causes and extent of any damages resulting from a serious nuclear accident, and to make public such findings except for information damaging to the national defense.

Pesticide Regulation

After months of delay and debate, Congress in November 1975 cleared legislation (HR 8841 — PL 94-140) extending the Environmental Protection Agency's (EPA) pesticide regulation program through March 1977.

Funding authority to carry out the Federal Insecticide, Fungicide and Rodenticide Act (FIFRA) had been set to expire June 30, 1975. But heavy lobbying by farm and chemical industry groups delayed action on the bill, and Congress twice passed temporary extensions that continued the program through Nov. 15 while it wrote the longer-term measure.

The farm and industry spokesmen complained that the EPA had been overzealous in protecting the environment and insensitive to their needs. They protested a wide range of EPA actions, including its moves to ban or limit the use of some potentially cancer-causing pesticides and a plan to require that farmers pass a test before using dangerous pesticides. EPA officials, backed by environmental groups, defended the agency's pesticide record and argued for the simple two-year extension the Ford administration originally had requested.

The final compromise bill satisfied neither side. The measure required the EPA to give the Agriculture Department a chance to comment in advance on major regulatory actions. The agency was prohibited from requiring farmers to pass examinations before using dangerous pesticides.

A dispute about the length of the authorization was resolved by extending FIFRA for 18 months, until March 1977. Critics argued for a one-year extension on grounds that Congress should keep the EPA on a short leash. The agency's defenders said it needed more time to implement the sweeping 1972 amendments to the 1947 pesticide law before undergoing another congressional grilling. *(1972 law, p. 148)*

The 1975 bill postponed for one year, until October 1977, the final deadline for implementation of the 1972 amendments to the pesticide law (PL 92-516), which called for a new system of registration and classification for all pesticides and greatly strengthened the EPA's authority to control pesticide use.

Provisions

As signed into law, major provisions of HR 8841 (PL 94-140):

- Authorized funds for implementation of the Federal Insecticide, Fungicide and Rodenticide Act in amounts of $47,868,000 through Sept. 30, 1976; and $23,600,000 from Oct. 1, 1976 through March 31, 1977.
- Extended to Oct. 21, 1976, from Oct. 21, 1975, the deadline for EPA approval of state plans for certification of pesticide users; extended to Oct. 21, 1977, from Oct. 21, 1976, the deadline for final EPA regulations on registration and reclassification of pesticides and implementation of restrictions on use of dangerous pesticides.
- Directed EPA to notify the secretary of agriculture at least 60 days before acting publicly to suspend, cancel or change the classification of a pesticide registered for use under the law. The Agriculture Department would have 30 days to comment on the action, and EPA would be required to publish the comment in the *Federal Register.* If the department did not comment within 30 days, EPA could proceed with the action. EPA would have to include in the notification an analysis of the impact the action would have on agricultural production and prices and the agricultural economy in general. The agency could waive the notification requirement when suspending or canceling the use of a pesticide to prevent an "imminent hazard to human health."
- Directed EPA to provide the agriculture secretary with copies of proposed pesticide regulations 60 days in advance of publication and to publish the department's comment if it is received within 30 days. The same requirement also would apply to final regulations but with deadlines of 30 and 15 days, respectively. For both proposed and final regulations, EPA would be required to notify the public through the *Federal Register* and the House and Senate Agriculture committees at the same time.
- Allowed EPA and the agriculture secretary to waive the notification requirements for specific regulations or cancellation or suspension actions.
- Required EPA to establish a scientific advisory panel to which the same 60-day notification and comment procedure would apply.
- Permitted EPA to approve state certification programs that allowed individuals to be certified to use dangerous ("restricted use") pesticides by signing a "self-certification" form instead of passing an examination to test their competence. EPA could approve a state program that required such an examination, however.
- Stipulated that a company submitting data gathered by another firm in support of a pesticide registration be required to compensate the donor firm only if the data originally was submitted to EPA on or after Jan. 1, 1970. In addition, the bill affirmed that the compensation requirement applied to all applications for registration or reregistration submitted on or after Oct. 21, 1972, when amendments to the law took effect.

DES Controversy

The Senate voted in September 1975 to suspend the use of diethylstilbestrol (DES) as a growth stimulant in livestock until the government determined that the drug did not pose a serious cancer threat to humans. But the House never acted on the legislation (S 963), which also would have increased the independence of the Food and Drug Administration (FDA). It was the second time the Senate had passed such a ban. *(1972 action, p. 149)*

FDA finally announced a ban on the manufacture and use of DES as a growth stimulant for cattle and sheep; the ban took effect in late 1979. However, in early 1980 FDA reported widespread violations of the ban.

OSHA Consultation

Employer groups made some headway in 1975 in their attempt to obtain on-site advice from the Department of Labor on federal health and safety regulations when the House passed such a measure. But the legislation died when the Senate failed to act on the bill.

Employers — particularly heads of small businesses — argued that they often found the rules vague, contradictory or highly technical and that they could not afford to hire their own consultants. Because OSHA compliance officers inspected businesses at random and had to issue citations for whatever violations they found, employers claimed they could be penalized for things they knew nothing about.

The U.S. Chamber of Commerce opposed the bill, contending it would compound rather than alleviate businesses' problems of complying with OSHA standards. The Chamber of Commerce principally objected to provisions that allowed OSHA to require the correction of certain potentially dangerous violations found during the consultation visits; under the bill, the consultant could report any situation that posed an imminent danger or substantial probability of death or serious injury to OSHA's enforcement division.

The bill also ran into opposition from labor unions, which saw it as a device to undermine the federal enforcement effort by "siphoning off" OSHA staff for consultation duties.

In related action, Congress did add an amendment to the fiscal 1976 appropriations bill for the Departments of Labor and Health, Education and Welfare (HR 8069 — PL 94-206) directing OSHA to fully develop the state advisory program and provided another $9 million for it. Congress had earmarked $5 million for the program in 1974.

At the same time, Congress also called on OSHA to simplify its regulations, upgrade compliance inspectors' skills, shift the focus of inspections from worker safety to worker health and concentrate enforcement efforts on industries with the most severe health and safety problems.

1976

Industry and Ford administration opposition contributed to the last-minute defeat of the major environmental bill of the year — a compromise measure amending the 1970 Clean Air Amendments.

Congress approved a long-debated toxic substances control bill and expanded solid waste management programs. But it let stand President Ford's veto of a pesticide regulation bill.

A Ford administration plan to permit private industry to produce enriched uranium was killed in the Senate. A Senate-passed food safety measure died when the House failed to act on it.

Clean Air Amendments

A complex and heavily lobbied bill (S 3219) amending the 1970 Clean Air Amendments (PL 91-604) was killed on the last day of the 94th Congress by a Senate filibuster.

The bill would have made the first comprehensive revision of the 1970 act, which initiated an ambitious federal-state clean-up effort directed by the Environmental Protection Agency (EPA). The agency, in cooperation with the states, was charged with establishing and enforcing national standards for major air pollutants within specific time limits — mid-1975 or 1977 in most cases.

By 1975, when Congress began to work on S 3219, affected industries — auto, steel, electric utilities and many others — were calling for modifications in the 1970 law to take account of the energy pinch and related economic problems such as unemployment and capital shortages.

Environmentalists resisted those appeals, insisting that new evidence about the effects of air pollution on human health made strict enforcement of the law more important than ever.

The Senate filibuster was directed at the final version of S 3219, which extended deadlines for compliance with auto and industrial emission limits and established a new system for regulating industrial growth in areas of the country with relatively pure air (known as the "no significant deterioration" policy).

Non-deterioration

It was these non-deterioration provisions that leaders of the Senate filibuster assailed, claiming that they would shut off development of important new energy supplies in many states and generally harm the economy. The filibuster was led by Jake Garn, R-Utah.

The provisions also were opposed by the Ford administration, electric utilities, oil and paper companies, real estate and construction interests, and business groups such as the U.S. Chamber of Commerce and the Business Roundtable.

Defeat of S 3219 left the non-deterioration policy in the hands of the EPA, which had issued regulations in 1974 to carry it out in response to a 1973 Supreme Court decision interpreting the Clean Air Act to intend that "no significant deterioration" of air quality should be allowed.

Auto Emission

The other big controversy over the final clean air bill involved the auto emissions timetable. S 3219 delayed the final standards somewhat but not as long as the auto industry, the Ford administration or a majority of the House had recommended. The major U.S. auto companies opposed the final bill and some sponsors gave them major responsibility for its defeat.

The industry was left with the timetables in existing law, imposing strict emission limits for all three controlled tailpipe pollutants on model-1978 cars, which would appear in showrooms in the fall of 1977. Industry spokesmen were confident that they could convince Congress to grant them an extension early in 1977, warning that otherwise they would be forced to produce illegal cars or close their factories.

Noise Control

Putting off a comprehensive review, Congress in 1976 approved a bill (HR 5272 — PL 94-301) authorizing fiscal 1976-77 funds for Environmental Protection Agency programs under the Noise Control Act of 1972 (PL 92-574). *(1972 law, p. 143)*

HR 5272 authorized \$13.3 million for fiscal 1976, \$3.3 million for the budgetary transition period and \$14.6 million for fiscal 1977.

Solid Waste Management

While legislation on air and water pollution was getting most of the attention, Congress cleared in late 1976 a bill (S 2150 — PL 94-580) expanding the federal solid waste program and authorizing new funds for state and local efforts to cope with garbage and sludge.

Sponsors called the vexing solid waste problem "the stepchild of the environmental movement," and warned that without increased efforts to solve it almost half the nation's cities were expected to run out of waste disposal sites by the early 1980s.

Unlike the 1976 clean air and water bills, which stirred great controversy and died in the final days of the session, the solid waste measure sailed through Congress with little opposition.

The "Resource Conservation and Recovery Act of 1976" amended the 1965 Solid Waste Disposal Act (PL 89-272), which was strengthened in 1970 by the Resource Recovery Act (PL 91-512). The titles reflected the growing sophistication of solid waste management concerns — from simple disposal to recycling to cutting down on the amount of wastes generated. *(1970 law, p. 138)*

The 1976 bill authorized a total of \$365.9 million for solid waste programs, mostly in fiscal 1978-79. That included \$80 million in those two years for general use by the Environmental Protection Agency (EPA), \$70 million to finance state solid waste management programs, \$50 million for state hazardous waste programs and \$35 million to help finance demonstration projects on new methods of recycling, extracting resources from or disposing of solid wastes.

The bill also established a federal permit program to

regulate hazardous wastes and required states receiving federal grants to ban all open dumping within five years of enactment.

Provisions

As signed into law, major provisions of S 2150 (PL 94-580):

EPA Solid Waste Program

• Directed the EPA to establish an Office of Solid Waste to administer the law. (This provision gave legal status to an existing EPA office.)

• Required that all solid waste regulations be reviewed and revised if necessary at least once every three years.

• Directed the EPA to establish a series of expert panels to advise state and local governments on solid waste programs. At least 20 percent of the annual appropriation for solid waste would have to be used for these panels.

• Authorized $750,000 annually in fiscal 1978-79 for grants covering 5 percent of the cost of tire shredders.

• Authorized $35 million in fiscal 1977, $38 million in fiscal 1978 and $42 million in fiscal 1979 to administer the solid waste law.

Hazardous Wastes

• Required the EPA, within a year and a half of enactment, to issue regulations defining the term hazardous waste and listing specific hazardous wastes. All hazardous waste handlers (manufacturers, transporters, etc.) would have another three months to notify the agency of their operations.

• Authorized state governors to petition the EPA to add substances to the hazardous waste list and gave the agency three months to respond.

• Required the EPA, within a year and a half of enactment, to issue regulations setting safety standards for producers and transporters of hazardous wastes and for operators of hazardous waste treatment, storage and disposal facilities. The regulations were to include requirements for record keeping, reporting, storage, labeling and disposal.

• Required the EPA, within a year and a half of enactment, to issue regulations requiring permits to operate hazardous waste treatment, storage or disposal facilities.

• Required the EPA, within a year and a half of enactment, to issue guidelines to help states set up hazardous waste programs. States authorized by the agency could take over administration of the permits and safety rules.

• Authorized the EPA and state officials to inspect the premises and records of hazardous waste handlers.

• Established a civil penalty of up to $25,000 a day for hazardous waste violations that took place after state or federal compliance deadlines; set a criminal penalty of up to $25,000 a day and/or one year in prison for knowing violations.

• Permitted states to issue hazardous waste regulations more stringent than federal regulations.

• Authorized $25 million annually in fiscal 1978-79 for grants to states for hazardous waste programs. The EPA would allot the funds according to a formula based on the volume of hazardous waste, extent of human exposure and other factors. At least 30 percent of each year's solid waste appropriation would have to be used for these grants.

• Authorized the EPA to seek a court injunction to control a hazardous waste that presented an imminent danger to health or the environment.

State and Regional Solid Waste Plans

• Required the EPA, within six months of enactment, to publish guidelines for state solid waste management plans.

• Authorized states to enter into agreements to carry out joint solid waste management programs.

• Established a timetable for states to develop state or regional solid waste management plans. To win EPA approval, a plan had to phase out all open dumps within five years, require that all solid waste be recycled or disposed of safely, and provide for the closing or upgrading of existing open dumps.

• Required the EPA, within one year of enactment, to issue regulations distinguishing sanitary landfills from open dumps. One year later the agency would be required to publish an inventory of all open dumps in the nation.

• Authorized $30 million in fiscal 1978 and $40 million in fiscal 1979 for grants to states for development and implementation of solid waste management plans.

• Authorized $15 million annually in fiscal 1978-79 for grants to states, counties, cities and local agencies for solid waste programs — including resource recovery, resource conservation and hazardous waste management. EPA would allot the funds according to a formula based on population size.

• Authorized $2.5 million annually in fiscal 1978-79 for grants to small cities with severe solid waste problems caused by disposal from outlying areas.

• Authorized $25 million annually in fiscal 1978-79 for special grants covering 75 percent of the cost of solid waste management facilities in rural communities.

Research, Development and Demonstration

• Directed the EPA, in cooperation with other federal agencies, to provide financial aid to government agencies and private firms for research and demonstration projects on solid waste — including experimental plants producing fuel from solid waste.

• Authorized $8 million in fiscal 1978-79 for the EPA to conduct 10 studies on solid waste including recovery of glass and plastic waste, sludge problems and aviation hazards caused by airport landfills.

• Authorized $2 million for a Resource Conservation Committee, headed by the EPA administrator and composed of top administration officials, to study all aspects of resource conservation.

• Directed the EPA to do studies and demonstration projects on solid waste recovery and conservation issues such as the need for surcharges on consumer products to cover the cost of disposal.

• Authorized $35 million in fiscal 1978 for grants covering 75 percent of the cost of resource recovery demonstration projects or construction of new or improved solid waste disposal facilities. The funds would be used for research, not commercial, projects.

Other Provisions

• Forbade EPA officials and employees to "lobby for or otherwise represent an agency position in favor of resource recovery or resource conservation" as part of state or local laws, regulations or policies.

• Required federal officials administering the solid waste law to file annual financial disclosures of all interests in individuals or companies receiving federal solid waste funds.

• Directed the Labor Department to investigate allegations that employees were fired or discriminated against for participating in enforcement of the solid waste law, and to take remedial action on valid complaints.

• Directed the EPA to monitor the law's effect on employment and to investigate plant closings and layoffs attributed to solid waste regulations.

• Authorized private citizens to sue violators of the law and the EPA for failure to enforce it.

• Authorized private citizens to petition the EPA to issue, amend or repeal a solid waste regulation.

• Required all federal facilities to comply with solid waste regulations, except when the president made an exception in the national interest.

• Required government agencies to purchase items composed of the highest possible percentage of recycled materials consistent with reasonable price and performance; directed them to use fuel generated from recovered materials as often as possible.

Uranium Enrichment

President Gerald R. Ford's plan to open up the uranium enrichment industry to private enterprise died in the Senate in 1976. The proposal (HR 8401) was passed by the House after a series of close votes. But opponents kept it off the Senate floor until late in the session when a motion to bring it up was rejected.

HR 8401 would have permitted private industry to begin production of enriched uranium, ending 30 years of government monopoly over the technology. Uranium must be enriched to serve as fuel in nuclear power plants. The private nuclear power industry had been seeking such authority since 1969 with the support of the Nixon and Ford administrations.

As passed by the House Aug. 4, the bill authorized the Energy Research and Development Administration (ERDA) to make tentative contract agreements with private firms to produce enriched uranium. Such tentative contracts would be submitted to Congress, which would have to approve any contract within 60 days in order for it to take effect.

ERDA would have been authorized under HR 8401 to guarantee domestic investors that the government would assume all assets and liabilities, including debt, if a private uranium enrichment venture failed prior to the end of a year of commercial operation. Foreign investment would not be protected under the guarantee.

ERDA would have been limited to $8 billion in contract authority, a figure estimated by the administration to be the maximum potential cost to the government if up to four private ventures covered by cooperative agreements with the government failed. The money was to cover costs of assuming assets and liabilities of the ventures, including takeover of the plants.

HR 8401 also directed ERDA to expand the federally owned enrichment facility at Portsmouth, Ohio.

The controversial nature of HR 8401 was reflected by House floor votes on an amendment by Jonathan B. Bingham, D-N.Y., that would have dropped all of the bill's provisions except expansion of the federal facility at Portsmouth. The amendment was originally accepted 170-168, but was then rejected, 192-193. The Senate's Sept. 29 vote against bringing the bill to the floor was also close, 30-33.

Toxic Substances Control

The House and Senate reconciled past differences and cleared a toxic substances control bill (S 3149 — PL 94-469) in September 1976. The measure expanded federal regulation of industrial and commercial chemicals and for the first time required pre-market testing for potentially dangerous chemicals.

President Ford signed it despite earlier administration opposition to some provisions. The compromise bill was not entirely satisfactory to either side, but it retained the support of the environmental, labor and consumer forces who favored a strong bill as well as that of the Manufacturing Chemists Association (later renamed the Chemical Manufacturers Association), a trade organization of large companies that originally had endorsed a more limited bill.

The environmentalists were relieved to have a toxic substances program in place after five years of debate and hoped to strengthen it in the future. The industry promised to keep an eye on the Environmental Protection Agency (EPA) as it put the law into effect, hoping the regulations would not be burdensome.

With a toxic substances law in effect, backers said, chemical hazards such as vinyl chloride and fluorocarbons could have been detected earlier.

The bill singled out for special attention a class of chemical compounds known as PCBs (polychlorinated biphenyls), used as insulators in electric transformers and capacitors, and in many other commercial and industrial products.

Like the banned pesticide DDT, PCBs persisted in the environment, could accumulate in human tissues and were a serious health hazard. High levels of PCBs were discovered in the Great Lakes, the Hudson River in New York and other U.S. waters in 1976, damaging the commercial fishing industry and giving impetus to the push for federal controls. The new law called for a complete ban on the manufacture and distribution of PCBs by early 1979.

The most debated issue during consideration of the measure was how much power the EPA should have to hold new chemicals off the market. The compromise version allowed the EPA to issue an order holding up the marketing of a chemical beyond the pre-market notice period to gather more information or banning its manufacture altogether for health or environmental reasons. If a manufacturer objected to such an EPA order, the EPA could either rescind the order or seek a court injunction to keep the chemical off the market.

Provisions

As signed into law, major provisions of S 3149 (PL 94-469):

• Set a national policy that adequate data should be developed on the health and environmental effects of chemicals, and that this should be the responsibility of the manufacturers and processors.

• Directed the EPA to require testing of chemical substances and mixtures that "present an unreasonable risk of injury to health or the environment" if there was insufficient data to predict the product's effects or if the product would be produced in substantial quantities and distributed widely.

• Required the EPA to establish standards for testing and to review them at least once a year. Companies producing the same chemicals could work out cost-sharing or reimbursement arrangements and the EPA could exempt a company from performing tests if the company reimbursed another firm for the work.

• Set up a committee of eight federal officials with scientific and regulatory expertise to prepare a list of chemicals to which the EPA would give priority in issuing testing requirements. The first list would be published within nine months of enactment and revised every six months. For the top 50 chemicals on the list, the agency would have one year from the time a chemical first appeared on the list to begin proceedings to require testing or publish reasons for not doing so.

• Required companies to notify the EPA 90 days before manufacturing any new chemical or before manufacturing or processing any chemical for a "significant new use" as defined by the agency. The notice would include test data and other information about the product. The agency could extend the notification period for an additional 90 days.

• Authorized the EPA to issue an order banning or regulating the use of any chemical that came to its attention through the notice procedure if there was insufficient evidence about its safety and it would be produced in substantial quantities and distributed widely, or if there was insufficient evidence and the product presented a health or environmental hazard. If a company objected to such an order, the agency would have to seek a court injunction to enforce it.

• Required the EPA to issue regulations taking effect immediately to control the marketing of chemicals that came to its attention under the notice procedure if they presented an unreasonable health or environmental risk. For a complete ban on manufacturing, however, the agency would be required to issue an order subject to objection by the company as in the other cases.

• Required the EPA to publish its reasons for not taking regulatory action on chemicals during the notice period.

• Required the EPA to issue regulations prohibiting the manufacture, limiting the amount manufactured, prescribing labeling or disposal requirements, or otherwise regulating any chemical substance or mixture that presented an unreasonable risk of injury to health or the environment. The agency was required to hold informal hearings on proposed regulations, giving interested parties a chance to testify or submit written arguments, although regulations could become effective immediately in cases of extreme hazard. The agency could pay the attorneys' fees and other costs of participating for groups that would contribute to the proceedings but otherwise could not afford to take part.

• Authorized the EPA to seek a court injunction halting the sale and distribution of any chemical that presented an imminent hazard.

• Required the EPA to ban or restrict the use of any chemical presenting a serious risk of cancer, gene mutations or birth defects.

• Prohibited the manufacture, sale or distribution of polychlorinated biphenyls (PCBs) not in "enclosed systems," beginning one year after enactment, unless the EPA found that continued use of PCBs in some other manner would not threaten health or the environment. Manufacture of all PCBs was prohibited two years after enactment and processing or distribution two and one-half years after enactment unless the agency made exceptions.

• Required the EPA, if it determined that any chemical risk could be controlled adequately under the authority of a law administered by another agency, to give that agency 90 days to begin regulatory action or determine that no action was necessary. The EPA would be required to use other laws under its jurisdiction to regulate chemicals if the laws were adequate, unless it decided using the toxic substances law instead would be in the public interest.

• Required chemical manufacturers and processors to keep records and file reports as prescribed by the EPA. Small companies and makers of chemicals in small quantities for research purposes would be exempt from some of the requirements.

• Required the EPA to keep an up-to-date list of all chemicals manufactured and processed in the United States.

• Required all chemical manufacturers and processors to keep for five years records of reported environmental or health problems connected with their products and for 30 years all records of employee health problems.

• Exempted from regulation under the law pesticides, cigarettes and other tobacco products, firearms and ammunition, foods, food additives, drugs, cosmetics, medical devices and nuclear materials. Chemicals intended for export were exempted from all but the reporting requirements, but imported chemicals were subject to the law.

• Set a civil penalty of up to $25,000 a day for violations of the law, and a criminal penalty for knowing or willing violations of $25,000 a day and/or one year in prison.

• Authorized the EPA to issue subpoenas and to inspect the premises and records of chemical manufacturers and processors.

• Authorized private citizens to sue companies for violations of the law and the EPA for failure to carry out mandatory provisions.

• Authorized private citizens to petition the EPA to begin a proceeding to issue, amend or repeal toxic substances regulations.

• Authorized the EPA to waive compliance with any provision of the law if the president requested it on national defense grounds.

• Prohibited companies from firing or discriminating against employees who participated in enforcement of the toxic substances law.

• Directed the EPA to monitor the effect of toxic substances regulations on employment and to investigate allegations that a company threatened to fire or lay off workers because of the regulations.

• Authorized the Department of Health, Education and Welfare to finance projects aimed at developing inexpensive and efficient methods for testing chemicals.

• Authorized $1.5 million annually in fiscal 1977-79 for EPA grants to states covering up to 75 percent of the cost of programs to reduce risks from chemicals.

• Authorized $10.1 million in fiscal 1977, $12.6 million in fiscal 1978 and $16.2 million in fiscal 1979 for administration of the law.

• Stipulated that the law would take effect Jan. 1, 1977, and required the EPA to submit an annual report on its administration to the president and Congress.

Food Safety

For the second Congress in a row, the Senate passed a comprehensive food safety and labeling bill (S 641) that died without House action. The proposed "Consumer Food Act" was similar to an earlier food safety bill (S 2373) passed by the Senate in 1974. *(p. 153)*

The measure imposed new safety requirements on food processors and increased the Food and Drug Administration's (FDA) food safety enforcement powers. It also required more information on food labels and provided legal authority for FDA regulations on nutritional, ingredient and data labeling.

The bill was referred to the House Interstate and Foreign Commerce Subcommittee on Health and the Environment, headed by Paul G. Rogers, D-Fla. Rogers preferred to develop his own food safety legislation but did not get around to the task in the 93rd or 94th Congress.

Related Development. The Senate in 1976 also approved a measure (S 1681) tightening federal regulation of the cosmetics industry, but it died without House action.

The bill would have required cosmetic makers to document the safety of their products before marketing them. It also would have given the FDA new authority to require additional testing of suspicious products and ban dangerous ones.

Pesticide Regulation

A bill (HR 12944) extending funding for Environmental Protection Agency (EPA) pesticide control programs for six months, through September 1977, died at the end of the session when Congress let stand President Ford's Aug. 13 veto.

Ford vetoed the measure because he opposed as unconstitutional a provision authorizing either chamber of Congress to invalidate any pesticide regulation issued by the EPA. The legislative veto amendment was added to the bill on the House floor with the support of farm state legislators who considered the agency's pesticide regulations too strict.

Congress had revised the pesticide program in 1975 after much debate about the EPA's performance. HR 12944 was a stopgap measure designed to postpone detailed oversight hearings until 1977. Sponsors made no attempt to override the veto, since in the meantime fiscal 1977 pesticide funds were appropriated under a procedure waiving the requirement for separating authorizing legislation. *(1975 bill, p. 154)*

Toxic Chemical Indemnities

The Senate March 10, 1976, passed a bill (S 2578) to authorize low-interest government loans to help farmers who suffered losses when their commodities or livestock were contaminated by toxic chemicals. The measure died when the House took no action.

The Senate Agriculture and Forestry Committee cited 17 incidents of chemical contamination of poultry since 1968 and seven involving livestock, with losses totaling more than $97 million. The report detailed the case of the accidental shipment in 1973 of a fire retardant chemical, polybrominated biphenyl (PBB), to Michigan dairy farmers for use as a feed supplement. More than 500 farms in that state were quarantined as a result; and more than 1 million animals and many tons of feed of dairy products had to be destroyed, the committee said.

The Agriculture Department opposed the bill, saying that other loan programs were available to aid farmers with such losses.

OSHA Exemptions

Critics of OSHA managed to chip away at the agency's power in 1976, as Congress voted to limit its authority over farms and businesses in certain instances.

Congressional attempts to exempt small businesses from OSHA health and safety regulations were turned down both in 1974 and 1975, but in 1976 the first exemption for small businesses was enacted. The exemption was added to the fiscal 1977 Labor-HEW appropriations bill and applied only to farms with 10 or fewer employees. Another amendment approved that year prohibited inspectors from fining a business for health and safety violations the first time they were detected unless the violations numbered 10 or more or involved serious hazards to workers. The $56.6 billion appropriation bill (PL 94-439) became law Sept. 30 when Congress overrode Ford's veto of it.

Black Lung Disease

Time ran out for legislation (HR 10760) that would have made more coal miners eligible for black lung disease benefits and shifted the cost of the benefit program to the coal industry. Passed by the House in March 1976, the bill did not reach the Senate floor until Sept. 30. But the Senate never got around to acting on the bill before adjournment Oct. 2.

The first section of the controversial House-passed bill made persons who had worked a certain number of years in coal mines automatically eligible for black lung disease benefits. Under existing law, miners had to prove they had the disease to collect benefits.

Black lung disease (pneumoconiosis) was caused by inhaling coal dust and led to severe breathing problems and premature death.

A second part of the bill established an industry-financed trust fund to pay benefits for miners who filed future claims.

This proposal was part of an ongoing effort to shift the cost of the program, created in 1969, from the federal government to coal mine operators. Since the program was last amended in 1972, the government had tried to foot the bill only as a last resort.

But coal companies continued to challenge claims for which they were found liable and assumed support in only about 100 cases. In contrast, the government paid benefits for 360,000 claims at a cost of close to $1 billion a year.

The measure had the strong support of the United Mine Workers of America, but was opposed by the administration and coal mine operators.

The administration argued that relaxing eligibility rules would cost too much and preferred improvement of state workers' compensation programs to the trust fund proposal.

Congress liberalized the program and established an industry trust fund in 1978. *(1972 amendments, p. 149; 1978 amendments, p. 173)*

1977

Four important environmental health bills were passed in 1977 and Congress all but completed action on two others. Probably the two most significant were extensions of the 1970 Clean Air Amendments and the 1972 water pollution control law. In passing the clean air extension, Congress once again delayed deadlines by which auto manufacturers and industries had to clean up car exhausts and industrial pollutants. Congress also permitted some delays in water pollution control deadlines. But in both cases, the basic goals of the legislation — to clean up the nation's air and water — remained intact.

Congress also acted to extend the safe drinking water law and to strengthen enforcement of federal health and safety regulations applied to mining operations.

A bill to make it easier for the Environmental Protection Agency to register pesticides neared completion, as did legislation to liberalize black lung benefits. Both bills were enacted in 1978.

Congress voted to delay imposition of a federal ban on the synthetic sweetener saccharin, which had been found to cause cancer in laboratory animals. President Carter vetoed a bill that continued funding for construction of a fast breeder nuclear reactor on Tennessee's Clinch River. Although Congress made no attempt to override that veto, the dispute over the Clinch River project would continue throughout Carter's term.

Clean Air Amendments

Congress barely beat a deadline Aug. 4 when it gave final approval to the Clean Air Act Amendments of 1977 (HR 6161 — PL 95-95).

Pressured by both the White House and the automobile industry, conferees negotiated for eight days before Congress began its summer recess. They finally reached agreement after a seven-hour session that ended at 2:20 a.m. Aug. 3, and both chambers adopted that agreement Aug. 4. President Carter signed the bill into law Aug. 7 with a promise to enforce it, particularly the controversial provisions to control automobile exhausts.

The law amended and extended the 1970 Clean Air Amendments (PL 91-604). Its passage completed a major job left over from the 94th Congress. At the end of the 1976 session a Senate filibuster led by Jake Garn, R-Utah, killed a conference report produced after months of hearings, committee meetings and debate. *(1970 act, p. 135; 1976 legislation, p. 156)*

Taken together, the 1970 act and the 1977 amendments formed the nation's most complex and far-reaching environmental law. It affected virtually all industrial and transportation activities, the production and use of energy, and real estate development. Its fundamental purpose was to protect public health by cleaning the air.

In its major provisions PL 95-95 did the following:

- Delayed existing standards for automobile emissions for two more years, but tightened standards for the 1980 models and again for 1981.
- Set new standards to protect clean-air areas, including national parks, but authorized variances and some development near such areas.
- Extended the deadline for cities to meet national air quality standards until 1982, and in some cases until 1987. The previous deadline was 1977.
- Gave most industrial polluters up to three additional years to comply before facing heavy fines.
- Directed the Environmental Protection Agency (EPA) to review criteria for ambient air quality standards before 1981 and required subsequent reviews every five years thereafter.
- Provided for continuing research into the effects of various substances and activities on the stratospheric ozone layer, and authorized EPA to regulate such substances.
- Established a National Commission on Air Quality.
- Required more than a dozen studies concerning air pollution.

Auto Emissions. The most difficult task Congress faced in writing the 1977 amendments concerned new standards and deadlines for three pollutants from automobile exhausts — hydrocarbons (HC), carbon monoxide (CO) and nitrogen oxide (NOx). The lowest-level "statutory standards" under the 1970 act were to have been met by the 1975-model cars. But three postponements — two by EPA and one by Congress — delayed the standards until the 1978-model year.

The car manufacturers, who requested the three delays, claimed they still could not meet the standards. As the 1978 cars were readied for production in August and September 1977, industry leaders threatened to shut down their assembly lines rather than produce "illegal" cars subject to fines of up to $10,000 each.

President Carter then urged Congress to act to avoid potential damage to the nation's economy. Congressional leaders took steps to delay the recess, scheduled to begin Aug. 5, until conferees agreed on a bill.

Non-deterioration. The second most difficult issue was "non-deterioration." The term meant preventing significant deterioration of air quality in areas where the air was cleaner than national ambient standards. That was the issue that killed the 1976 bill, and it created problems again in the 1977 conference.

PL 95-95 established three categories for clean-air areas, and set maximum allowable increases of particulates and sulfur dioxide for each class. It allowed a variance above the sulfur dioxide increments for up to 18 days a year in Class I areas, which included pristine areas such as national parks.

Non-attainment Areas. The third major issue in the 1977 amendments turned out to be not so controversial as anticipated. It regulated industrial development in "non-attainment" areas — primarily cities that had not attained national ambient standards by the mid-1977 deadline set in the 1970 act. The issue held up Senate committee action but did not cause lengthy anticipated floor fights.

The final provision solved the problem by extending the deadline and by allowing new sources only if the pollution they caused would be offset by reducing emissions from existing sources.

Provisions

HR 6161 (PL 95-95) amended most sections of the 1970 Clean Air Act. As signed into law, PL 95-95 contained the following major provisions:

Title I — Stationary Sources

Non-attainment Areas. Under the original law, all areas of the nation were to have attained national ambient air standards by mid-1977. The amendments extended the deadline to Dec. 31, 1982, except that cities with especially severe oxidant and carbon monoxide problems were given an extension to Dec. 31, 1987. States with non-attainment areas were required to submit revised implementation plans in 1979 and again in 1982.

The plans of states seeking extension to 1987 had to include alternative site analyses for proposed major sources of pollution, a schedule for implementing a vehicle inspection and maintenance program, and plans to improve public transportation. States with auto-related problems could adopt emission standards identical to California's. (California planned to reduce in 1982 the nitrogen oxide level from 1 gram per mile to 0.4 gram — stricter than national standards.)

All revised implementation plans had to contain a permit program for new or modified major facilities. Permits could be issued only if pollution offset requirements would be met or the new source would not exceed the new growth allowance. Prior to 1979, the EPA offset policy of Dec. 21, 1976, would be in effect in most non-attainment areas. New or expanded facilities would be required to use the best control technology and processes available.

Conferees on HR 6161 dropped the House provision to require equal reductions in emissions every two years. But they reported their intention that "regular, consistent emission reductions will be demonstrated through the mechanism of the implementation plan" up to the attainment deadline.

Governors were given authority, until they submitted revised plans, to suspend portions of existing transportation control plans dealing with on-street parking restrictions, gas rationing and retrofit of non-commercial vehicles.

Industrial Compliance. Stationary sources that directly emitted pollution could obtain delayed compliance permission from the state or EPA allowing them to continue operations temporarily even though they violated emission limitations. Orders were limited to not more than a three-year delay. No orders could be issued after July 1, 1979, unless they established delayed compliance penalties.

There were exceptions. Sources using innovative technology to control pollution were given up to a five-year delay. Sources ordered to convert to coal were given until Dec. 31, 1980, to comply with state implementation plans, with authority for an additional delay up to five years. Primary non-ferrous smelters operating at the time of enactment could be given two delayed compliance orders, the first until Jan. 1, 1983, the second until Jan. 1, 1988.

Penalties were designed to make non-compliance more expensive than compliance. Assessments had to be no less than the quarterly equivalent of the capital costs of compliance and debt service over a normal amortization period, operation and maintenance costs foregone as a result of non-compliance, and the additional economic value gained by delay in compliance beyond July 1, 1979.

Non-Deterioration. The legislation established three categories for areas having air cleaner than national ambient standards. They were labeled Class I, II and III, with Class I having the cleanest ("pristine") air.

Mandatory Class I areas were all international parks regardless of size, national memorial parks and wilderness areas exceeding 5,000 acres, and national parks exceeding 6,000 acres. Class II initially included all other clean-air areas, and they could be redesignated. Class III areas would be designated following hearings and studies, but several types of public lands exceeding 10,000 acres would not be eligible for Class III designation.

The legislation set increments for the maximum allowable increases of particulates and sulfur dioxide for each of the three classes. Within two years EPA was to propose increments or other means for preventing significant deterioration from nitrogen oxides, hydrocarbons, carbon monoxide and oxidants. These regulations would take effect in one year, when revision of state plans would begin. States could adopt control strategies other than increments for the four pollutants.

A variance above the sulfur dioxide increments only could be granted for up to 18 days a year in Class I areas, with different increments for high- and low-terrain areas as defined by the act. A violation of three hours in one day was considered a violation for the entire day. The governor could grant the variance only after public hearings. If the secretary of interior or other Cabinet officer in charge of the lands opposed the variance, the president would have to decide the issue within 90 days.

State plans had to require permits for pollution sources in clean-air areas, with conditions specified in the law. Indian tribes were authorized to redesignate tribal reservation lands as Class I or Class II.

Visibility Protection. The legislation included major parts of a House provision to reduce visible pollution in mandatory Class I areas.

Within six months the interior secretary was to identify all federal Class I areas where visibility was an important value. Interior and EPA would list such areas and recommendations for improvement within one year and periodically when appropriate.

States had to identify the sources that impaired visibility, and set emission limitations based on the best available retrofit technology for each source. Requirements of this section had to be included in state implementation plans.

New Source Standards. Performance standards for new sources of pollution were revised.

Boilers fired by fossil fuels were required to use "the best technological system of continuous emission reduction," no matter if they used untreated low-sulfur coal as a step toward compliance. Standards for such sources included both performance standards for emissions and a percentage reduction in pollution from untreated fuel. EPA was permitted to set a range of pollutant reductions to reflect varying fuel characteristics.

Waivers from the new source performance standards could be granted on a unit-by-unit or source-by-source basis to permit use of innovative continuous emission control technology. But the cumulative period of all waivers could not exceed seven years after the first waiver was granted to that unit or four years after the unit began operating, whichever occurred earlier.

Enforcement. The law authorized the courts to impose civil penalties of up to $25,000 a day for violations of the act. Knowing violations of the delayed compliance penalty provisions were made subject to criminal sanctions.

Implementation Plans. States were directed to revise implementation plans to meet new requirements of the law. Plans had to include air quality maintenance measures and pre-construction permit requirements.

EPA was prohibited from requiring indirect source review programs, except with respect to certain federally funded projects. However, state and local governments were allowed to adopt and enforce such programs.

This section also:

- Required that pre-construction reviews of direct sources include consideration of energy, environmental and economic impacts.
- Provided that implementation plans require the payment of permit fees by the owner or operator of major stationary sources.
- Prohibited owners or operators of stationary sources from making employees bear the costs of periodic shutdowns or production curtailments undertaken as supplemental or intermittent control measures.

Control Regions. Each state was required to send to EPA, within 120 days of enactment of the law, a list identifying air quality levels within its control regions. EPA was given 60 days to approve each list.

Governors were authorized to revise the boundaries of air quality control regions within their states to improve management.

Air Quality Standards. EPA had to review criteria for ambient air quality standards by Dec. 31, 1980. Subsequent reviews of standards were required at least once every five years thereafter. The EPA administrator had to appoint an independent scientific committee of seven members to recommend new standards.

Within one year of enactment, EPA had to set a national primary standard for nitrogen dioxide concentrations over a period of not more than three hours.

Other Provisions. Other sections of Title I did the following:

- Gave the governors authority to temporarily suspend state implementation plans when there was a presidential finding of an energy or economic emergency in the nation or region. However, only the president was authorized to suspend federal standards or requirements.
- Authorized EPA to establish design, equipment or operational standards when it was not feasible to set emission standards for hazardous air pollutants.
- Abolished the president's Air Quality Advisory Board.
- Classified radioactive substances as air pollutants, and required EPA to study several unregulated pollutants for possible inclusion under the act.
- Stated that tall stacks were not a means of emission limitation under the act, but made one exception for a 20-year-old steam plant operated by the TVA.
- Provided that the president or governor might require the use of local coal by certain plants to prevent severe economic disruption or unemployment.

Title II — Mobile Sources

Auto Emissions. The 1977 standards of 1.5 grams per mile of hydrocarbons (HC), 15 grams of carbon monoxide (CO) and 2 grams of nitrogen oxide (NOx) were extended through model years 1978 and 1979. The 1980 standards were tightened to .41 HC, 7 CO and 2 NOx. In 1981 and beyond they were set at .41 HC, 3.4 CO and 1 NOx. However, the CO standard for 1981 and 1982 could be waived up to 7 grams by the EPA if public health did not require the statutory standard and if technology to meet it did not exist.

Other waivers were permitted for NOx. Small manufacturers, including American Motors Corp., that depended on emissions technology produced by other companies were given a two-year waiver until 1983 to meet 1 gram NOx. A waiver to 1.5 grams NOx for any four-year period after 1980 was permitted for certain innovative technology on up to 50,000 vehicles or engines produced by one company. A four-year waiver to 1.5 grams NOx was permitted for light-duty diesel engines as well, but only for model years 1981-84.

Auto Emission Timetables

The following table compares the national standards and schedules for automobile exhaust pollutants as set by the 1970 Clean Air Act and relaxed by the 1977 amendments to that act. The standards are stated in grams per mile of hydrocarbons (HC), carbon monoxide (CO) and nitrogen oxide (NOx).

Model	1970 Act (PL 91-604)			1977 Amendments (PL 95-95)		
Year	HC	CO	NOx	HC	CO	NOx
'77	1.5	15.0	2.0	1.5	15.0	2.0
'78	.41	3.4	.4	1.5	15.0	2.0
'79	.41	3.4	.4	1.5	15.0	2.0
'80	.41	3.4	.4	.41	7.0	2.0
'81	.41	3.4	.4	.41	3.4*	1.0**
'82	.41	3.4	.4	.41	3.4*	1.0**

*EPA could waive the 3.4 gram CO standard for 1981 and 1982 if public health did not require it and if the technology to achieve it did not exist.

**A four-year waiver of up to 1.5 grams NOx was authorized for diesel engines (1981-84 only) and for innovative technology having potential air quality and fuel economy benefits.

High-Altitude Vehicles. Existing high-altitude regulations were suspended until 1981. Models 1981-1983 had to meet standards based on percentage reduction no greater than those for all cars, based on emissions from 1970 cars operating at high altitudes. For 1984 and thereafter, cars had to meet statutory standards at all altitudes.

Trucks, Buses and Motorcycles. EPA had to set interim standards for HC and CO through 1982, with statutory HC and CO standards becoming effective in 1983 and statutory NOx standards in 1985. Statutory standards for heavy-duty vehicles mandated a 90 percent reduction from base line for HC and CO, and a 75 percent reduction from base line for NOx. Revision of any statutory standard required four years of lead time.

Tampering. The measure prohibited removal of or tampering with emission control systems by manufacturers and dealers, independent repair and service businesses; and selling, leasing, trading or fleet operations. Civil penalties of up to $2,500 per vehicle were authorized.

Warranties and Parts. The legislation set a performance warranty of 24 months or 24,000 miles, during which the car manufacturer would have to bring into compliance with emissions standards any vehicle that failed an inspection and maintenance test. Catalytic converters, thermal reactors and other emission control devices had to have a warranty for five years or 50,000 miles.

Within two years of enactment, EPA was to provide regulations to certify parts made by other than the car manufacturer. Repairs and maintenance could be performed at any service shop using certified parts. The cost of any major part used principally for emission control and scheduled for replacement during the useful life of the vehicle had to be borne by the manufacturer. Car owners were made responsible for properly maintaining vehicles and equipment.

Production Line Test. The final legislation did not include the Senate bill's provision for a production line test. But conferees recognized existing authority for EPA to test or require testing of new cars to see whether they complied with emission standards. The bill directed EPA to revise test procedures to provide a short production line test that would "assure reasonable statistical certainty that each car produced will be able to pass an emissions inspection."

Fuels and Additives. The measure directed EPA to require manufacturers of fuels and fuel additives to test the potential health effects of their products, including the effect of a substance on emission control performance. Fuels or additives introduced into commerce or increased in concentration between Jan. 1, 1974, and March 31, 1977, had to be removed no later than Sept. 15, 1978.

The legislation relaxed standards on lead levels in gasoline produced by small refineries and directed EPA to set new standards for the period beyond Oct. 1, 1982.

California Waiver. EPA was authorized to grant a waiver from automobile standards for California if EPA determined that the state standards in the aggregate were as protective of public health and welfare as the federal standards.

Title III — Miscellaneous Provisions

The legislation contained miscellaneous provisions that:

- Authorized the EPA administrator to issue emergency orders in a public health emergency and required him to bring civil suit within 24 hours of such orders. Violators could be fined up to $5,000 a day.
- Allowed citizens to bring suit against sources to force compliance with emission standards or limitations, to prevent construction or modification of a major emitting facility without a permit, and to stop violation of conditions or requirements specified by the state or EPA under several provisions of the law.
- Retained existing provisions giving the Department of Justice primary responsibility for controlling and supervising civil litigation involving EPA.
- Required EPA to prepare an economic impact assessment on proposed regulations, with required analysis of five items. But EPA rules could not be challenged on failure to comply with this section.
- Established a National Commission on Air Quality of 13 members, including four from Congress. The commission was directed to make five studies in three years with a total authorization of $10 million.
- Required financial disclosure by members of the Scientific Review Committee established in Title I, and prohibited conflicts of interest, one year after enactment, by officers and employees of EPA and officers of other organizations (including non-profit organizations) engaged in activities related to air quality.
- Directed EPA to investigate, report and advise on the potential loss or shifts of employment resulting from the Clean Air Act. Protected employees who believed they were fired or discriminated against as a result of their testimony or legal action under the act, and authorized the secretary of labor to award compensatory damages for violations.
- Authorized EPA to withhold, condition or restrict construction grants for sewage treatment plants under limited circumstances related to the Clean Air Act.
- Required EPA within one year of enactment to set regulations establishing a standard air quality index for monitoring and reporting by state and local governments.
- Required the owners of retail gasoline outlets to pay for vapor recovery equipment on fuel storage tanks and pumps within three years. Independent marketers selling less than 50,000 gallons of gasoline a month were not required to install and use the equipment, unless their state or local governments required it.
- Authorized $200 million each year for fiscal 1978-1981 to implement provisions not authorized elsewhere.

Title IV — Studies

Title IV of the legislation:

- Provided a uniform standard of proof for EPA regulation of air pollutants applied to national ambient air quality, new stationary source performance, hazardous stationary source emissions, auto emissions, regulation of fuels and additives, and aircraft emissions. Authorized EPA to regulate any future air pollution from these sources.
- Required creation within three months of enactment of the law of a Task Force on Environmental Cancer and Heart and Lung Disease, led by EPA and including representatives of the National Institutes of Health, to conduct research programs and report to Congress annually.
- Required EPA and other agencies to conduct several studies on the effects of several specific pollutants.

Water Pollution

Overcoming difficulties that thwarted passage of similar legislation in 1976, the House and Senate reached agreement late in 1977 on a number of difficult water pollution problems. Though some delays in cleanup were allowed on economic grounds, the measure cleared by Congress Dec. 15 kept intact the basic principles of the strong 1972 water pollution control law.

The changes made by the Clean Water Act of 1977 (HR 3199 — PL 95-217) were touted as only "mid-course corrections," when Congress began tinkering with the law. But in fact industry had hoped for a major rewrite and environmentalists had feared a damaging postponement of the goals in the 1972 Federal Water Pollution Control Act Amendments (PL 92-500).

As it turned out, the final compromises left no clear victor. Spokesmen for industry hailed the bill as a step toward reasonableness in pollution control, but admitted some disappointments.

Environmental groups were split, with some joining Environmental Protection Agency (EPA) officials in praising the conferees and others insisting the legislation was a step backwards.

The overriding objective of the 1972 act, which replaced pollution control laws going back to 1899, was to "restore and maintain the chemical, physical and biological integrity of the nation's waters." The law also set two additional goals: fishable and swimmable waters by 1983 and elimination of all polluted discharges into navigable waters by 1985. *(1972 law, p. 145)*

To achieve those goals, the law required all U.S. industries to use, by July 1, 1977, the "best practicable control technology currently available" for treatment of discharges. By July 1, 1983, industries were to use the "best available technology economically achievable."

Municipal waste treatment plants were directed to provide "secondary treatment" removing 85 percent of pollutants by July 1, 1977 — and to use "best practicable" technology by July 1, 1983. The law authorized $18 billion in federal funds to help construct new public waste-water treatment facilities and upgrade existing ones, with the federal government paying 75 percent of construction costs.

Deadlines Postponed

One of the key controversies between the House and Senate in 1977 was over postponement of the industry deadline to meet the "best available technology" requirement. An estimated 80 to 90 percent of the nation's industries had met the 1977 deadline for use of "best practicable technology." With that good record, industry officials argued forcefully for a postponement of the 1983 deadline. They contended that the expensive equipment needed to meet the requirement could cost industry $60 billion and would provide only incremental improvement in water quality.

The Senate agreed in part with these arguments and, in its bill, clarified the authority of the EPA administrator to waive 1983 requirements in some cases for conventional pollutants such as dirt, nitrogen and phosphorous. The Senate bill did not permit waivers for toxic pollutants.

The House bill did not contain any comparable provisions. However, the majority of House conferees felt that the Senate bill did not provide industry enough relief. They suggested that EPA require industry to use the best available technology only for toxics or when the water quality of a certain stream demanded it. Best practicable technology would continue to be the standard for other types of pollutants.

The issue was not resolved until the last week of the conference, when conferees created three different categories of pollutants with different requirements for each. For conventional pollutants, conferees created a new standard called the "best conventional technology." EPA was required to define that standard, but Congress stipulated that it had to be at least the best practicable technology. Moreover, best conventional technology effluent limitations could not violate water quality standards or require other dischargers on the waterway to upgrade their equipment.

Conferees took several steps to increase EPA control over toxic pollutants. They allowed no waivers from cleanup requirements and postponed the deadline to meet best available technology standards for one year, to July 1, 1984, solely to give EPA additional time to develop regulations.

The third category was unconventional pollutants, those that were neither conventional nor known to be toxic. The compromise gave industry until 1987 to comply with the best available technology requirement and allowed waivers under certain conditions.

Wetlands

The other major controversy, and one that helped kill the 1976 legislation, involved Section 404 of the 1972 law, which required the Army Corps of Engineers to issue permits for dredge and fill operations in waters and wetlands. Under the 1972 law the program applied to traditionally navigable waters and their adjacent wetlands.

However, a March 1975 federal district court decision held that the law applied to all U.S. waters. Farmers and foresters complained, claiming that the Corps of Engineers might require them to obtain permits for routine activities, such as digging a ranch stock pond or dumping soil in a farm ditch.

As a result, the House restricted the federal jurisdiction over wetlands and waters only to traditionally navigable waters, their adjacent wetlands and coastal wetlands. A similar amendment by Sen. Lloyd Bentsen, D-Texas, lost on the Senate floor, 45-51.

The Senate, however, did change the permit program to give qualified states the opportunity to administer permits for all but traditionally navigable waters. The Senate version also exempted routine farming and forestry activities from needing specific permits.

The House agreed to the general principles of the Senate provisions, but held fast to their amendment exempting federal activities, such as Army Corps of Engineers projects, from the permit requirement. The Senate finally consented to compromise language that exempted federal projects specifically authorized by Congress so long as the project's environmental impact statement included information on the effects of dredged or fill material equivalent to that required by the permit system.

Construction Grants

In provisions everyone could agree on, the final version of HR 3199 authorized major funding for the sewage treatment construction program — $4.5 billion in fiscal 1978 and $5 billion annually for fiscal years 1979 through 1982. The final version also permitted the states to set their own priorities for construction, which meant that some funds would be spent on extension or expansion of systems to handle new growth or treatment of storm water. The Senate and President Carter had sought to limit that sort of project. The major limitation in the final version gave EPA the right to hold a public hearing on the state's priority list and then to remove a project if it would not contribute to the clean water goals in the act.

Provisions

As signed into law Dec. 27, HR 3199 (PL 95-217):

- Authorized $471.5 million annually in fiscal 1978-80 for various water treatment programs, including $150 million to EPA for non-research programs and grants to states for enforcement, $150 million to aid planning of areawide waste treatment and $60 million for programs to clean up polluted lakes.
- Clarified state jurisdiction over water rights and authorized EPA to report by July 1, 1978, on coordination of water resources management and pollution control.
- Established a national clearinghouse for information on alternative treatment.
- Directed EPA to require applicants for grants for waste treatment to show why alternative treatment that recycled water had not been selected as the treatment system.

• Authorized grants for privately owned treatment works serving one or more existing principal residences or small commercial establishments when a public body had applied for the federal grants and shown why a publicly owned system was not feasible.

• Authorized funding for alternative treatment that was not the most cost-effective so long as its life cycle costs did not exceed those of the most cost effective substitute by more than 15 percent.

• Authorized federal grants of 85 percent for alternative wastewater treatment while continuing the share for conventional treatment works at 75 percent.

• Allowed municipalities to use *ad valorem* taxes instead of meters to charge for sewage treatment so long as the charges reflected actual use by different classes of users.

• Exempted from industrial cost recovery requirements those industries discharging 25,000 gallons or less a day into municipal treatment plants so long as the effluent did not contain toxic chemicals or other materials that would contaminate or reduce the utility of the resulting sludge.

• Allotted water treatment construction grants to states based on population and needs, with small states receiving a minimum of 1/2 of 1 percent of the total construction grant funding and $75 million a year authorized to cover costs of paying the minimum, subject to annual appropriations.

• Authorized use of 2 percent or $400,000, whichever was greater, of a state's construction allotment for grants to states for their administrative costs.

• Directed EPA to set aside 4 percent of the allotment for states with rural populations of 25 percent or more to pay for alternatives to conventional sewage treatment works in small towns (population of 3,500 or less) or sparsely settled suburbs. Governors of other states could also request the allotment.

• Provided a ceiling for the 85 percent grants for alternative treatment by limiting funding of the additional 10 percent to 2 percent of the construction grants in each of fiscal years 1979 and 1980 and 3 percent in fiscal 1981.

• Authorized $1 billion in construction grants for fiscal 1977, $4.5 billion for fiscal 1978 and $5 billion annually for fiscal years 1979-82.

• Authorized grants of 100 percent of costs for two years to states for developing areawide waste treatment management planning processes if the grant were made before Oct. 1, 1977; the grant would be 75 percent of costs thereafter.

• Exempted from controls on point source discharges the return flows from irrigation of agricultural lands.

• Provided authority to EPA to oversee and reject any state plans for requiring use of best management practices by farmers and others whose activities indirectly polluted water through, for example, agricultural runoff.

• Authorized $200 million in fiscal 1979 and $400 million for fiscal 1980 for aid to farmers to use soil conservation practices that would reduce runoff of soil, fertilizers and pesticides into streams. The funds could pay for up to 50 percent of the costs of the controls when the farmer had entered a five- to 10-year contract with the Department of Agriculture that allowed the federal government to oversee his pollution control practices.

• Required that states set the priority for funding of treatment works, but with EPA given the right, after holding public hearings, to veto a state's priority list and request a revised list.

• Required that states use at least 25 percent of their construction funds for major sewer system rehabilitation, new collector sewers, new interceptors and correction of combined sewer overflows.

• Created a new treatment standard, best conventional technology, that dischargers of conventional pollutants, such as suspended solids or those usually found in sanitary wastes, would have to meet by July 1, 1984.

• Extended the deadline for compliance with 1983 requirements for control of toxic pollutants with best available technology from July 1, 1983, to July 1, 1984.

• Extended the deadline for compliance with best available technology requirements for dischargers of non-conventional pollutants (those not on the toxics list and not defined as conventional) from 1983 to July 1, 1987, at the latest.

• Allowed EPA to modify requirements for non-conventional pollutants so long as the modification would not degrade the water quality, require other dischargers to upgrade controls or allow possibly toxic pollutants to enter the water supply.

• Reduced secondary treatment requirements for cities such as Los Angeles that discharged their wastes through outfall pipes into deep ocean waters.

• Extended municipal deadlines from 1977 to July 1, 1983, on a case-by-case basis for those cities where compliance was held up by construction delays or lack of promised federal funds.

• Extended the 1977 deadlines to July 1, 1983, for industrial dischargers that had planned to tie in to municipal treatment systems that qualified for the municipal extension.

• Extended the 1983 deadline to July 1, 1987, for industries installing innovative treatment systems when the system had the potential for industry-wide application.

• Required EPA to base criteria for setting best conventional technology requirements on whether the costs of adding the pollution control equipment were reasonable when compared to the improvement in water quality.

• Made the 65 toxics and classes of toxics derived from the *Flannery* court settlement the existing list of toxic pollutants in water and allowed EPA to either add or subtract from that list depending on test results.

• Allowed EPA to use informal rule-making procedures to establish effluent limitations for toxic pollutants.

• Set national standards for industrial treatment of wastes that would be discharged into a publicly owned treatment system. Local governments could ask for a waiver from the standard for a local industry, but would have to show that the public system, either alone or in combination with industrial treatment, so cleaned the discharge that it would meet toxic standards for direct discharges from industry.

• Extended the 1977 industrial deadlines to April 1, 1979, for those industries that had attempted "in good faith" to attain them and had begun construction of pollution control facilities.

• Extended controls on oil pollution from 12 miles from shore to 200 miles from shore by making the law apply to pollution that might affect natural resources managed under the Fishery Conservation and Management Act of 1976.

• Removed the ceiling of $14 million on liability for oil spill cleanup and increased the liability limit for oil spill cleanup to $150 per gross ton for tankers, or a minimum liability of $250,000; to $125 per gross ton for inland barges, or a minimum of $125,000; and to $50 million for onshore and offshore facilities.

• Required commercial vessels on the Great Lakes to treat discharges at a level at least equal to secondary treatment requirements.

• Required federal facilities built after Sept. 30, 1979, to use alternative systems for waste treatment unless such a system was more than 15 percent more expensive than the most cost effective alternative.

• Required federal compliance with water pollution laws.

• Allowed the U.S. Army Corps of Engineers to issue general, five-year permits for activities that discharged dredged or fill material when the activities were routine farming, forestry or dam and canal maintenance operations that would have only minimal cumulative adverse effect on the environment.

• Allowed EPA to give states administrative responsibilities for the permit program for dredge or fill activities on waterways that were not traditionally navigable if the state requested it and had an acceptable program description.

• Gave EPA authority to take back from the states the administrative aspect of the permit program if, after public hearing, EPA found the state was not operating the program as approved.

• Required that states give EPA a copy of every permit issued and that EPA give a copy to the Fish and Wildlife Service of the Department of Interior. The public would also have access to the permits.

• Exempted federal activities that discharged dredged or fill materials from the permit requirements when the project was specifically authorized by Congress, when an environmental impact statement on the project contained information equivalent to that required in permits and when Congress had seen the impact statement prior to either the authorization or appropriation of construction funds.

• Placed an 18-month moratorium on municipal charges to industry for construction costs related to their discharges, known as industrial cost recovery, so that EPA could study the efficiency of the program and its impact on small communities.

Safe Drinking Water

President Carter Nov. 16, 1977, signed a bill (S 1528 — PL 95-190) amending and extending the Safe Drinking Water Act (PL 93-523).

S 1528 authorized $71 million for fiscal 1978 and $81 million for fiscal 1979. The largest share was in grants to the states for public water supervision programs, $35 million in 1978 and $45 million in 1979. Other authorizations were: studies, technical assistance and training, $17 million each year; grants for underground water source protection, $10 million each year; special emergency assistance, $8 million annually; and survey of rural drinking water supplies, $1 million a year.

The bill granted a waiver of the law's requirement that states must assume primary enforcement responsibility for public water systems, thus allowing them to receive up to 75 percent of their grants, and extended for an additional 270 days the time limit for states to implement underground injection control programs to protect drinking water sources.

Other amendments to the act provided for Environmental Protection Agency training grants to state and local personnel; extended until Sept. 30, 1979, the expiration date for certificates of need for water treatment chemicals, by which states could receive chemicals that were not readily available; applied the act and state and local regulations to federally owned or maintained public water systems; and authorized 80 new super-grade positions.

Ocean Dumping

Congress in 1977 amended the 1972 Marine Protection Act (PL 92-532) to prohibit ocean dumping of most leftovers from municipal sewage treatment plants. The dumping was to stop by Dec. 31, 1981, or earlier if possible.

That action was intended to give more force to an identical Environmental Protection Agency (EPA) regulation issued in January 1977. Because a statutory version would foreclose extensions beyond the cutoff date for any reason, EPA opposed a legislative ban. The agency had been issuing "interim" permits that allowed dumping to continue until municipalities could come up with alternative disposal methods.

Dumping of sludge contaminated ocean waters with potentially lethal metals such as cadmium and mercury and other harmful materials, proponents of the ban argued. Nearly 20 percent of shellfish waters had been closed to harvesting because of "intolerable levels of pollution," Robert L. Leggett, D-Calif., told the House. "We cannot continue to expect the oceans to act as a food resource, recreation center and cesspool." A firm deadline was needed, and the prime offenders — Camden, N.J., Philadelphia and New York — could find alternatives, Leggett said.

The dumping ban was the only substantive revision of the 1972 law contained in a fiscal 1978 authorization bill (HR 4197) for marine protection. The bill authorized $11.8 million for fiscal 1978; the funds were divided between EPA and the Commerce Department.

Clinch River Reactor

As 1977 ended, a bill authorizing the Department of Energy to devote as much as $6.2 billion to civilian energy research and development in fiscal 1978 was left for dead on Capitol Hill.

The bill was a victim of the ongoing dispute between President Carter and Congress over the future of the not-yet-built Clinch River Breeder Reactor Plant, once the nation's No. 1 nuclear power project.

The energy research bill (S 1811 — S Rept 95-328; H Rept 95-349, Parts I, II and III) passed the Senate July 12 and the House Sept. 23. It was cleared for the White House Oct. 20. President Carter vetoed it Nov. 5, casting the first veto of his administration. The veto came primarily because buried deep within the $6,161,445,000 authorization was an $80 million item for continued work on the controversial breeder plant.

No attempt was made during the remaining weeks of the 1977 session to override the veto.

In December the House approved a Senate-passed bill (S 1340), which it had amended to be identical to S 1811

Joint Atomic Energy Committee Quietly Eliminated in 1977

The Joint Atomic Energy Committee, once described as "the most powerful congressional committee in the history of the nation" quietly died in 1977. The committee's all-inclusive jurisdiction over matters involving atomic energy was divided among standing committees in each chamber.

Background

The Atomic Energy Act of 1946 (PL 79-585) created both the Atomic Energy Commission (AEC) and the joint committee to foster development of the new power of atomic energy.

It was the only permanent joint committee ever created that received continuing authority to report legislation. Granted unique oversight powers in its chartering act, the committee soon dominated policy formation to an extent unprecedented for a legislative panel. Sen. Henry M. Jackson, D-Wash., a longtime committee member, asserted as far back as 1953 that "the committee made the decisions, with the advice and consent of the executive branch," instead of the reverse, as was more usual.

For most of its life, the joint committee functioned almost as a unicameral legislature within the bicameral Congress. It usually reported identical bills simultaneously to each chamber, and when presented with floor amendments, resolved differences between House and Senate versions by functioning as its own conference committee.

Controversy and Challenge

As nuclear power became more and more a matter of public controversy in the 1970s, however, the joint committee drew increasing criticism for its protective attitude toward the subject and the industry.

In 1976 for the first time, opponents of the committee were able to block several major committee initiatives.

The full Senate killed a joint committee bill proposing to allow private investment in the uranium enrichment business, until that time a government monopoly. The committee's bill authorizing fiscal 1977 funds for the Energy Research and Development Administration died on the Senate floor late in the session. And committee opponents also blocked the appointment of a veteran member of the joint committee staff to the Nuclear Regulatory Commission.

Six of the committee's 18 members retired at the end of the 94th Congress or were defeated in the November 1976 elections. With one-third of the seats on the panel vacant, it was clearly a propitious time for its opponents to move.

That move came in early December 1976. Rep. Jonathan B. Bingham, D-N.Y., proposed to the House Democratic Caucus that the House strip the joint committee of virtually all its legislative power, the key factor that had made it so unique among joint committees in the history of Congress. On Dec. 8, the House Democrats agreed to back that proposal.

1977 Action

The full House formally adopted a package of House reforms (H Res 5) on Jan. 4, the opening day of the 95th Congress. Among the changes in House rules made by this package, adopted by a vote of 256-142, was elimination of the legislative authority of the Joint Committee on Atomic Energy. The jurisdiction of the joint committee was then divided among five standing committees, as follows:

- Military nuclear concerns to the Committee on Armed Services;
- General regulation of the nuclear industry to the Committee on Interior and Insular Affairs;
- Nuclear export questions to the Committee on International Relations;
- Research and development questions to the Committee on Science and Technology;
- Facilities regulation and oversight to the Committee on Interstate and Foreign Commerce.

Opponents of nuclear power hailed the reform as providing nuclear power critics with access to policy questions from the subcommittee stage on up for the first time. Also, they welcomed the entry of the Interior Committee, headed by liberal environmentalist Morris K. Udall, D-Ariz., into direct nuclear power policy-making. Finally, the reforms seemed to put nuclear power on an equal footing with other energy technologies.

The Senate concurred in the action of the House Feb. 4, when it approved a major overhaul of the Senate committee structure that included abolition of the Joint Atomic Energy Committee. The Senate resolution (S Res 4) reallocated the joint committee's responsibilities among three standing committees:

- Military nuclear matters to the Senate Armed Services Committee.
- Non-military development of nuclear energy to the new Committee on Energy and Natural Resources.
- Non-military environmental regulation of nuclear energy to the new Committee on Environment and Public Works.

The Senate followed that action with passage March 31 of a bill (S 1153 — PL 95-110) amending the Atomic Energy Act of 1954 (PL 83-703), by abolishing the joint committee. The House passed an amended version of S 1153 by voice vote Aug. 5. The Senate cleared the measure the same day, completing the formal interment of the Joint Atomic Energy Committee.

except for the Clinch River provisions, which were deleted. The Senate did not act on the revised bill before adjournment but cleared the measure Feb. 8, 1978.

Nuclear Plant Dispute

Consideration of S 1811 in both chambers was dominated by debate over President Carter's proposal to terminate the nuclear power plant, which was to be built on the Clinch River in Tennessee near Oak Ridge to show that the plutonium-fueled and plutonium-producing "breeder" reactors were a feasible source of electricity and nuclear fuel.

The original budget request for the plant for fiscal 1978 was $150 million. After Carter decided to terminate the project — because of his concern that increasing the use of plutonium would enlarge the risk of nuclear proliferation — he asked Congress to provide only $33 million in termination costs.

Congress eventually decided on $80 million, enough to keep the project going in fiscal 1978 while Congress studied Carter's termination proposal.

Neither the veto of S 1811 nor congressional inaction spelled final doom for the plant. The fiscal 1978 supplemental appropriations bill (HR 9375) left pending at the end of the 1977 session contained $80 million for the reactor, which could be spent even without enactment of the authorizing legislation.

The supplemental funding bill containing the $80 million appropriation was signed into law (PL 95-240) early in 1978.

Programs Continued

The total authorized in the vetoed bill included about $3.2 billion for nuclear power projects and $1.8 billion for non-nuclear programs. The projects were to be administered by the research division of the Department of Energy, formerly the Energy Research and Development Administration (ERDA).

Because the regular ERDA appropriations bill (HR 7553 — PL 95-96) had moved through Congress ahead of the authorizing legislation, language allowing expenditure of the appropriated funds, even without authorizing legislation in place, was included in that bill.

The presidential veto of S 1811 therefore had no effect on spending for any ongoing ERDA programs, including the Clinch River project. Only programs for which the initial authority was included in or revised by S 1811 were affected by the veto.

New Bill

S 1340 (PL 95-238), the bill that cleared Feb. 8, 1978, was identical to the vetoed measure it replaced except that it omitted authorization for the Clinch River project and language revising uranium pricing agreements to which Carter also had objected.

As signed into law Feb. 25, PL 95-238 provided $6,081,400,000 for energy research programs in fiscal 1978. Of that total, just over half — $3.2 billion — was for nuclear programs, while $1.8 billion was authorized for non-nuclear research and development. The remaining amounts would be used for environmental and safety research, basic research and program management. (Authorization totals include operating expenses and plant and capital equipment costs.)

Saccharin Ban Delay

Congress Nov. 4, 1977, cleared legislation (S 1750 — PL 95-203) delaying a proposed Food and Drug Administration (FDA) ban on the artificial sweetener saccharin.

The FDA had proposed the ban March 9 because of scientific evidence linking saccharin with an increased risk of bladder cancer. Congress was forced into the issue because of an avalanche of complaints from angry constituents who said they needed saccharin because of illness or obesity. Some members reported receiving more mail and phone calls on this than on any other issue in years.

Congress voted to delay the ban 18 months, pending new studies of saccharin and the whole question of carcinogenicity in food products.

In 1980, Congress cleared legislation extending the ban through June 30, 1981. In August 1981 the ban was again extended, until June 30, 1983.

The Saccharin Controversy

The FDA proposed the saccharin ban after Canadian studies showed that high dosages of the food additive produced bladder cancer in rats. Five years earlier FDA had expressed doubts about saccharin's safety.

The proposed ban was based on both the general Food, Drug and Cosmetic Act of 1938 and its controversial Delaney clause, which prohibited use of food additives found to induce cancer in animals. The FDA proposal would have permitted the sale of saccharin as an over-the-counter drug — temporarily, and with a warning label. Manufacturers would have been given six months to prove that it was an effective drug for diabetics and the obese. "All hell broke loose" after the FDA proposal, one member of Congress recalled. A 1969 FDA ban on cyclamates, another form of artificial sweetener, had been relatively uncontroversial because there was an alternative — saccharin. But the proposal to eliminate the last non-caloric sweetener provoked very strong protests.

Major Provisions

As signed into law, S 1750:

- Prohibited the HEW secretary from banning or restricting for 18 months the sale or distribution of saccharin or any product containing it on the basis of any studies or tests available before the date of enactment of the bill. The provision would not prohibit the secretary from banning saccharin due to new information discovered during the 18-month moratorium.
- Stipulated that the secretary's new authority to require labels and warning signs about the risks associated with saccharin would not be considered as restricting or prohibiting the sale or distribution of saccharin.
- Required that any food product containing saccharin introduced into interstate commerce beginning 90 days after enactment of the bill would be considered misbranded under the Food, Drug and Cosmetic Act if it did not contain the following label in conspicuous and legible type: "Use of this product may be hazardous to your health. This product contains saccharin which has been determined to cause cancer in laboratory animals."
- Authorized the secretary to revise or remove labeling and information requirements if new information about saccharin warranted it.
- Required manufacturers of products containing sac-

charin to provide retail establishments selling those products with warning signs informing consumers of the health risks associated with saccharin. Food sold in a store that did not display such signs would be considered misbranded.

- Authorized the secretary to require vending machines containing saccharin products to display in a conspicuous place on the machine a warning of the health risks associated with saccharin usage.
- Required the secretary to conduct studies and report to Congress within 15 months on a number of subjects, including existing technical capability to determine the carcinogenicity of substances added to or normally occurring in food, the health benefits and risks to humans from carcinogenic substances in food, and federal food regulatory policy as it related to carcinogenic substances.
- Required the secretary to report to Congress within one year on the chemical identity of any impurities found in saccharin, their toxicity and carcinogenicity, and the health benefits resulting from the use of artificial sweeteners in general and saccharin in particular.

Toxic Substances

Victims of chemical spills could be compensated for their out-of-pocket losses under a bill (S 1531 — S Rept 95-202) approved by the Senate in 1977.

By voice vote the Senate Oct. 31 amended the 1976 Toxic Substances Control Act (PL 94-469) to set up a state-administered indemnity fund. Farmers forced to slaughter condemned livestock, supermarkets forced to dump contaminated food or individuals with medical problems attributable to a chemical spill could recover up to 75 percent of their expenses from the fund.

The bill also raised the fiscal 1978 authorization under the toxic substances statute from $12.6 million to $50 million although the Environmental Protection Agency (EPA) had indicated earlier that it could not absorb the extra funding. *(1976 Toxic Substances Act, p. 158)*

The House took no action in 1977 but in 1978 killed legislation that simply would have increased the authorization for the Toxic Substances Control Act to $50 million in fiscal 1979. The House measure contained no indemnity provisions.

Pesticides Regulation

Both the House and the Senate passed bills in 1977 making changes in the way the Environmental Protection Agency (EPA) registered pesticides, but conferees did not complete action on the measure until 1978. *(Details, p. 173)*

The bills (HR 7073, S 1678) were designed to make it easier for the EPA to complete the enormous task of evaluating the safety of the tens of thousands of pesticides currently on the market.

The sheer volume of the project, together with extended court fights over control of test data, had made it impossible for the EPA to meet the Oct. 21, 1977 deadline mandated in the 1972 pesticide control law. Some experts said it could take 15 years to complete the job.

Mine Safety Standards

Resisting heavy pressure from industry, Congress approved legislation Oct. 27, 1977, to toughen enforcement of mine health and safety standards.

Key provisions of the bill (S 717 — PL 95-164) transferred regulatory authority over all types of mining activities from the Department of the Interior to the Department of Labor. Unions and their supporters had long advocated such a shift, claiming that competing functions led the Interior Department to take a lax approach to job health and safety matters.

"We have, for too long, paid for our energy and minerals in a dreadful currency of human suffering and death," said Harrison A. Williams Jr., D-N.J., chairman of the Senate Human Resources Committee. "This new mine safety law . . . will go a long way toward assuring the safety and health of our miners."

The bill applied a single statute — the Federal Coal Mine Health and Safety Act of 1969 — to both coal and non-coal mines, repealing a more lenient 1966 law covering metal and mineral mines. Without requiring identical standards for all types of mining, the consolidation assured uniform regulatory procedures in each case.

Though the new framework was mainly intended to upgrade conditions in metal and non-metal mines, the bill revised the coal act as well, to expedite procedures for setting standards, imposing penalties and collecting fines from mine operators. The cumbersome processes of the past, sponsors believed, had done much to discourage the industry from voluntarily complying with the law.

The Carter administration joined organized labor in pushing for the bill, including the transfer of regulatory functions from Interior to Labor. Similar legislation failed to clear Congress in 1976 when the Senate ran out of time to act on it.

Provisions

As signed into law Nov. 9, the Federal Mine Safety and Health Act of 1977 (S 717 — PL 95-164):

- Amended the Federal Coal Mine Health and Safety Act of 1969 (PL 91-153) to apply to metal and non-metal mining, repealing the Federal Metal and Non-metallic Mine Safety Act of 1966 (PL 89-577).
- Transferred enforcement functions of the Mining Enforcement and Safety Administration (MESA) from the Department of the Interior to the Department of Labor; placed such responsibilities within a new office called the Mine Safety and Health Administration, separate from the Occupational Safety and Health Administration (OSHA), headed by an assistant secretary.
- Assigned health research functions to the Department of Health, Education and Welfare (HEW) and left mine safety research under the jurisdiction of the Interior Department.
- Increased to $60 million, from $30 million, the annual authorization for mine safety research.
- Retained existing coal mine standards as well as all existing mandatory standards applicable to metal and non-metal mines.
- Established expedited procedures for reviewing and modifying those regulations and for promulgating new standards; required that new standards be at least as strict as existing ones.
- Required stiffer standards on toxic substances; re-

quired operators to periodically examine miners for adverse effects of exposure and reassign them to less hazardous duties if necessary.

- Required at least four unannounced federal inspections of each underground mine every year; required at least two unannounced inspections of each surface mine every year.
- Required one spot inspection of especially hazardous or gassy mines every five working days, and somewhat less frequent spot inspections in other dangerous situations.
- Permitted miners — through their representatives — to request additional inspections and to accompany federal inspectors on their rounds; barred companies from retaliating against miners who filed complaints, refused to work under unsafe or unhealthful conditions, or participated actively in any aspect of the enforcement process.
- Required the closing of a mine where there is imminent danger or a "pattern of violations."
- Required operators to compensate miners for work lost during such closures.
- Provided a system of mandatory penalties for mine violations: specified fines of up to $10,000 for each violation by an operator and up to $1,000 for each day of operation in defiance of an order.
- Empowered the secretary of labor to obtain court injunctions against hazardous mining activities in cases of repeated health and safety violations.
- Established a five-member Mine Safety and Health Review Commission, independent of the Department of Labor, to handle disputes arising under the act.

Black Lung Benefits

Congress in 1977 all but completed work on two measures to liberalize the black lung benefits program for coal miners. Both measures were cleared early in 1978.

The bills (HR 4544 — PL 95-239; HR 5322 — PL 95-227), dealing respectively with eligibility and tax provisions, made permanent the federal program guaranteeing assistance to coal miners suffering from the debilitating disease. *(Details, p. 173)*

1978

Congress enacted no new major initiatives in the environmental health field in 1978, but it took some significant actions. A measure liberalizing black lung benefits and shifting much of the burden for paying for those benefits to the coal industry was passed, as was a bill to make it easier for the Environmental Protection Agency to register pesticides.

Congress extended and expanded the federal noise control program, although legislation to provide federal aid to help airlines install quieter engines on their commercial airplanes was killed when the two chambers could not agree on a passenger surcharge to help finance the cost.

A measure to clean up several million tons of uranium mill wastes was also cleared but the House defeated a proposal to increase the authorization for the toxic substances control bill.

Noise Control Program

Legislation directing the Environmental Protection Agency (EPA) to encourage state and local noise control programs and to conduct a research and technical assistance program on noise was cleared by Congress Oct. 13, 1978.

The bill (S 3083 — PL 95-609) also extended for one year the Noise Control Act of 1972 (PL 92-574), which required the EPA to set maximum noise levels that could be tolerated without adversely affecting health, establish noise emission standards for commercial products such as motors or air conditioners, study the effects of noise on humans and develop improved noise control methods. *(1972 law, p. 143)*

Provisions

As cleared by Congress, S 3083:

- Directed EPA to conduct and finance research on such topics as the psychological and physiological effects of noise, noise control technology, equipment for noise control programs, the economic impact of noise and the use of economic incentives (including emission taxes) on noise control.
- Required EPA to administer a program of grants to state and local governments and regional planning agencies to identify noise problems, develop noise control programs and evaluate techniques for controlling noise.
- Directed EPA to provide technical assistance to state and local noise control programs, including lending them monitoring equipment.
- Mandated a joint EPA/Transportation Department study of how noise from airports affected communities located in adjoining states.
- Provided civil penalties of up to $10,000 a day for manufacturers who distributed new products in violation of EPA noise emission standards.
- Authorized appropriations of $15 million in fiscal 1979 for activities other than research and development. The EPA research and development fiscal 1979 authorization included $4 million for noise control research.

Aircraft Noise Control

Congress did not complete action in the 95th Congress on legislation that would have provided commercial airline companies with federal aid to help them pay for quieter planes.

Although the House and Senate passed differing versions of the bill (HR 8729, S 3279) in 1978, an attempt in the last days of the session to complete action on a compromise that would be acceptable to a majority of both houses foundered.

The main stumbling block was a House provision to allow the airlines to impose a 2 percent surcharge on passenger tickets and freight rates and then use the surcharge to replace or retrofit noisy engines. The Senate deleted the surcharge provisions.

Airline and airport operators argued that the legislation was needed to placate communities located near noisy airports and to ensure that financially strapped airlines would be able to meet the federal noise control standards. When the measure was introduced in early 1977, airline revenues had been lagging. But by the summer of 1978, revenues had risen to all-time highs, and the bill's critics wanted the airlines to meet federal noise control standards with their own funds. They branded the bill a "rip-off" and a "giveaway."

Both the Senate and House versions would have authorized grants to airports to help them reduce their noise levels. They also contained provisions to increase funding from the Airport and Airway Trust Fund for general airport operations and maintenance.

In 1980 Congress cleared a noise control bill that abandoned the surcharge approach and instead delayed implementation of some of the federal noise control standards. *(1979-80 action, p. 183)*

Uranium Mill Waste

A program to clean up some 25 million tons of potentially hazardous uranium wastes was cleared by Congress Oct. 15, 1978.

The bill (HR 13650 — PL 95-604) mandating the cleanup also provided for stricter controls on future handling and disposal of wastes resulting from uranium processing.

Under the legislation, the federal government would pay 90 percent of the costs of cleaning up the wastes; the affected states would pay 10 percent. The Carter administration had recommended that the federal-state split be 75-25, while members of Congress from the affected states advocated that the federal government pay the entire cost.

Existing law gave no federal agency explicit authority to regulate or dispose of the wastes at 24 mills located in eight Western states and Pennsylvania. The mills originally were operated under federal contracts for the production of uranium for nuclear weapons. The wastes — called tailings — at first were considered harmless and often were used in building construction. However, scientists and environmentalists had grown increasingly concerned about the potential health hazards of the radioactive tailings.

Clinch River Reactor

Congress adjourned in 1978 without completing action on legislation authorizing the non-military programs administered by the new Department of Energy in fiscal 1979.

Failure of Congress to complete action left in limbo the future of the controversial breeder reactor plant planned for construction on the Clinch River in Tennessee.

Three authorization bills (S 2692, HR 12163, HR 11392) were reported by committees. Two of them, S 2692 and HR 11392, never reached a floor vote. The third measure, HR 12163, was passed by the House July 17 but was not taken up by the Senate.

The legislation languished when the Democratic leadership in both houses refused to bring it up for fear it would become the vehicle for several controversial attempts to remove or modify price controls on oil.

The leaders wanted to avoid a major floor flight on energy until after Congress had completed action on President Carter's energy policy package.

But the energy bill did not clear until the final day of the session, which did not leave enough time before adjournment for action on the Energy Department authorization.

Authorization of $2.97 billion for military energy programs administered by the Energy Department was contained in separate legislation (HR 11686 — PL 95-509).

Spending Continued

Because Congress failed to act, spending for the Clinch River reactor project — which was opposed by the administration — continued at the rate of about $15 million a month.

Without a new bill providing authority to modify or terminate the plutonium breeder, the Energy Department had to continue to operate under existing authority, which required construction. The $172 million appropriated for the project in fiscal 1979 in the public works appropriations bill (HR 12928 — H J Res 1139) had to be spent on new parts, engineering, design and other scheduled work on the $2.56 billion reactor.

Carter wanted the project killed because he said it was too expensive, its design was obsolete and it would lead to the spread of nuclear weapons. The reactor would produce plutonium, a nuclear fuel that could be used to make bombs.

Throughout the year, the administration attempted to work out some sort of compromise that would end the project.

But in July, the House voted twice to refuse to allow the administration to terminate the breeder. The two votes were on amendments to HR 12163.

The Senate Energy Committee, on the other hand, in its bill (S 2692) gave Carter authority to end the Clinch River project. But the full Senate did not vote on that bill during the session.

Toxic Substances

What began as a non-controversial authorization for toxic substances control was defeated by the House June 12, 1978, as members protested government spending and federal controls on business.

The bill (HR 12441 — H Rept 95-1163) would have increased the authorization for implementation of the Toxic Substances Control Act of 1976 to $50 million, from $16 million, for fiscal 1979.

The funding would have allowed the Environmental Protection Agency (EPA) to start enforcing the act, which was designed to evaluate the safety of chemicals before they entered the marketplace.

Rejection of HR 12441 also doomed a more ambitious Senate bill passed in 1977 that increased authorizations for toxic substances control and set up an indemnity program for victims of chemical spills. Congress also failed to extend the law in the 96th Congress. *(1977 action, p. 161; 1979-80 action, p. 181)*

Pesticides Registration

Legislation to end the bureaucratic snarls tying up registration and marketing of pesticides was cleared by Congress Sept. 19, 1978.

The legislation (S 1678 — PL 95-396) left intact the basic philosophy that the public should be protected from harmful poisons. But it speeded up the process by which the Environmental Protection Agency (EPA) evaluated the safety of pesticides and thus made it easier for farmers to obtain effective and safe pesticides.

Registration Backlog

The pesticide registration problem began in 1972 when Congress passed a law (PL 92-516) setting strict new standards for pesticide safety. The law required that all pesticides used in the United States be registered with the EPA and be backed by extensive test data on safety and efficacy. *(Details, 1972 law, p. 148)*

The 1972 law also mandated re-registration according to the new criteria of all pesticide products already on the market. An Oct. 21, 1977, deadline for completion of the re-registration process was set. But the sheer volume of the project, together with extended court fights over control of test data, made it impossible for the EPA to come even close to completing its task within the allotted time. Experts estimated that it would take up to 15 years to finish the job.

Thus, S 1678 represented an attempt at compromise between the conflicting interests of chemical manufacturers, pesticide formulators, farmers, environmentalists and the EPA, all with an important stake invested in the outcome.

Farmers were angry because registration delays made it impossible for them to buy products to stop new pest outbreaks. Environmentalists were worried that the slowdown in safety checks of existing pesticides would lead to more disasters like the one that hit Virginia in 1976, when workers were sickened and the James River closed to fishing because of contamination by poisonous Kepone.

To calm those concerns, S 1678 hastened the process by allowing the EPA to register pesticides according to their chemical composition instead of by their product name. This change, known as "generic" registration, allowed the agency to focus its efforts on determining the safety of about 1,400 basic substances.

The measure also dropped the existing requirement that the EPA consider the efficacy of a product for which registration was sought. Congress decided that, in the case of agricultural pesticides, most farmers were perfectly able to determine for themselves how well a particular product worked.

Exclusive Use

Of particular concern to chemical manufacturers was the related issue of access to test data, and this issue was not so easily resolved.

Requests for pesticide registration with the EPA had to be accompanied by submission of great quantities of test data. Only the largest firms had the resources to undertake the necessary tests. Small companies formulating pesticides for particular uses were forced to rely on test data generated by other firms.

In 1972 Congress required the companies to pay "reasonable compensation" for use of data developed by other companies to support registration. This led to extensive litigation that further slowed down registration.

Large chemical companies wanted to amend the 1972 law to provide that companies generating test data be given a 10-year period of "exclusive use" of information filed to support their registrations. During that period other firms could not make use of the data to justify their own registrations.

Representatives of those corporations asserted that a period of exclusive use was the best way to protect their research investment, since compensation was unlikely to repay them fully for their research outlays. Only a lengthy monopoly on the information necessary for registration, the producers argued, would provide the unique position in the marketplace that alone could serve as adequate incentive for further research and development.

The EPA opposed exclusive use on the grounds that the agency needed to be able to look at all relevant information relating to a pesticide, even if the information was controlled by a firm other than the one seeking registration.

The final version gave those who developed new chemicals in the future 10 years of exclusive use of the safety data and an additional five years of compensation from others who used the data. The period of exclusive use coincided with the time during which a patent protected the product; as a result, the pesticides laws did not give an extra competitive edge to the large companies that developed new products.

For extra health and safety data on products already on the market, a company could not claim exclusive use, but would be compensated by other companies using the data for 15 years after the data was submitted.

Other Provisions

In addition to the generic registration and exclusive use provisions, S 1678 (PL 95-396):

- Extended the Federal Insecticide, Fungicide and Rodenticide Act of 1975 (PL 94-140) through fiscal 1979 and authorized $54.5 million in fiscal 1978 and $70 million in fiscal 1979 to carry it out.
- Gave the public access to information about the effect of a pesticide on human health and the environment.
- Gave the states new authority to enforce controls on pesticides once they met standards designed to maintain minimum nationwide controls on the substances; retained existing EPA authority to veto a state registration.

Black Lung Benefits

Congress early in 1978 completed action on two measures liberalizing the black lung benefits program and establishing a new financial mechanism to pay for it.

Conferees reached agreement on the legislation late in the 1977 session, but final action was deferred until 1978. Congress cleared HR 5322 Jan. 24 and HR 4544 Feb. 15.

A top priority of the United Mine Workers (UMW), the bills (HR 4544, HR 5322) made the black lung program permanent by repealing its 1981 expiration date. While less sweeping than proponents originally intended, the revisions in HR 4544 relaxed eligibility rules in various ways, guaranteeing benefits to survivors of miners with lengthy work experience and applying a more lenient definition of disability to recent claims.

HR 4544 did not go as far as the UMW wished, however. Supporters of union-backed automatic entitlement provisions granting benefits to all those who had worked 30 years in the mines (25 years in anthracite coal mines) were forced to drop the idea in the face of substantial opposition.

The second bill (HR 5322) sought to shift a major portion of program costs from the federal government to the coal companies, creating an industry-financed trust fund to handle claims filed after 1973 for which no particular operator could be considered responsible. Operators who could be identified as responsible for individual miners' disabilities would pay the total cost of claims through a separate tax-exempt trust.

Background

Black lung disease, clinically known as "pneumoconiosis," was caused by continued inhalation of coal dust. Afflicted miners could suffer severe breathing difficulties and premature death.

The black lung benefits program was established in 1969 to compensate miners, their survivors and dependents when death or total disability resulted from the disease. Under revisions made in 1972, the federal government took responsibility for claims filed before Dec. 31, 1973. After that, coal companies were supposed to pay the costs of new claims through state worker compensation programs. *(1972 law, p. 149)*

But, since none of the state programs met federal standards, the government generally had to pick up the tab. Infrequently, the Labor Department held companies liable for individual cases, but the operators tended to challenge such findings in court.

Under the pre-1974 program (known as Part B), the government had paid about $1 billion a year to more than 500,000 beneficiaries. The more recent (Part C) claims cost the government an additional $30 million a year. Only about 200 Part C claims had been paid by the companies.

In 1976 the House passed legislation automatically granting black lung benefits to miners who worked a certain number of years in the mines and establishing an industry-financed trust fund to pay future claims. But the measure ran into opposition from the administration and coal mine operators, and the Senate never completed action on it.

Major Provisions

Eligibility Standards. As signed into law, HR 4544 (PL 95-239):

- Stipulated that continued employment in a mine was not conclusive evidence that a miner was not totally disabled. Miners whose conditions of work had changed, indicating a reduced ability to do mine work, and the survivors of miners who were employed at the time of death, might thus become eligible for benefits.
- Provided that the survivors of miners who had worked more than 25 years in the mines before June 30, 1971, would be eligible for benefits, unless there was conclusive evidence that the miner did not have black lung problems.
- Required the Labor Department to accept as proof of lung impairment X-rays performed by certified radiologists.
- Permitted miners to substantiate their disability claims by means of a complete pulmonary examination.
- Provided that the "interim" eligibility standards developed by HEW were to remain in effect until the Labor Department could promulgate permanent standards.
- Required HEW and the Labor Department to undertake reviews of claims previously denied, in light of changes in eligibility requirements made by the bill. HEW would review "Part B" claims, which were filed before 1974, while Labor would handle "Part C" claims, which were filed beginning in 1974.
- Required the departments of HEW and Labor to undertake broad informational campaigns to inform prospective beneficiaries of changes in the law.
- Authorized establishment of an insurance fund to assist mine operators in meeting their individual obligations to afflicted employees.
- Provided that affidavits as to the prior health of a deceased miner would be sufficient to establish eligibility unless there was medical evidence to the contrary.

Financing. As signed into law, HR 5322 (PL 95-227):

- Established a federal excise tax on coal sales, at the rate of 50 cents per ton on underground-mined coal and 25 cents per ton on surface-mined coal. Limited the amount of tax to 2 percent of the sale price.
- Established a Black Lung Disability Trust Fund, with an appropriation equal to the revenue from the coal tax, to pay black lung disability claims in cases where no operator could be found to be responsible for the miner's disability.
- Permitted an operator to establish a tax-exempt trust fund to cover its obligations in cases where it was found to be responsible for payment of benefits to afflicted miners.
- Established rules governing the tax-exempt status of the operator trusts and the deductibility of contributions to those trusts.

1979

The March accident at the Three Mile Island nuclear reactor in Pennsylvania focused congressional attention on problems associated with development of nuclear power. Despite the accident, Congress refused to impose a six-month moratorium on construction of new nuclear power plants, but committees did begin to work on nuclear waste disposal legislation.

The Senate passed a bill to extend federal solid waste disposal legislation but the House did not act. Nor did the House act on a Senate-passed measure to extend the Toxic Substances Control Act. And a bill to extend the pesticide regulation program died after House-Senate conferees were unable to agree on legislative veto provisions.

Congress sought to preserve the nation's diminishing wetlands by making several million acres eligible for federal wetland funding.

The Senate also passed a bill to re-allocate federally irrigated land in the West, primarily in the rich agriculture fields of California. The House did not take action on that measure in 1979.

Congress finally succeeded in adding several amendments to restrict the scope of the Occupational Safety and Health Act, exempting from inspection certain small businesses with low incidences of safety problems.

Hazardous Waste Disposal

The Senate in 1979 approved a bill (S 1156 — S Rept 96-172) extending for three years the Solid Waste Disposal Act (PL 89-82) as amended by the Resource Conservation and Recovery Act of 1976 (PL 94-580). The bill, passed by voice vote June 4, authorized $524 million in fiscal 1980-82 for programs to study, plan and control the handling of solid waste — including, but not limited to, hazardous waste.

Although a House committee reported a one-year extension bill (HR 3994 — H Rept 96-191), the full House did not act until 1980, when the legislation was cleared. *(Details, p. 180)*

Toxic Substances

The Senate May 22 passed by voice vote a bill (S 1147 — S Rept 96-162) to extend the Toxic Substances Control Act (PL 94-469) for three years through fiscal 1982. The measure authorized a total of $284.3 million for the three years. A House committee reported a one-year extension bill (HR 2606 — H Rept 96-174), but the full House never acted on the bill. *(1980 action, p. 180)*

Wetlands Funding

Congress completed action Dec. 20, 1979, on a bill (HR 2043 — PL 96-182) that made up to 20 million acres of wooded and swamp land located primarily in several Southern states eligible for wetlands funding under the Water Bank Act of 1970.

Wetlands are low-lying, frequently flooded areas, such as swamps, marshes and river banks, that provide nesting and breeding areas for dozens of species of waterfowl. The areas also help control floods, recharge ground water supplies and control pollution and sediment.

Under the Water Bank Act (PL 91-559), the federal government paid landowners between $5 and $20 an acre to leave their wetlands in a natural state. Since the program began, some 589,000 acres had been protected from drainage and development.

Most of these wetlands were located in the "prairie pothole" region of the upper Midwest, where ducks and other waterbirds bred and nested in heavily wooded areas surrounding prairie ponds.

But wetlands were being lost at a rate of 35,000 to 60,000 acres a year because rising land prices encouraged farmers either to drain and farm the land, or sell or lease it to developers. That was particularly true of wetlands not eligible for water bank funding. Those lands most seriously in need of protection were in California, the Southeast and the lower Mississippi Valley.

In addition to increasing the types of lowlands eligible for funding under the national wetlands conservation program, the bill tripled — from $10 million to $30 million — the amount available for conserving those wetlands beginning in 1981.

It also allowed the secretary of agriculture to adjust Water Bank payment rates every five years to reflect prevailing land and crop values.

Despite Carter Veto Dioxins Study Is Ordered

President Carter Jan. 2, 1980, vetoed a bill (S 2096) requiring the Department of Health, Education and Welfare (HEW) to study the health effects of dioxins, the chemicals used in Agent Orange and other herbicides. Congress had cleared the bill Dec. 19, 1979.

Carter said he supported efforts to investigate the effects of dioxins, but disapproved S 2096 because it required that HEW's design for the study be approved by Congress' Office of Technology Assessment (OTA). Such a "legislative veto device" was an "unconstitutional intrusion" into the executive branch's administrative authority, he said. The bill was unnecessary anyway, he added, because HEW already planned to conduct a study of dioxins.

Carter signed another bill (HR 3892 — PL 96-151) that contained an identical provision with regard to a Veterans Administration (VA) study of dioxins, because that bill also extended authorizations for veterans' health benefits and contained provisions on staffing of VA hospitals that had been worked out in lengthy negotiations with Congress. However, Carter said he would tell the VA administrator not to consider the provision requiring OTA approval of its study legally binding.

S 2096 was the result of a compromise between the House and Senate Veterans' Affairs committees on what agency should study the health effects of Agent Orange, a defoliant used in Vietnam, on U.S. soldiers who served there. The House panel insisted the VA should do it, and that was authorized in HR 3892.

In return, the House committee agreed to S 2096, which required HEW to study the health effects of dioxin exposure on agricultural, Forest Service and chemical workers and other civilians who had come in contact with dioxins, and to review existing scientific studies of the long-range health effects of dioxin exposure. The Senate passed the bill Dec. 6, the House Dec. 19. There was no attempt to override the veto.

Western Water-Use Reform

The 96th Congress revived but did not resolve a bitter struggle over who should receive federally subsidized irrigation water in the West.

The Senate in 1979 passed legislation to increase fourfold the amount of federally irrigated land a small farmer could own, but it exempted from the acreage limits several of the largest agribusiness operations in California.

Another version of the legislation was reported by the House Interior Committee in 1980, but it never reached the House floor, and the legislation died at the end of the year.

The age-old battle pitted giant agribusiness conglomerates and absentee landlords — some with holdings of more than 100,000 acres — against family farmers who were unable to buy federally irrigated land because it was controlled by the large corporations.

The question facing Congress was who should benefit from the $11.5 billion worth of dams and irrigation systems built by the federal government in the 17 Western states.

Should it be the family farmers living on or near the land, who were the intended beneficiaries of the 1902 Reclamation Act that authorized the system? Or should the heavily subsidized water continue to be concentrated in the hands of the large but relatively few farm corporations?

The 1902 Reclamation Act limited to 160 acres per person — or 320 per man and wife — the amount of land a farmer could own and irrigate with water from federal public works projects. There were no limits on leasing additional irrigated land, but the law specified that a farmer had to live on the land in order to receive reclamation water.

The original purpose of the act was plainly stated by its sponsor, Rep. Francis G. Newlands, D-Nev. (House 1893-1903, Senate 1903-1917), who said:

"The very purpose of this bill is to guard against land monopoly and to hold this land in small tracts for the people of the entire country, to give to each only the amount of land that will be necessary for the support of a family."

Farmers could own more than the 160 acres of federally irrigated land and continue receiving water, as long as the owner signed a "recordable contract" with the Interior Department, promising to sell the excess land within a specified period, usually 10 years. The farmer also had to agree to sell the excess land at a "dry land" price that excluded the value added to the land because of the irrigation water it received.

But the department's Bureau of Reclamation in many cases simply did not enforce the recordable contracts or the acreage limitations, and it dropped the residency requirement. Thus, over the years huge agricultural conglomerates developed — most of them in California — where there had once been only arid land.

With the bureau's blessing, the agricultural giants literally turned the desert into the nation's hothouse, using cheap, federally subsidized water from billion-dollar dams thousands of miles away in the Rocky Mountains.

In many cases the landowners were merely "paper farmers" — absentee real estate investors and railroad and oil companies.

In 1976, the department was sued by a small farmers' group, National Land for People, for not enforcing the law. And a federal district court that year ordered the department to draw up a set of regulations to enforce the act.

When the regulations were issued in 1977, the large landowners were infuriated. The department intended to enforce the acreage limitation, forcing the companies to divest themselves of huge chunks of farmland.

The large landowners promptly sued, claiming the department had not done an environmental impact statement before issuing the regulations. While the impact statement was being completed, the department was prohibited from enforcing the new regulations and a moratorium on the sale of excess lands under recordable contracts was imposed.

Meanwhile, the landowners formed the Farm/Water Alliance, a well-financed lobby group made up of landowners, farmers, water districts and banking and real estate associations. They lobbied heavily to get the act amended in Congress.

The Carter administration supported legislation to retain the reclamation law's original intent to promote the family farm.

Nuclear Plant Moratorium

Notwithstanding the national alarm over nuclear safety that followed the Three Mile Island accident in March 1979, both chambers of Congress decisively rejected proposals to impose a six-month moratorium on permits for constructing new nuclear power plants.

Those permits were issued by the Nuclear Regulatory Commission (NRC), which blunted the force of the moratorium proposal by voluntarily halting issuance of new permits and licenses. The commission said it would resume licensing after the accident had been fully studied.

The moratorium requirement was proposed as an amendment to the NRC authorization bill for fiscal 1980 (HR 2608, S 562). At year's end that measure was still in conference. Congress completed action on the measure in mid-1980.

The major point of difference between the House and Senate bills was a Senate provision requiring a shutdown of all nuclear power plants in states that lacked an approved plan for dealing with a nuclear emergency such as Three Mile Island. This provision faced stiff House opposition.

NRC Moratorium. The senior staff of the NRC decided May 21 not to issue new construction permits or operating licenses for plants until August. That delay would allow the commission to evaluate the results of investigations of the Three Mile Island accident. The commission subsequently approved the decision. In November the commission extended its self-imposed moratorium into 1980.

Nuclear Waste Disposal

Late in 1979, the Senate Energy Committee approved legislation (S 2189) requiring the Energy Department to come up with a design and site for a long-term nuclear waste storage facility within one year. The panel admitted that its action was intended to force Congress to solve the longstanding problem of what to do with nuclear waste.

Congress in 1980 approved a weakened version of S 2189 (PL 96-573) giving the states responsibility for disposing of nuclear wastes generated by nuclear power plants, hospitals and industry. But it could not agree on what should be done about disposal of spent nuclear fuel and wastes created from reprocessing nuclear reactor fuels. *(Story, p. 184)*

The intent of S 2189 as approved by the Senate committee was to force the government to design a giant, concrete vault-like facility from which nuclear waste could eventually be retrieved and placed in permanent storage. The waste would be monitored and could be stored there for decades or longer.

In the meantime, the government would continue its studies of and planning for permanent storage, probably in an underground site that could isolate the waste for the centuries during which it would be radioactive.

The nuclear industry supported the committee bill as an interim solution to the nuclear waste problem. But critics charged that the bill would only distract government planners from the effort to develop permanent storage. They also argued that the giant vaults could mislead the public into thinking the waste disposal question had been solved.

The Carter administration opposed the plan to use concrete vault storage, favoring instead efforts to develop geologic disposal.

Nuclear Defense Programs

Nuclear waste disposal was the central issue during consideration of the fiscal 1980 authorization for nuclear weapons programs. S 673 (PL 96-164) authorized $3,053,968,000 for those programs, which were administered by the Energy Department for the Department of Defense.

The final version reduced by $140 million the budget request for long-term storage of nuclear waste generated by the weapons programs. More than $100 million of that savings was then added to the administration requests for weapons development and for manufacturing the raw material used in nuclear bombs, programs Congress thought the Carter administration had systematically underfunded.

Nuclear Waste

Nuclear waste disposal, an issue that had long bedeviled the civilian nuclear power program, was the most controversial issue confronting Congress during consideration of S 673. At the center of the dispute was the Waste Isolation Pilot Plant (WIPP) that had been authorized by Congress as a demonstration project to dispose of the types of waste produced by the Energy Department's nuclear defense plants.

Subsequently, the scope of the project was expanded to include permanent storage of waste from civilian reactors. At the same time, officials in New Mexico, where the plant was to be located, began to demand a say in the design and operation of it, citing potential safety threats to the surrounding area.

Both the House and Senate versions of the nuclear defense bill insisted that the project be restricted to its original, solely military purposes. But the Senate approved $26.5 million of the $55 million requested in fiscal 1980 for the plant while the House bill denied the request and further recommended that $30 million of the $68 million previously authorized for WIPP be rescinded. The House bill also barred any state veto of the project.

The final version of S 673 authorized $20 million for WIPP in fiscal 1980. It also directed the secretary of energy to agree with New Mexico by Sept. 30, 1980, on a formal system for consulting with state officials on aspects of the project affecting local health and safety. The bill did not provide any remedy in case state and federal officials could not agree on a procedure. But in their report, conferees were insistent that WIPP construction proceed on schedule and that state officials not be given a veto over the project.

Pesticide Regulation

The fiscal 1980 reauthorization bill for the federal pesticide control law was allowed to die Dec. 18, 1979, after House-Senate conferees deadlocked on the issue of a one-house legislative veto of environmental regulations.

Because fiscal 1980 funds for the program already had been appropriated (HR 4394 — PL 96-103), conferees decided there was no need to complete action.

Several House conferees were not happy with the fact that the program was funded without a new authorization having been passed first; they had wanted to clamp down on Environmental Protection Agency (EPA) pesticide regulations through the one-house veto provision.

That provision was included in the House version (HR 3546 — H Rept 96-147) of the $66.5 million pesticide control bill, which was passed Nov. 28. It was not part of the Senate bill (S 717 — S Rept 96-146), passed May 22. The House provision would have allowed either chamber of Congress to veto an EPA pesticide regulation within 60 days after it became final.

Another potential controversy was averted when the House overruled its Agriculture Committee and voted to continue a ban on the pesticide mirex. EPA had banned the pesticide in June 1978 because it found mirex to be carcinogenic; the pesticide had been used to control fire ants in Southern states.

The Federal Insecticide, Fungicide and Rodenticide Act was last extended in 1978. President Ford had vetoed a 1976 extension because it contained the one-house veto provision. *(1978 extension, p. 173; 1976 veto, p. 160)*

OSHA Restrictions

Opponents of the Occupational Safety and Health Administration (OSHA) succeeded in 1979 in adding a number of amendments restricting the agency's powers to the fiscal 1980 Labor-Health, Education and Welfare appropriations bill (HR 4389). Although the controversy over federal funding of abortions prevented final passage of that bill, the OSHA restrictions were added to a continuing funding resolution for fiscal 1980 (H J Res 440 — PL 96-123).

Most of the amendments exempted small operations from OSHA inspections or regulations. The amendments:

- Prohibited OSHA from inspecting businesses with 10 or fewer employees if they were in industries with injury rates of less than seven per 100 employees. Exceptions were made to allow OSHA to investigate health hazards or when employers were deemed to be engaging in activities involving substantial hazards, an employer requested consultation, a worker made a complaint, there was an imminent danger or there had been an accident leading to hospitalization or death.
- Prohibited OSHA from issuing civil fines for first-time health and safety violations of a non-serious nature unless the establishment involved was cited for 10 or more serious violations on first inspection.
- Prohibited OSHA from issuing civil penalties for non-serious violations by an employer of 10 or fewer employees if the employer was making a good faith effort to eliminate a hazard found by a consultant.
- Exempted from OSHA regulation all farms with 10 or

fewer employees that did not maintain a labor camp.

- Prohibited OSHA from inspecting any business within six months of the time the establishment had been investigated by a state safety and health agency, with certain exceptions, including catastrophe and fatality.

1980

In the final days of the 1980 session, Congress passed legislation to create a $1.6 billion "superfund" to clean up toxics dumped into the environment. The bill, however, did not cover oil spills. The legislation authorized the federal government to clean up chemical spills that threatened public health and to sue those responsible for the spills to recover the costs. Most of the fund would come from the chemical industry. In separate legislation, Congress also made it easier for the Environmental Protection Agency to go after people who deliberately dumped hazardous wastes rather than disposing of them safely.

Nuclear safety continued to demand congressional attention. Authorizing fiscal 1980 funds for the Nuclear Regulatory Commission almost a year late, Congress approved the first federal safety reforms adopted since the 1979 Three Mile Island accident. Congress also passed legislation giving states most of the responsibility for disposing of low-level nuclear wastes; it was unable to agree on how high-level wastes, including those resulting from weapons production, should be handled.

In other action, Congress postponed the effect of several federal measures to improve the environment. After three years of wrangling, Congress finally approved a measure delaying imposition of noise control standards on commercial airlines. The legislators also gave some cities an additional three years to meet safe drinking water standards, and Congress again postponed imposition of a ban on the artificial sweetener saccharin. A provision of the water control act that required industries using municipal sewage treatment facilities to pay part of the cost of constructing those plants was repealed.

Toxic Spills 'Superfund'

In the waning days of the 1980 session, the 96th Congress resurrected and cleared a drastically scaled-down version of President Carter's 1979 proposal to establish a $1.6 billion emergency "superfund" to clean up toxic contaminants spilled or dumped into the environment.

The House cleared the measure (HR 7020 — PL 96-510) Dec. 3, when it grudgingly accepted the Senate-passed version of the bill by a 274-94 vote under suspension of the rules. A minimum of 246 votes was needed to pass the bill under suspension.

Neither environmentalists nor the chemical industry were entirely happy with the final bill. But the administration gave it reluctant support, and President Carter made several 11th-hour telephone calls to Capitol Hill urging House passage.

However, the final bill contained weaker liability provisions than the president had sought. It also did not cover oil spills, as Carter had proposed and as the House had done in its $1.9 billion superfund package (HR 7020, HR 85).

Carter signed the bill Dec. 11, after noting that congressional leaders had promised to deal with oil spills in the 97th Congress.

The omission of oil spills had led several House sponsors to try to kill the measure at the last minute, but their efforts failed when a majority of the House agreed with proponents that some bill — no matter how flawed — was better than no bill.

As cleared, HR 7020 gave the federal government the authority and the money to act in emergencies to clean up spilled or dumped chemicals threatening public health or the environment. And the government could sue the persons or companies responsible for the damage — if they could be found — to recoup the cleanup costs.

The fund was to be set up over five years, with $1.38 billion coming from the chemical industry and the oil companies that produced chemicals and the rest coming from general revenues.

The measure had been in the drafting stages for two Congresses. It was the congressional response to environmental disasters such as the 1977 discovery in Niagara Falls, N.Y., that the Love Canal subdivision had been built on top of a former chemical dump and that chemicals leaking from the discarded drums were poisoning the residents.

However, the final bill did not allow the superfund to compensate victims injured by such chemical incidents. That controversial proposal, added by the Senate Environment Committee, was deleted before the measure ever reached the Senate floor.

Environmentalists immediately vowed to try again in the next Congress to pass a bill to compensate victims of chemical disasters.

Background

After the Love Canal disaster came to light in 1977, dozens of other chemical wastelands were discovered throughout the nation. Hardly a state was unscathed. But no one really knew how extensive the hazardous waste problem was.

EPA also estimated that 90 percent of the waste being generated was dumped in "an environmentally unsound manner." That included dumping at municipal landfills that did not meet EPA standards and dumping in vacant lots, open pits and lagoons or in barrel-filled tractor-trailers left by the side of the road. Much of the improper disposal was blamed on infamous "midnight dumpers" who operated without permits.

Despite the enormity of the problem, EPA was forced to use a mishmash of existing laws to start cleaning up the most dangerous waste problems. It said the laws were inadequate to do the job. The statutes included:

- Section 311 of the Clean Water Act (PL 92-500), which provided money to clean up spills of oil and 297 toxic chemicals.

But the money could be used only to clean up spills into navigable waters. It did not cover pollution of air, land or ground water. And it did not provide cleanup money for hazardous wastes that were not one of the 297 designated chemicals.

The fund also was far too small to handle the huge

hazardous waste problem. Only $35 million could be appropriated each year, and that had to be shared with the Coast Guard's oil spill cleanup program.

- Section 504 of the same law. It authorized the government to spend up to $10 million a year to clean up any hazardous substance causing any type of pollution. But no appropriations had ever been sought under that section, primarily because the law did not include any controls over how the money would be spent.
- Section 7003 of the Resource Conservation and Recovery Act (PL 94-580). It allowed EPA to sue to require cleanup if an abandoned waste site was posing an "imminent and substantial" hazard to public health. But EPA had to prove in court that the hazard was significant, thus preventing immediate action. The law also did not provide for cleanup of abandoned sites where the owner was unknown or could not afford the cleanup.

House Action

Because of restrictions on committee jurisdictions, the House superfund package was made up of two measures: a bill to clean up abandoned chemical dumps (HR 7020) and a measure to clean up oil and chemicals spilled into navigable waterways (HR 85).

As reported first by the Interstate and Foreign Commerce Committee, HR 7020 (H Rept 96-1016, Part I) provided for a $600 million fund, with half the money coming from industry and half from general revenues. That version was substantially weaker than the original legislation (HR 5790) introduced in 1979; that version had been buried in a subcommittee.

HR 7020 then went to the House Ways and Means Committee (Part II), which increased the amount available in the fund to $1.2 billion and raised industry's share to 75 percent, reducing the government's contribution to 25 percent.

That version received broad bipartisan support when the measure reached the House floor Sept. 19. It was passed, 351-23, on Sept. 23. Before approving the bill, the House rejected an amendment that would have given state environmental agencies the authority to clean up most abandoned chemical dumps. But it adopted amendments tightening the liability provisions, which held companies liable for all cleanup costs resulting from the release of a hazardous waste unless they could prove they had exercised due care or that the release was caused solely by a third party.

HR 85 (H Rept 96-172, Parts I, II and III), the companion bill, was reported first by the House Merchant Marine and Fisheries Committee in 1979. It provided for a $200 million fund dealing only with oil spills in navigable waters.

The version reported by the Public Works and Transportation Committee May 16, 1980, added a $100 million fund to clean up chemical spills in navigable waters.

The Ways and Means Committee version, reported June 20, increased the size of the two funds to $375 million each, financed solely by industry taxes. The committee later agreed to some changes to accommodate the other two committees, and that amended version was sent to the House floor.

The House passed HR 85 Sept. 19 by a 288-11 vote after agreeing to an amendment that limited industry's liability for cleanup costs and damages to those spills of a quantity that EPA determined "may be harmful."

Senate Action

The broadest version of the superfund bill was reported by the Senate Environment Committee May 11. That measure (S 1480 — S Rept 96-848) established a $4.1 billion fund to clean up all types of toxic chemicals in the environment. It also allowed compensation for victims of chemical disasters under certain limited conditions.

There was no Senate action on S 1480 before the election recess, and the bill appeared to be dead following the Republican's election landslide. Republican Senate leaders — who would control the Senate in 1981 — said they wanted to wait until then to give the new administration an opportunity to review the proposal.

But President-elect Reagan indicated to Senate Minority Leader Howard H. Baker Jr., R-Tenn., that he would not object if the lame-duck Congress completed action on the controversial measure before he took office.

Despite that go-ahead, sponsors still had to make major concessions to overcome the objections of other Senate Republicans who threatened to filibuster the Environment Committee bill. After several closed-door sessions, sponsors brought a stripped down version to the Senate floor. The $1.6 billion substitute was passed Nov. 24 by a 78-9 vote. The substitute required industry to contribute 86 percent of the cleanup fund. Although it covered many more types of incidents than the House bills, it did not cover spills involving oil, as did HR 85. Nor did it provide compensation to victims of chemical spills.

The Senate then substituted S 1480 for HR 7020, returned HR 7020, as amended, to the House with a warning that the House should accept the Senate version without change because opponents would kill the bill if it came back to the Senate.

The "take-it-or-leave-it" attitude of the Senate incensed some House sponsors of HR 85. It was the second House-passed oil spill measure that the Senate had refused to act upon. In the 95th Congress, the House twice had passed oil spill measures, but the Senate would not act because they did not contain provisions for chemical spill cleanups.

Nonetheless, other proponents of the superfund legislation urged their colleagues to accept the Senate version of HR 7020, which did not include HR 85, claiming that any problems could be corrected in a later Congress. "This is the proverbial bird in the hand," said Thomas J. Downey, D-N.Y., of the Senate bill.

The Senate version came to the House floor Dec. 3 under suspension of the rules, which prohibited any floor amendments. The House passed the measure with 28 votes more than the two-thirds needed under this procedure. That vote cleared the bill for the president.

Provisions

As signed into law Dec. 11, HR 7020 (PL 96-510) contained the following major provisions:

The Fund

- Established a $1.6 billion Hazardous Substance Response Trust Fund covering fiscal 1981-85, with $1.38 billion (86 percent) coming from fees on the chemical and oil industries and $220 million (14 percent) coming from general revenues appropriated by Congress.
- Provided that the fees would be collected on 45 specified substances, based initially on the quantity of such substances produced by an individual company and ad-

justed later to reflect the number of incidents in which the fund had to clean up each of the particular substances.

• Provided that the fund could pay for the following losses resulting from spills of hazardous chemicals: 90 percent of the operation and maintenance costs of any remedial action taken at the site of the spill (states would pay the other 10 percent); loss of natural resources and costs of restoring lost resources up to $50 million; and costs of health studies and diagnostic examinations for persons injured by chemical spills, but not other medical expenses.

Liability

• Imposed liability equivalent to that in the Clean Water Act (PL 92-500) for government cleanup costs and damage to natural resources of up to $50 million on anyone releasing hazardous substances into the environment.

• Provided that the only defenses to liability were an act of God, an act of war or the act of a third party.

• Exempted from the bill's liability spills and dumps that were in compliance with permits issued under the Clean Water Act, Solid Waste Disposal Act (PL 94-580), 1972 Marine Protection, Research, and Sanctuaries Act (PL 92-532), Safe Drinking Water Act (PL 93-523), the Clean Air Act (PL 95-95) and Atomic Energy Act of 1954 (PL 84-141).

Emergency Response

• Authorized the president to order a company to remove or control hazardous substances threatening the public health, welfare or environment.

• Authorized the president to order whatever emergency cleanup action he deemed necessary — by either the government or the responsible party — to protect the public whenever a pollutant was released or there was "the substantial threat" of such a release.

• Provided that government measures could include cleanup and temporary or permanent provision of alternative water supplies and housing.

Scope

• Defined hazardous substances as any toxic substance identified under certain sections of the Clean Water Act, the Solid Waste Disposal Act and the Toxic Substances Control Act (PL 94-469).

• Exempted spills or releases of petroleum, natural gas and synthetic fuels and their derivatives, unless identified in another act as hazardous.

• Authorized the president to designate as hazardous other substances that could present substantial danger to public health, welfare and the environment.

• Provided that the law applied to release of hazardous substances into the air, land, navigable waters, ground water or public water supplies, at disposal sites, facilities and vessels.

• Defined "release" as "any spilling, leaking, pumping, pouring, emitting, emptying, discharging, injecting, escaping, leaching or dumping" into the environment, or any other release "which presents or may present" a substantial danger to the public.

• Exempted releases in the workplace and releases of nuclear materials or byproducts, normal field applications of fertilizers and engine exhausts.

Legislative Veto

• Provided that if within 60 days of promulgation of any agency regulation written to carry out the act either the House or the Senate passed a resolution disapproving the regulation, or if both houses adopted such a resolution within 90 days, the regulation would not become effective.

Penalties

• Required anyone in charge of a facility found to have released a hazardous substance to notify immediately the appropriate federal agency or face up to $10,000 in fines.

• Required owners or operators of facilities where hazardous substances were stored or disposed of to notify the administrator of the appropriate government agency of the existence of the facility or site, and to specify the amount and type of hazardous substances there and any likely discharges from that facility. Provided that failure to comply could result in a fine of up to $10,000 and/or imprisonment for up to one year.

• Required deeds for hazardous waste disposal sites to disclose the location of toxic chemicals on the site. Provided that violators would be subject to a $10,000 fine and/or up to a year in prison and would be liable for any damage resulting from chemical releases.

Hazardous Waste Disposal

Legislation (S 1156 — PL 96-482) giving the Environmental Protection Agency (EPA) tougher enforcement powers to control "midnight dumpers" of hazardous wastes was cleared by Congress in October 1980.

S 1156 made it a felony for anyone to "knowingly" endanger human life when disposing of hazardous wastes. Under existing law, violators of waste handling regulations could be charged only with a misdemeanor.

The legislation also allowed EPA to go to court to seek a cleanup order if a hazardous waste "may" present an imminent or substantial danger to the health or environment. Under existing law, the agency had to prove that a waste actually threatened life or the environment before the agency could take action.

The bill also expanded some of EPA's toxic waste enforcement powers, but curtailed others — primarily EPA's authority to regulate oil and gas drilling residues.

The measure did not mandate specific solutions to problems of abandoned waste sites or of transportation of wastes.

Congress in 1980 passed "superfund" legislation that enabled the government to clean up hazardous waste sites immediately upon determining that they posed a serious threat to health or the environment. The government then could sue the person or company responsible for the dump to recoup the cleanup costs. *("Superfund" legislation, p. 178)*

S 1156 extended the Solid Waste Disposal Act (PL 89-272), as amended by the 1976 Resource Conservation and Recovery Act (RCRA — PL 94-580), for three years. It authorized $514.5 million during fiscal 1980, 1981 and 1982 to administer the act, plus another $36 million (for certain groups) through fiscal 1985.

RCRA was passed in 1976, partially to stop "midnight dumping" of chemical wastes into vacant lots and along roadsides.

The act gave EPA authority to promote the safe disposal of both solid and hazardous wastes and to encourage recycling and conservation of wastes. Besides writing regulations on how wastes should be handled, EPA was authorized to provide grants to states and cities to plan and manage their own waste control programs.

Legislative Action

The versions of S 1156 approved by the House and Senate were similar. The Senate approved S 1156 (S Rept 96-172) on June 4, 1979. That bill authorized $524 million over three years for programs under the Solid Waste Disposal Act. And it suspended for two years EPA's authority to regulate as hazardous wastes residues from the production of oil, natural gas, coal and geothermal energy.

The House version (HR 3994 — H Rept 96-191), passed Feb. 10, 1980, with only 10 dissenting votes, extended the act for only one year. It added a number of wastes, including those from phosphate and uranium mining, to the list that EPA could not regulate as hazardous wastes.

Further action on the measure was put on hold until late in the year, primarily because conferees were working on the "superfund" legislation. When they met on S 1156 Sept. 30, conferees had little trouble resolving the differences between the two versions. They agreed to a three-year extension at $514.6 million. Conferees also dropped the House amendment on EPA regulation of uranium and phosphate mining wastes, but they retained a House provision authorizing $20 million to develop a list of hazardous waste dumps and to assess the threats those dumps posed to human health.

The Senate adopted the conference report (H Rept 96-1444; S Rept 96-1010) Oct. 1; the House adoped it Oct. 2, clearing the measure.

Provisions

As signed into law Oct. 21, PL 96-482:

- Authorized $514.5 million during fiscal 1980, 1981 and 1982 for administering the Solid Waste Disposal Act, as amended by RCRA, and $36 million during fiscal 1983-85 for certain state and local grant programs.
- Stipulated that the secretary of the interior would regulate all coal mining wastes under the Surface Mining and Reclamation Act of 1977.
- Established an inter-agency committee to coordinate federal resource conservation and recovery efforts, and programs for recovering energy from solid wastes.
- Suspended EPA regulation of oil and gas drilling wastes until after EPA had studied the adverse effects of such wastes and provided that EPA could not promulgate regulations to control such wastes without prior congressional approval.
- Suspended EPA regulations of "special wastes," such as fly ash, bottom ash, slag waste and flue gas wastes, until studies were completed on the toxicity of those wastes.
- Authorized EPA to develop regulations relating to radioactive phosphate and uranium mining wastes after studying the adverse effects of such wastes.
- Required EPA "where appropriate" to establish different waste disposal requirements for older waste treatment plants than for newer facilities.
- Allowed EPA to issue compliance orders to violators of the act immediately upon discovering the violations.
- Created a new "knowing endangerment" offense, punishable by either five years in prison or up to a $250,000 fine for breaking the law with "extreme indifference" to human life, or two years in prison and up to a $250,000 fine for "unjustified and inexcusable" disregard for human life.
- Authorized $20 million for states to make an inventory of chemical dumps.
- Authorized $5.5 million for cities to relocate toxic dumps located above drinking water supplies.
- Authorized EPA to order cleanup of a dump that "may" present an imminent threat to health or the environment.

Toxic Substances

The House killed an extension of the Toxic Substances Control Act of 1976 when it failed to act on reauthorizing legislation approved by the House Commerce Committee (HR 7126 — H Rept 96-968).

Nor did it act on a similar Commerce bill (HR 2606) reported in 1979 or on a three-year reauthorization measure (S 1147) approved by the Senate in 1979. *(1979 action, p. 175)*

Waste Treatment Plant Costs

Congress in 1980 sent to the president a bill (S 2725 — PL 96-483) repealing a controversial requirement that industries discharging waste into municipal sewage treatment plants pay some of the cost of building those plants.

Revocation of the 1972 Clean Water Act's industrial cost recovery (ICR) provision was included in legislation authorizing fiscal 1981 and 1982 funds to administer nine expiring portions of the act (PL 92-500). *(Clean Water Act, p. 145; 1977 amendments, p. 164)*

The ICR provision had been included in the Clean Water Act at the urging of Sen. Edmund S. Muskie, D-Maine (1959-80). He had argued that without ICR, the federal government would be providing industry with massive subsidies. But industry and the municipalities contended that the provision was unworkable and not cost effective.

Muskie had successfully held off many attempts to repeal the provision. But because of the difficulties municipalities experienced in recovering the charges and because of fears of the effect the charges would have on employment in economically depressed areas, Congress in 1977 exempted small industrial users and granted an 18-month moratorium on other collections. In December 1979 Congress extended the moratorium for six months, through June 30, 1980.

Then, on May 8, 1980, only 15 hours after Muskie left the Senate to become secretary of state, the Senate Environmental Pollution Subcommittee, which Muskie had chaired, voted to repeal the ICR provision.

"It was wrongheaded in concept then [in 1972], and it is wrongheaded today," Rep. James C. Cleveland, R-N.H. (1963-81), said of the ICR provision just before the House passed the compromise version of the bill.

Cleveland and Don H. Clausen, R-Calif., said during the House debate that they expected the Environmental Protection Agency (EPA) to direct municipalities to reimburse companies for any ICR collections they had made, but the final compromise did not include language directing the agency to do that.

In place of the disputed ICR requirement, the final bill included an amendment by Sen. Robert T. Stafford, R-Vt., prohibiting the use of federal money to construct facilities for treating industrial discharges of more than 50,000 gallons a day.

House members had opposed the Stafford amendment, but the Senate insisted on it. Eventually, senators agreed to a House proposal postponing the effective date of the Stafford amendment until Nov. 15, 1981.

In the meantime, the EPA was instructed to conduct an analysis by March 15, 1981, on the impact of the Stafford amendment.

Other Compromises

As enacted, the $987.5 million bill was a compromise between a $618.7 million Senate-passed measure and a $1.7 billion House proposal.

In other compromises, the House accepted a Senate amendment that allowed states and cities to pay more than their traditional 25 percent share of federal/state sewer grants, if their governors chose to do so.

House members also agreed to a Senate amendment allowing New York State to use up to $20 million of its sewer grant funds to dredge highly toxic PCBs (polychlorinated biphenyl) that were dumped into the Hudson River. The House added a stipulation that the state must try to incinerate the dredged PCBs, or destroy them chemically, before dumping them in a landfill. Landfills were not considered safe disposal spots for PCBs.

In addition, the bill included a compromise extending from two years to three years the time a state had to spend its 1979 sewer construction grant allotment. However, a House-passed provision giving cities two extra years to comply with the Clean Water Act was dropped.

Provisions

As signed into law Oct. 21, PL 96-483:

- Reauthorized nine expiring portions of the Clean Water Act, with a total authorization of $987.5 million in fiscal 1981 and 1982.
- Repealed the industrial cost recovery provision.
- Made the portion of sewage treatment plant construction costs attributable to the treatment of industrial discharges in excess of 50,000 gallons a day ineligible for federal funding after Nov. 15, 1981.
- Extended from two to three years the period during which 1979 construction grants would be available to states for obligation before they had to be returned to the EPA to be disbursed to other states.
- Authorized New York to use $20 million of its construction funds for a demonstration project to dredge PCBs from the Hudson River, provided that incineration and chemical destruction were considered as methods of disposal before landfill disposal.
- Allowed the federal government to pay less than its traditional 75 percent share of federal/state sewer grants, as long as the lower share was uniform on a statewide basis.
- Authorized EPA to disburse $30 million to the states for use in paying up to 90 percent of the cost of demonstration programs to clean up state-owned abandoned mines that could be used as hazardous waste disposal sites, and mandated that, at a minimum, such projects be undertaken in Ohio, Illinois and West Virginia.
- Allowed states to be reimbursed for money they spent on sewage treatment plants before the federal grants for such purposes had become available.
- Raised the construction cost limits applicable to small cities (up to 25,000 population) receiving combined planning and construction grants from $2 million to $4 million, and from $3 million to $5 million in states with unusually high construction costs.

Safe Drinking Water

President Carter in 1980 signed into law a bill (HR 8117 — PL 96-502) giving some cities three extra years to meet federal standards for cleaning up cancer-causing substances in public drinking water supplies.

Less than two weeks later, the Council on Environmental Quality (CEQ) released a report that contained new evidence of a possible link between chlorinated drinking water and certain kinds of cancer in humans.

The bill gave states authority to extend from Jan. 1, 1981, to Jan. 1, 1984, the deadline for cities to meet the interim safe drinking water standards established under the 1974 Safe Drinking Water Act (PL 93-523). *(1974 act, p. 151)*

At least 13,600 water systems, most of them serving fewer than 2,500 persons, were in violation of one or more of those standards and could not meet the Jan. 1 deadline. The interim standards, which became effective in 1977, were scheduled to be replaced by permanent standards to be proposed in June 1982.

Cities planning to regionalize their water treatment systems were also given an additional three years, until Jan. 1, 1986, to comply with the act.

The study issued Dec. 17 by the CEQ strengthened previous reports that had linked rectal, colon and bladder cancer to the practice of using chlorine to disinfect public water supplies. Chlorine combines with natural organic matter in water to produce chemicals — trihalogenated methanes — that had been shown to cause cancer at high doses in laboratory animals.

The measure gave the Environmental Protection Agency the discretion to approve state underground oil and gas injection programs, without subjecting them to federal regulations prepared under the act, if those plans adequately protected underground water supplies. The bill also exempted natural gas storage wells from the underground injection control program mandated by the act.

Coastal Zone Management

Congress cleared for the president in 1980 legislation (S 2622 — PL 96-464) to revamp the Coastal Zone Management program.

The final bill cut back existing authorizations for coastal planning grants by $75 million a year, but established new state grant programs to revitalize urban waterfronts and help coastal cities adversely affected by energy development.

As cleared, S 2622 authorized $161 million annually for five years (fiscal 1981-85), for a total of $805 million. Of that amount, $240 million would be divided among 25 states that voluntarily participated in the basic program, which provided 80 percent federal funding for coastal area development planning.

Maintaining that it was time to phase out federal participation in the coastal management program, the administration had requested $405 million over eight years, with the federal share of grants to the states dropping from 80 percent to 33 percent by the end of the period.

Noise Control Programs

The House and Senate passed differing versions of legislation to reauthorize the Environmental Protection Agency's noise control programs in fiscal 1980 and 1981, but the 96th Congress did not complete action on the measure.

The law was last reauthorized in 1978. *(Story, p. 171)*

Airplane Noise Control

Ending three years of debate and disagreement, Congress Feb. 5, 1980, sent to the president legislation to allow domestic airlines to delay meeting federal noise control standards on some passenger planes.

President Carter, whose threat of a veto helped force a compromise that greatly restricted the scope of the exemptions originally contemplated, signed the bill (HR 2440 — PL 96-193) Feb. 18.

Federal Aviation Administration (FAA) standards issued in 1969 required all commercial passenger jets manufactured afer 1974 to comply with federal noise standards. In 1976 the FAA required airlines to bring their older planes into compliance with those standards, either by retrofitting their engines or replacing the planes altogether. Some two- and three-engine aircraft were to meet the noise reduction standards by 1981, others by 1983. Four-engine jets had to comply by 1985.

When the FAA issued its 1976 order, the Ford administration recommended that Congress approve federal aid to airlines to help them defray the costs of muffling or replacing their noisy jets.

In 1978 the House approved legislation that would have levied a 2 percent tax on passenger fares and freight rates to subsidize the airline noise control programs. The Senate rejected the subsidy approach and the session adjourned before any compromise could be reached. *(Details, p. 171)*

In HR 2440 Congress decided instead to delay some of the noise control deadlines airlines were ordered to meet.

As signed into law, HR 2440 exempted two-engine jets with 100 or fewer seats until 1988 and two-engine jets with more than 100 seats until 1985. Two-engine aircraft with more than 100 seats were exempt until 1986 if the airlines signed a contract by 1983 to replace the planes with jets meeting even more stringent standards than required by the FAA. This was known as the "new technology waiver." Three-engine aircraft would be eligible for the waiver until 1985 if the airline contracted by 1983 for replacements meeting the more stringent standards. No waivers were allowed for four-engine aircraft.

Proponents of the bill claimed the system of exemptions and waivers would encourage airlines to purchase even quieter craft. They contended that retrofitting existing planes to meet the standards would be extremely expensive and provide little significant noise relief.

On the other hand, opponents charged that the exemptions and waivers were a sham that would permit noisy planes to fly despite the FAA standards.

The final version of the bill also authorized funds for noise and land use compatibility programs and for airport development.

1980 NRC Funds

Almost a year late, Congress in June 1980 sent to the White House a bill (S 562 — PL 96-295) authorizing $426.8 million for the Nuclear Regulatory Commission (NRC) in fiscal 1980. PL 96-295 also contained the first statutory reforms concerning nuclear power plant safety since the March 1979 accident at the Three Mile Island nuclear plant. *(Accident, p. 176)*

PL 96-295 made plain the feeling of Congress that all states should have federally approved plans for responding to emergencies such as the Three Mile Island incident. The law forbade the NRC to issue any new operating licenses to power plants in any state that lacked such a plan.

The law also required the NRC to develop a plan for a federal response to such a crisis and standards requiring that all new power plants be located a certain distance from large population centers. In addition, the measure substantially increased the penalties that could be imposed upon plant operators who violated safety regulations, removing the existing ceiling of $25,000 per month in fines for such violations.

S 562 was approved by the Senate in mid-1979 and the House in December 1979. Final action was delayed for six more months, however, as conferees wrangled over a Senate provision requiring the shutdown of all nuclear power plants in states lacking approved plans for dealing with a nuclear plant emergency.

Provisions

As signed into law, PL 96-295 authorized a total of $426,821,000 in fiscal 1980 for the NRC. Within that grand total, $213 million was allocated to nuclear regulatory research, $66.5 million to nuclear reactor regulation, $15.9 million to standards development, $42.4 million to inspection and enforcement, $32.4 million to nuclear materials safety and safeguards, $18.1 million to program technical support, and $38.4 million to program administration and direction.

In addition, PL 96-295 contained provisions that:

- Required that no new operating licenses be issued in a state unless the state had an NRC-approved plan for evacuations and other steps in case of a nuclear emergency. If a state were uncooperative, then a utility could draft an emergency response plan and submit it to the NRC for approval. The NRC was directed to write standards that states and utilities would follow in drafting their plans.
- Required the NRC to develop by Sept. 30, 1980, a plan for federal government response to nuclear accidents.
- Required that a proposed reactor meet new federal standards for siting away from population centers before it

Reorganizing the NRC

With congressional approval, President Carter in 1980 reorganized the Nuclear Regulatory Commission to place more authority in the hands of its chairman. This restructuring was Carter's solution to the problems that had impeded the NRC from responding effectively to the Three Mile Island accident in 1979.

In October 1979, the Kemeny Commission, which Carter had appointed to investigate the accident, called for the abolition of the NRC. Carter answered in December 1979 with some less drastic proposals, which were set out in detail in Reorganization Plan No. 1 for 1980, sent to Congress in March 1980.

Even before proposing the reorganization at the NRC, Carter had removed Joseph M. Hendrie as chairman. Hendrie, whom Carter had placed on the commission as chairman in 1977, remained a member. As acting chairman, Carter chose John Ahearne, a former Energy Department official whom Carter had appointed to the NRC in 1978.

Carter in 1980 nominated Harvard professor Albert Carnesale to a vacant seat on the NRC, indicating that he would name him its chairman once he was confirmed. But political considerations in an election year worked against Carnesale's confirmation, and the seat remained vacant for most of 1980. Ahearne continued to act as chairman through the last months of the Carter administration.

Reorganization Approved

Reorganization Plan No. 1 substantially upgraded the authority of the NRC chairman, making clear that he was the principal executive officer and spokesman for the commission. The plan further authorized the chairman to act for the commission in an emergency.

Carter modified his initial proposals, sending amendments to the plan to Congress in May. Those amendments were in response to criticism that the chairman would wield too much power, leaving little for the other members of the commission to do. The amendments clarified the roles that the other commissioners would have.

Had Congress wished to block the proposed changes, it would have had to demonstrate its disapproval by June 11.

On May 22, the Senate tacitly gave its approval to the plan when the Senate Governmental Affairs Committee recommended against passage of a resolution of disapproval (S Res 397 — S Rept 96-790).

A week later, on May 30, the House by voice vote rejected a resolution (H Res 624 — H Rept 96-1043) disapproving the plan.

could be issued a construction permit. The NRC was directed to write the standards, which would have to specify allowable population density and other criteria.

- Directed the NRC to list for Congress all safety-related rules and regulations that were not being met by individual nuclear reactors.
- Made it a federal crime to sabotage nuclear facilities or murder, assault, intimidate or otherwise interfere with NRC personnel on a project licensed by the NRC.
- Set criminal penalties of $25,000 a day or two years in jail for any director, officer or employee of a firm constructing or supplying components of a nuclear facility who knowingly and willfully violated the Atomic Energy Act. On a second conviction, the fine would increase to $50,000 a day.
- Authorized the NRC to assume control of emergency response actions, thus pre-empting state responsibility, if the NRC determined that a state had failed to protect the public health and safety. However, conferees stated in the report that they intended the NRC to exercise that authority "only as a last resort."
- Increased civil penalties for safety violations at nuclear plants from $5,000 to $100,000 per violation. The cap in existing law of $25,000 in fines per month was removed.
- Exempted from the Freedom of Information Act any nuclear data whose release "could reasonably be expected to have a significant adverse effect on health and safety of the public."
- Required the NRC to notify governors in advance of shipments of nuclear wastes through their states except when shipments would not pose a hazard to public health and safety because of the type of waste or quantity.
- Prohibited the storage of any nuclear wastes in oceans.
- Required the NRC to develop within six months a plan for improving operator training.

1981 NRC Funds

Congress adjourned in 1980 without completing action on the fiscal 1981 authorization bill for the Nuclear Regulatory Commission (NRC).

The Senate easily approved its version (S 2358 — S Rept 96-767) of the $445 million measure July 31. But the House never considered its version (HR 6628).

A main point of contention appeared to be whether the NRC should provide funding to public interest groups, individuals and others who wished to intervene in NRC licensing and rule-making procedures. The Senate and the House Interior Committee rejected the administration's request for a demonstration intervenor program; the House Commerce Committee supported the proposal.

Nuclear Waste Disposal

Unable to reach agreement upon a national policy for disposing of nuclear waste, the 96th Congress late in 1980 passed the task of finding a solution to the 97th Congress. As a step in that direction, Congress in December 1980 approved legislation (S 2189 — PL 96-573) giving the states the primary responsibility for disposing of low-level radioactive wastes.

Low-level wastes were produced by power plants, hospitals and industrial plants in every state. They could be paper, plastics, construction materials, tools, clothing, vials or other items contaminated by radioactivity. The term "low-level" was in some sense misleading, for it referred to the source of the radioactivity, not the degree of radioactivity of the waste. Low-level waste was the phrase used to describe all radioactive waste except that produced in nuclear reactors or in the reprocessing of nuclear fuels.

Background

When the 96th Congress convened, both the nuclear industry and its critics were hoping that the legislators would act to resolve some of the long-standing questions regarding the future of nuclear power. One of those key issues was nuclear waste. Despite decade-old accumulations of nuclear waste materials, the nation was still without any comprehensive policy to guide the management or long-term storage of those hazardous substances. Most of those wastes were stored in 1980 in pools of water at the reactor sites where they were produced.

The Three Mile Island nuclear accident in March 1979 rearranged any plans the 1979 session had for considering nuclear waste disposal, but late in that year the Senate Energy Committee ordered reported legislation (S 2189 — S Rept 96-548) calculated to force action on the matter. As reported, S 2189 required the Energy Department to find a site and produce a design for a long-term nuclear waste storage facility within one year of the bill's enactment. *(1979 action, p. 176)*

High-Level Waste: 1980 Stalemate

In mid-summer 1980, the Senate approved S 2189, which directed the federal government to build aboveground vaults in which high-level radioactive waste could be stored for as long as a century. The Senate bill, approved July 30 by a key vote of 88-7, was backed by the nuclear industry and utilities. It was clearly a temporary solution to the problem of containing those wastes, most of which would remain active for hundreds of years.

S 2189 provided for federal storage of spent nuclear fuel produced by commercial reactors at sites away from those reactors. It also gave the states the power to veto a federal decision to deposit such waste within the state's boundaries, so long as one chamber of Congress agreed with the state's opposition. If the waste involved was generated by military nuclear activities, however, and the president decided that storage in a particular state was essential to the national security, a state's veto of that decision would hold only if it was supported by both chambers of Congress.

S 2189 stated that federal policy was to require each state to be responsible for the low-level waste generated by non-federal activities within its borders. The bill suggested that states might enter into compacts or other regional agreements for developing multi-state plans and facilities for disposing of such waste.

House Action. Three House committees — Science, Commerce and Interior — reported five versions of two bills dealing with nuclear waste disposal in 1980 (HR 7418 — H Rept 96-1156, Parts I-III; HR 6390 — H Rept 96-1382, Parts I-II).

In mid-November, members of the Commerce and Interior committees agreed on a compromise (HR 8378) that the House considered and passed by voice vote on Dec. 3.

NRC Membership

The Nuclear Regulatory Commission (NRC), which came under sharp criticism during the Carter administration, underwent a number of changes in its membership during the 1977-80 period.

President Carter had the opportunity to name three of the commission's five members in his first year in office, but only two of his choices won confirmation. Those two were Joseph M. Hendrie, chairman of the department of applied science at the Brookhaven (N.Y.) National Laboratory, whom Carter named as chairman of the NRC; and Peter A. Bradford, a member of the Maine Public Service Commission.

Carter also named Kent F. Hansen, a professor of nuclear engineering at the Massachusetts Institute of Technology, to a seat on the commission, but his nomination was rejected by the Senate Environment and Public Works Committee. Lack of experience in policy matters and a possible conflict of interest were cited as the reasons for the committee's action.

In 1978 Carter filled the vacant seat on the commission, naming John F. Ahearne, who had served on the White House energy policy staff and in the Department of Energy before moving to the commission. In December 1979, after the Three Mile Island incident, Carter removed Hendrie as chairman (although he remained a commissioner) and named Ahearne acting chairman, a post he retained for the remainder of the Carter administration, due in part to the refusal of the Senate to confirm Carter's choice of a new chairman.

Two of the original members of the NRC, Victor Gilinsky and Richard T. Kennedy, served in those posts during the Carter administration. Gilinsky was nominated by Carter to a second term in 1979, and was confirmed. His new term expired in June 1984. Kennedy's term expired in June 1980, at which time he left his post.

In July 1980, Carter named Albert Carnesale as Kennedy's successor, indicating his intention to designate Carnesale as chairman of the commission, once he was confirmed. Carnesale, a nuclear engineer and professor of public policy at Harvard's John F. Kennedy School of Government, served from 1969 until 1972 as chief of defense weapons at the Arms Control and Disarmament Agency.

After Carter lost his bid for re-election and after several key Republican senators voiced reservations about Carnesale's position on the controversial issues of nuclear reprocessing and breeder reactors, the Senate Environment Committee shelved the nomination, letting it die with the end of the 96th Congress.

The House bill, substituted for the Senate-approved text of S 2189, was radically different from the Senate measure. The House bill set out a timetable for federal decisions on siting and building permanent repositories in natural rock and other geologic formations for high-level nuclear waste by the mid-1990s. A site would have to be chosen by 1987.

Unlike the Senate bill, the measure did not give the federal government responsibility for away-from-reactor storage of spent nuclear fuel used by utilities. Nor did the House measure make any provision for above-ground storage of nuclear wastes.

The House bill, however, did contain language allowing a state to veto the storage of nuclear waste within its boundaries so long as one chamber of Congress passed a resolution supporting that veto. By a key vote of 161-218, the House rejected an amendment that would have allowed a state veto to stand unless both chambers voted to override it.

The House version of the bill also contained language giving states the primary responsibility for disposing of their own low-level wastes.

Compromise Negotiations. As soon as the House approved its version of S 2189 Dec. 3, key members sought to work out a compromise with the Senate, meeting in the back room of the Capitol beyond public view. But by Dec. 12, it was clear that a compromise would not be reached before adjournment. The critical issue was the power of states to veto the storage within their boundaries of nuclear waste generated by federal military activities, such as the production of nuclear weapons.

Senate Energy Committee Chairman Henry M. Jackson, D-Wash., insisted that the states should not be permitted to veto storage of military nuclear waste. But other key senators, led by John Glenn, D-Ohio, and backed by members of the House committees dealing with the issue, argued that the states should have some voice in such decisions. Faced with that impasse, Jackson and Glenn agreed to defer further consideration of the matter until the 97th Congress.

Low-Level Waste: 1980 Action

Only three states had dumps in which commercial low-level wastes could be buried in 1980 — Washington, Nevada and South Carolina. But the first two had already moved to close their dumps to out-of-state nuclear waste, and the third had indicated it would curtail the amount it would accept from out-of-state sources in the future.

When the comprehensive nuclear waste bill appeared dead for the 96th Congress, South Carolina Gov. Richard W. Riley, D, let it be known that the state's dump could be closed to all out-of-state waste if Congress did not pass at least some measure dealing with low-level wastes.

Rep. Butler Derrick, D-S.C., then began a forceful effort to win enactment of the provisions of the House and Senate measures concerning low-level waste. He camped on or just off the Senate floor for more than nine hours Dec. 13, working persistently to convince senators to approve that portion of S 2189. He was successful, and the Senate approved the low-level provisions on Saturday, Dec. 13. The House cleared the bill a few hours later, approving the Senate amendments.

As enacted, S 2189 made the disposal of commercial low-level waste a state responsibility. States could decide whether to build dump sites or form regional compacts with other states to establish a mutual dump site. Waste generated by the federal government would not be a state responsibility, and the compacts could not make policies affecting federal waste.

Nuclear Fusion

Hoping to have a commercial demonstration plant using nuclear fusion to generate an infinite supply of clean, safe energy by the year 2000, Congress in 1980 accelerated the federal nuclear fusion development program.

HR 6308 (PL 96-386) was intended to speed up current Energy Department fusion work by 15 to 20 years; it envisioned the spending of as much as $20 billion by the year 2000.

Existing nuclear reactors produced heat to make electricity by a process called fission, which involved splitting atoms of uranium. Nuclear fusion involved combining hydrogen atoms, which could be extracted from water, to form helium. That process released vast amounts of energy. To make it occur, it was necessary to heat the hydrogen gas to more than 100 million degrees centigrade while confining it within a very strong magnetic field; thus the process was known as magnetic fusion.

The administration supported the legislation.

Provisions

PL 96-386 declared that it was U.S. policy to "accelerate the national effort" on fusion. The bill did not authorize specific funding, but called for a doubling of present funding within seven years, increasing spending by 25 percent in fiscal 1982 and again in fiscal 1983.

The fiscal 1981 appropriations bill for energy and water resources (PL 96-367 — HR 7590) provided $393 million for fusion research.

The bill also required the secretary of energy to:

- Maintain a broadly based fusion research program.
- Establish a national magnetic fusion center.
- Initiate design of a fusion engineering test device, to be operational no later than 1990.
- Initiate as soon as practicable all activities required to meet the national goal of operating a nuclear fusion demonstration plant by 2000.
- Establish a comprehensive fusion development program by Jan. 1, 1982.

Nuclear Weapons

Congress completed action in 1980 on legislation (S 3074 — PL 96-540) authorizing $3.97 billion in fiscal 1981 for nuclear weapons research and development programs administered by the Energy Department for the Pentagon. The final bill contained language reiterating Congress' insistence that the issue of storing radioactive waste generated by nuclear weapons plants be insulated from the political controversy over the storage of waste products from commercial nuclear projects. S 3074 authorized $34 million to continue construction of the Waste Isolation Pilot Plant (WIPP) in New Mexico, which was to be used only for waste from nuclear weapons plants. Carter had planned to halt the project.

The bill also incorporated a House provision ordering the Energy Department to place all weapons-related waste disposal activity under the purview of its assistant secretary for defense, rather than leaving it tied to commercial waste disposal activities in another division. *(Commercial nuclear waste disposal, story, p. 184)*

New York Nuclear Waste

To show that it could be done, Congress agreed in 1980 that the federal government would undertake, with the state of New York, to remove high-level radioactive liquid wastes from the site of a defunct nuclear reprocessing plant.

S 2443 (PL 96-368) obligated the U.S. government to demonstrate how large quantities of such wastes can be solidified and moved to a permanent storage site. The total cost of the project was estimated at $300 million, of which the United States would pay 90 percent and the state the remainder. The cleanup was expected to take a decade or longer to complete. PL 96-368 provided an initial authorization of $5 million for work in fiscal 1981.

The plant that generated this waste — the Western New York Nuclear Service Center — was a private venture, established with federal encouragement in the 1950s to turn spent fuel from nuclear reactors into additional fuel. It began operating in 1966; it was the only commercial reprocessing plant ever operated in the United States. Owned by the state of New York, the site was located 30 miles from Buffalo.

In the early 1970s the federal government changed the rules for such reprocessing, amending the standards concerning storage of liquid nuclear wastes. As a result of those changes, the operators of the Western New York plant found it impossible to operate profitably and shut down the plant in 1972.

About 580,000 gallons of high-level radioactive liquids remained at the site in 1980, contained in two carbon tanks. The liquids were corrosive and leaks were possible. Under PL 96-368, the liquids would be solidified and taken to a federal repository.

Pesticide Regulation

Congress late in 1980 cleared legislation (HR 7018 — PL 96-539) allowing Congress, by a majority vote of both chambers, to veto any proposed federal pesticide regulation.

The two-house veto provision was contained in a bill that extended the Federal Insecticide, Fungicide and Rodenticide Act (FIFRA — PL 94-940) for one year, through fiscal 1981, and authorized $77.5 million for its pesticide control programs.

Under the veto provision, any regulation proposed to implement the law could be killed if both the House and Senate passed a resolution of disapproval within 90 days of the date the regulation was proposed.

The fiscal 1980 FIFRA reauthorization bill died in 1979 when Senate conferees refused to go along with a one-house veto provision contained in the House version of the measure. *(Story, p. 177)*

The final bill contained two other provisions, which had been proposed by the House. These required the administrator of the Environmental Protection Agency (EPA) to submit to the Scientific Advisory Panel — a non-governmental board set up under FIFRA to review EPA's pesticide decisions — any data EPA used in making a decision to order an emergency suspension of a pesticide. It also directed the EPA administrator to require peer review of the design of scientific pesticides studies.

Saccharin Ban Moratorium

Legislation permitting the use of saccharin in soft drinks and diet foods until June 30, 1981, was signed into law June 17, 1980.

The bill (HR 4453 — PL 96-273) cleared Congress June 9, when the Senate by voice vote approved, unchanged, the bill passed by the House in 1979.

The Food and Drug Administration (FDA) had moved to ban saccharin in 1977, after laboratory tests linked it to cancer in rats. Under pressure from consumers and diet food and drink manufacturers, Congress placed an 18-month moratorium on the proposed ban. That moratorium (PL 95-203) expired May 23, 1979. *(1977 action, p. 169)*

HR 4453 also continued the 1977 moratorium's requirements that saccharin-flavored products bear health warning labels.

OSHA Restrictions

Intense lobbying by organized labor in 1980 succeeded in blocking legislation (S 2153) that would have exempted an estimated 90 percent of U.S. businesses from safety inspections by the Occupational Safety and Health Administration (OSHA).

S 2153, introduced by Sen. Richard S. Schweiker, R-Pa. (1969-81), was the latest in a series of moves in Congress to restrict the controversial agency's authority to enforce its safety regulations. The bill would have exempted from routine safety inspections businesses with records of no or low numbers of injuries. Health inspections would not have been affected by the legislation.

Supporters said that the bill would have permitted OSHA inspectors to spend their time on the 10 percent of businesses that had the worst safety records.

However, OSHA head Eula Bingham and other opponents of the measure argued that all businesses should remain under the agency's legal authority. The threat of inspection, no matter how unlikely, made every business conscious of safety, Bingham said, while a statutory exemption would leave many workers without any protection.

Black Lung Claims

The Senate in 1980 did not act on House-passed legislation shifting responsibility for the black lung disability claims of several thousand coal miners from individual operators to a trust fund financed by a tax on coal.

The two 1978 laws that established and regulated the trust fund (PL 95-239, PL 95-227) required a review, under liberalized criteria, of rejected disability claims filed by miners who had retired between 1970 and 1973. That review had made some 10,000 miners newly eligible for black lung benefits. Under the 1978 laws, those benefits were to be paid by the individual coal companies who had employed the miners. *(1978 laws, p. 173)*

The House bill (HR 7745), passed Dec. 1, would have shifted responsibility for paying those benefits to the trust fund. The legislation would have transferred "liability from coal operators individually to coal operators indirectly and proportionally. . . ," said Carl D. Perkins, D-Ky., chairman of the House Education and Labor Committee.

Selected Documents

Court decisions, agency reports, scientific studies and other documents frequently affect environmental health actions. Excerpts from a selection of such documents are published in the following section. All were issued since 1979.

The most recent document, the 1981 Supreme Court decision in *American Textile Manufacturers Institute* v. *Donovan,* concerned the controversy over the cost of safety regulations in the workplace. The court upheld the economic feasibility of cotton dust exposure standards mandated by the Occupational Safety and Health Administration (OSHA).

Justice William J. Brennan Jr. said in the majority opinion that "Congress itself defined the basic relationship between costs and benefits by placing the 'benefit' of worker health above all other considerations save those of making attainment of this 'benefit' achievable."

The National Commission on Air Quality's report, "To Breathe Clean Air," published in March 1981, was the result of a study authorized by the Clean Air Act Amendments of 1977. The report was expected to have a significant impact on debate over revision of the Act, scheduled to be completed in 1982.

In 1980 a chromosome study conducted by the Biogenics Corp. of Houston, Texas, indicated that residents of the Love Canal area near Niagara Falls, N.Y., might have suffered genetic damage from an old chemical dump. According to the study, Love Canal residents had chromosome aberrations that could lead to birth defects and cancer.

Also in 1980 the Supreme Court upheld a Department of Labor regulation giving workers the right to refuse dangerous jobs. The case, *Whirlpool* v. *Marshall,* was decided unanimously in favor of two maintenance men who refused to perform their regular tasks because of hazardous working conditions. The men had been sent home without pay and officially reprimanded by their company for their actions.

In a January 1980 report, "The Health Consequences of Smoking for Women," Dr. Julius B. Richmond, then U. S. surgeon general, offered figures to disprove the belief that women were less susceptible than men to health problems caused by smoking. The report said that lung cancer could overtake breast cancer as the leading cause of death among women.

In 1979 the president's commission on the accident at the Three Mile Island nuclear power plant near Harrisburg, Pa., recommended abolishing the Nuclear Regulatory Commission and improving the safety of nuclear plant construction and operation. The report to President Carter was the result of a six-month study headed by John G. Kemeny, president of Dartmouth College.

SUPREME COURT COTTON DUST DECISION

By a 5-3 vote the Supreme Court ruled June 17, 1981, that the regulations protecting textile workers from exposure to toxic substances must be upheld without regard to the balance between costs and benefits. Ruling on two cases, American Textile Manufacturers Institute *v.* Donovan, *and* National Cotton Council *v.* Donovan, *the court found that Congress had struck that balance itself when it enacted the 1970 Occupational Safety and Health Act. The law required the Occupational Safety and Health Administration (OSHA) to set standards that would assure "to the extent feasible" that no worker "will suffer material impairment of health" from exposure to a hazardous substance throughout his working life.*

Writing for the majority, Justice William J. Brennan Jr. stated, "Any standard based on a balancing of costs and benefits by the Secretary [of Labor] that strikes a different balance than that struck by Congress would be inconsistent with the command set forth in § 6 (b)(5) [of the 1970 Act]. Thus, cost-benefit analysis by OSHA is not required by the statute because feasibility analysis is."

The cotton dust standards had been upheld by the U.S. Court of Appeals for the District of Columbia, and the textile industry appealed that ruling to the Supreme Court. The textile industry had argued that the costs of 1978 OSHA regulations would force some companies out of business.

Justices William H. Rehnquist and Potter Stewart dissented, along with Chief Justice Warren E. Burger. Stewart stated that OSHA had not presented substantial evidence to justify the cost of the standard and that "feasibility" could not therefore be determined. Rehnquist, with whom Burger joined, said the "feasibility" test was no standard at all, but simply served to mask an unconstitutional delegation of legislative power to the executive branch.

The decision dealt a blow to the Reagan administration policy of subjecting regulations to cost-benefit analysis. The court heard arguments in the case Jan. 21, the day after President Reagan took office. Two months later, in a highly unusual move, the administration asked the court to delay ruling on the cases, but that request was ignored.

Following are excerpts from the majority opinion, written for the court by Justice Brennan, and from Justice Rehnquist's dissenting opinion:

Nos. 79-1429 and 79-1583

American Textile Manufacturers Institute, Inc., et al, Petitioners, 79-1429 *v.* Raymond J. Donovan, Secretary of Labor, United States Department of Labor, et al. National Cotton Council of America, Petitioner, 79-1583 *v.* Raymond J. Donovan, Secretary of Labor, United States Department of Labor, et al.	On Writs of Certiorari to the United States Court of Appeals for the District of Columbia Circuit.

[June 17, 1981]

BRENNAN, J., delivered the opinion of the Court, in which WHITE, MARSHALL, BLACKMUN, and STEVENS, JJ., joined. STEWART, J., filed a dissenting opinion. REHNQUIST, J., filed a dissenting opinion, in which BURGER, C. J., joined. POWELL, J., took no part in the decision of the cases.

JUSTICE BRENNAN delivered the opinion of the Court.

Congress enacted the Occupational Safety and Health Act of 1970 (the Act) "to assure so far as possible every working man and woman in the Nation safe and healthful working conditions. . . ." The Act authorizes the Secretary of Labor to establish, after notice and opportunity to comment, mandatory nationwide standards governing health and safety in the workplace. In 1978, the Secretary, acting through the Occupational Safety and Health Administration (OSHA), promulgated a standard limiting occupational exposure to cotton dust, an airborne particle byproduct of the preparation and manufacture of cotton products, exposure to which induces a "constellation of respiratory effects" known as "byssinosis." This disease was one of the expressly recognized health hazards that led to passage of the Occupational Safety and Health Act of 1970.

Petitioners in these consolidated cases, representing the interests of the cotton industry, challenged the validity of the "Cotton Dust Standard" in the Court of Appeals for the District of Columbia Circuit pursuant to § 6 (f) of the Act. They contend in this Court, as they did below, that the Act requires OSHA to demonstrate that its Standard reflects a reasonable relationship between the costs and benefits associated with the Standard. Respondents, the Secretary of Labor and two labor organizations [Industrial Union Department, AFL-CIO, and Amalgamated Clothing & Textile Workers Union, AFL-CIO], counter that Congress balanced the costs and benefits in the Act itself, and that the Act should therefore be construed not to require OSHA to do so. They interpret the Act as mandating that OSHA enact the most protective standard possible to eliminate a significant risk of material health impairment, subject to the constraints of economic and technological feasibility. The Court of Appeals held that the Act did not require OSHA to compare costs and benefits. We granted certiorari (1980) to resolve this important question, which was presented but not decided in last Term's *Industrial Union Department* v. *American Petroleum Institute* (1980), and to decide other issues related to the Cotton Dust Standard.

I

Byssinosis, known in its more severe manifestations as "brown lung" disease, is a serious and potentially disabling respiratory disease primarily caused by the inhalation of cotton dust. Byssinosis is a "continuum . . . disease," that has been categorized into four grades. In its least serious form, byssinosis produces both subjective symptoms, such as chest tightness, shortness of breath, coughing, and wheezing, and objective indications of loss of pulmonary functions. In its most serious form, byssinosis is a chronic and irreversible obstructive pulmonary disease, clinically similar to chronic bronchitis or emphysema, and can be severely disabling. At worst, as is true of other respiratory diseases including bronchitis, emphysema, and asthma, byssinosis can create an additional strain on cardiovascular functions and can contribute to death from heart failure. . . . One authority has described the increasing seriousness of byssinosis as follows:

> "In the first few years of exposure [to cotton dust], symptoms occur on Monday, or other days after absence from the work environment; later, symptoms occur on other days of the week; and eventually, symptoms are continuous, even in the absence of dust exposure." A. Bouhuys, Byssinosis in the United States.

While there is some uncertainty over the manner in which the disease progresses from its least serious to its disabling grades, it is likely that prolonged exposure contributes to the progression. It also appears that a worker may suddenly contract a severe grade without experiencing milder grades of the disease.

Estimates indicate that at least 35,000 employed and retired cotton mill workers, or 1 in 12 such workers, suffers from the most disabling form of byssinosis. The Senate Report accompanying the Act cited estimates that 100,000 active and retired workers suffer from some grade of the disease. One study found that over 25% of a sample of active cotton preparation and yarn manufacturing workers suffer at least some form of the disease at a dust exposure level common prior to adoption of the current Standard. Other studies confirm these general findings on the prevalence of byssinosis.

Not until the early 1960's was byssinosis recognized in the United States as a distinct occupational hazard associated with cotton mills. In 1966, the American Conference of Governmental Industrial Hygienists (ACGIH), a private organization, recommended that exposure to total cotton dust be limited to a "threshold limit value" of 1,000 micrograms per cubic meter of air (1000 $\mu g/m^3$) averaged over an 8-hour workday. The United States Government first regulated exposure to cotton dust in 1968, when the Secretary of Labor, pursuant to the Walsh-Healey Act promulgated airborne contaminant threshold limit values, applicable to public contractors, that included the 1000 $\mu g/m^3$ limit for total cotton dust. Following passage of the Act in 1970, the 1000 $\mu g/m^3$ standard was adopted as an "established Federal standard" under § 6 (a) of the Act, a provision designed to guarantee immediate protection of workers for the period between enactment of the statute and promulgation of permanent standards.

In 1974, ACGIH, adopting a new measurement unit of respirable rather than total dust, lowered its previous exposure limit recommendation to 200 $\mu g/m^3$ measured by a vertical elutriator, a device that measures cotton dust particles 15 microns or less in diameter. That same year, the Director of the National Institute for Occupational Safety and Health (NIOSH), pursuant to the Act, submitted to the Secretary of Labor a recommendation for a cotton dust standard with a permissible exposure limit (PEL) that "should be set at the lowest level feasible, but in no case at an environmental concentration as high as 0.2 mg lint-free cotton dust/cu. m.," or 200 $\mu g/m^3$ of lint-free respirable dust. Several months later, OSHA published an Advance Notice of Proposed Rulemaking, requesting comments from interested parties on the NIOSH recommendation and other related matters. Soon thereafter, the Textile Worker's Union of America, joined by the North Carolina Public Interest Research Group, petitioned the Secretary, urging a more stringent PEL of 100 $\mu g/m^3$.

On December 28, 1976, OSHA published a proposal to replace the existing Federal standard on cotton dust with a new permanent standard, pursuant to § 6 (b)(5) of the Act. The proposed standard contained a PEL of 200 μg/m³ of vertical elutriated lint-free respirable cotton dust for all segments of the cotton industry. It also suggested an implementation strategy for achieving the PEL that relied on respirators for the short-term and engineering controls for the long-term. OSHA invited interested parties to submit written comments within a 90-day period.

Following the comment period, OSHA conducted three hearings in Washington, D.C., Greenville, Miss., and Lubbock, Tex. that lasted over 14 days. Public participation was widespread, involving representatives from industry and the workforce, scientists, economists, industrial hygienists, and many others. By the time the informal rule-making procedure had terminated, OSHA had received 263 comments and 109 notices of intent to appear at the hearings. The voluminous record, composed of a transcript of written and oral testimony, exhibits, and post-hearing comments and briefs, totaled some 105,000 pages. OSHA issued its final Cotton Dust Standard — the one challenged in the instant case — on June 23, 1978. Along with an accompanying statement of findings and reasons, the Standard occupied 69 pages of the Federal Register.

The Cotton Dust Standard promulgated by OSHA establishes mandatory PELs over an 8-hour period of 200 μg/m³ for yarn manufacturing, 750 μg/m³ for slashing and weaving operations, and 500 μg/m³ for all other processes in the cotton industry. These levels represent a relaxation of the proposed PEL of 200 μg/m³ for all segments of the cotton industry.

OSHA chose an implementation strategy for the Standard that depended primarily on a mix of engineering controls, such as installation of ventilation systems, and work practice controls, such as special floor sweeping procedures. Full compliance with the PELs is required within 4 years, except to the extent that employers can establish that the engineering and work practice controls are infeasible. During this compliance period, and at certain other times, the Standard requires employers to provide respirators to employees. Other requirements include monitoring of cotton dust exposure, medical surveillance of all employees, annual medical examinations, employee education and training programs, and the posting of warning signs. A specific provision also under challenge in the instant case requires employers to transfer employees unable to wear respirators to another position, if available, having a dust level at or below the Standard's PELs, with "no loss of earnings or other employment rights or benefits as a result of the transfer."

On the basis of the evidence in the record as a whole, the Secretary determined that exposure to cotton dust represents a "significant health hazard to employees," and that "the prevalence of byssinosis should be significantly reduced" by the adoption of the Standard's PELs. In assessing the health risks from cotton dust and the risk reduction obtained from lowered exposure, OSHA relied particularly on data showing a strong linear relationship between the prevalence of byssinosis and the concentration of lint-free respirable cotton dust. Even at the 200 μg/m³ PEL, OSHA found that the prevalence of at least Grade ½ byssinosis would be 13% of all employees in the yarn manufacturing sector.

In enacting the Cotton Dust Standard, OSHA interpreted the Act to require adoption of the most stringent standard to protect against material health impairment, bounded only by technological and economic feasibility. OSHA therefore rejected the industry's alternative proposal for a PEL of 500 μg/m³ in yarn manufacturing, a proposal which would produce a 25% prevalence of at least Grade ½ byssinosis. The agency expressly found the Standard to be both technologically and economically feasible based on the evidence in the record as a whole. Although recognizing that permitted levels of exposure to cotton dust would still cause some byssinosis, OSHA nevertheless rejected the union proposal for a 100 μg/m³ PEL because it was not within the "technological capabilities of the industry." Similarly, OSHA set PELS for some segments of the cotton industry at 500 μg/m³ in part because of limitations of technological feasibility. Finally, the Secretary found that "engineering dust controls in weaving may not be feasible even with massive expenditures by the industry," and for that and other reasons adopted a less stringent PEL of 750 μg/m³ for weaving and slashing.

The Court of Appeals upheld the Standard in all major respects. The court rejected the industry's claim that OSHA failed to consider its proposed alternative or give sufficient reasons for failing to adopt it. The court also held that the Standard was "reasonably necessary and appropriate" within the meaning of § 3 (8) of the Act, because of the risk of material health impairment caused by exposure to cotton dust. Rejecting the industry position that OSHA must demonstrate that the benefits of the Standard are proportionate to its costs, the court instead agreed with OSHA's interpretation that the Standard must protect employees against material health impairment subject only to the limits of technological and economic feasibility. The court held that "Congress itself struck the balance between costs and benefits in the mandate to the agency" under § 6 (b)(5) of the Act and that OSHA is powerless to circumvent that judgment by adopting less than the most protective feasible standard. Finally, the court held that the agency's determination of technological and economic feasibility was supported by substantial evidence in the record as a whole.

We affirm in part, and vacate in part.

II

The principal question presented in this case is whether the Occupational Safety and Health Act requires the Secretary, in promulgating a standard pursuant to § 6 (b)(5) of the Act to determine that the costs of the standard bear a reasonable relationship to its benefits. Relying on §§ 6 (b)(5) and 3 (8) of the Act, petitioners urge not only that OSHA must show that a standard addresses a significant risk of material health impairment, see *Industrial Union Department* v. *American Petroleum Institute* (plurality opinion), but also that OSHA must demonstrate that the reduction in risk of material health impairment is significant in light of the costs of attaining that reduction. Respondents on the other hand contend that the Act requires OSHA to promulgate standards that eliminate or reduce such risks "to the extent such protection is technologically and economically feasible." To resolve this debate, we must turn to the language, structure, and legislative history of the Occupational Safety and Health Act.

A. The starting point of our analysis is the language of the statute itself. *Steadman* v. *SEC* (1981); *Reiter* v. *Sonotone Corp.* (1979). Section 6 (b)(5) of the Act, (emphasis added), provides:

> "The Secretary, in promulgating standards dealing with toxic materials or harmful physical agents under this subsection, shall set the standard which most adequately assures, *to the extent feasible,* on the basis of the best available evidence, that no employee will suffer material impairment of health or functional capacity even if such employee has regular exposure to the hazard dealt with by such standard for the period of his working life."

Although their interpretations differ, all parties agree that the phrase "to the extent feasible" contains the critical language in § 6 (b)(5) for purposes of this case.

The plain meaning of the word "feasible" supports respondents' interpretation of the statute. According to Webster's Third New International Dictionary of the English Language, "feasible" means "capable of being done, executed, or effected."... Thus, § 6 (b)(5) directs the Secretary to issue the standard that "most adequately assures ... that no employee will suffer material impairment of health," limited only by the extent to which this is "capable of being done." In effect then, as the Court of Appeals held, Congress itself defined the basic relationship between costs and benefits, by placing the "benefit" of worker health above all other considerations save those making attainment of this "benefit" unachievable. Any standard based on a balancing of costs and benefits by the Secretary that strikes a different balance than that struck by Congress would be inconsistent with the command set forth in § 6 (b)(5). Thus, cost-benefit analysis by OSHA is not required by the statute because feasibility analysis is. See *Industrial Union Department* v. *American Petroleum Institute,* (MAR-

SHALL, J., dissenting).

When Congress has intended that an agency engage in cost-benefit analysis, it has clearly indicated such intent on the face of the statute. One early example is the Food Control Act of 1936.

> "[T]he Federal Government should improve or participate in the improvement of navigable waters or their tributaries, including watersheds thereof, for flood-control purposes if the *benefits to whomsoever they may accrue are in excess of the estimated costs,* and if the lives and social security of people are otherwise adversely affected."

A more recent example is the Outer Continental Shelf Lands Act Amendments of 1978, providing that offshore drilling operations shall use:

> "the best available and safest technologies which the Secretary determines to be economically *feasible,* wherever failure of equipment would have a significant effect on safety, health, or the environment, except where the Secretary determines that the *incremental benefits are clearly insufficient to justify the incremental costs of using such technologies.*"

These and other statutes demonstrate that Congress uses specific language when intending that an agency engage in cost-benefits analysis. See *Industrial Union Department* v. *American Petroleum Institute,* (MARSHALL, J., dissenting). Certainly in light of its ordinary meaning, the word "feasible" cannot be construed to articulate such congressional intent. We therefore reject the argument that Congress required cost-benefit analysis in § 6 (b)(5)....

[Section B omitted]

C. The legislative history of the Act, while concededly not crystal clear, provides general support for respondents' interpretation of the Act. The congressional reports and debates certainly confirm that Congress meant "feasible" and nothing else in using that term. Congress was concerned that the Act might be thought to require achievement of absolute safety, an impossible standard, and therefore insisted that health and safety goals be capable of economic and technological accomplishment. Perhaps most telling is the absence of any indication whatsoever that Congress intended OSHA to conduct its own cost-benefit analysis before promulgating a toxic material or harmful physical agent standard. The legislative history demonstrates conclusively that Congress was fully aware that the Act would impose real and substantial costs of compliance on industry, and believed that such costs were part of the cost of doing business....

...Nowhere is there any indication that Congress contemplated a different balancing by OSHA of the benefits of worker health and safety against the costs of achieving them. Indeed Congress thought that the *financial costs* of health and safety problems in the workplace were as large or larger than the *financial costs* of eliminating these problems. In its statement of findings and declaration of purpose encompassed in the Act itself, Congress announced that "personal injuries and illnesses arising out of work situations impose a substantial burden upon, and are a hindrance to, interstate commerce in terms of lost production, wage loss, medical expenses, and disability compensation payment." The Senate was well aware of the magnitude of these costs:

> "[T]he economic impact of industrial deaths and disability is staggering. Over $1.5 billion is wasted in lost wages, and the annual loss to the Gross National Product is estimated to be over $8 billion. Vast resources that could be available for productive use are siphoned off to pay workmen's compensation benefits and medical expenses."
> S. Rep. No. 91-1281.

Senator Eagleton [Thomas F. Eagleton, D-Mo.] summarized, "Whether we, as individuals, are motivated by simple humanity or by simple economics, we can no longer permit profits to be dependent upon an unsafe or unhealthy worksite." Legis. Hist. 1150-1151.

III

B. After estimating the cost of compliance with the Cotton Dust Standard, OSHA analyzed whether it was "economically feasible" for the cotton industry to bear this cost. OSHA concluded that it was, finding that "although some marginal employers may shut down rather than comply, the industry as a whole will not be threatened by the capital requirements of the regulation." ... In reaching this conclusion on the Standard's economic impact, OSHA made specific findings with respect to employment, energy consumption, capital financing availability, and profitability. To support its findings, the agency relied primarily on RTI's [Research Triangle Institute, OSHA-controlled group that prepared a financial analysis of the standard] comprehensive investigation of the Standard's economic impact.

RTI evaluated the likely economic impact on the cotton industry and the United States economy of OSHA's original proposed standard, an across-the-board 200 $\mu g/m^3$ PEL. RTI had estimated a total compliance cost of $2.7 billion for a 200 $\mu g/m^3$ PEL, and used this estimate in assessing the economic impact of such a standard. ... OSHA estimated total compliance costs of $656.5 million for the final Cotton Dust Standard, a Standard less stringent than the across-the-board 200 $\mu g/m^3$ PEL of the proposed standard. Therefore, the agency found that the economic impact of its Standard would be "much less severe" than that suggested by RTI for a 200 $\mu g/m^3$ PEL estimate of $2.7 billion. Nevertheless, it is instructive to review RTI's conclusions with respect to the economic impact of a $2.7 billion cost estimate. RTI found:

> "Implementation of the proposed [200 $\mu g/m^3$] standard will require adjustments within the cotton textile industry that will take time to work themselves out and that may be difficult for many firms. In time, however, prices may be expected to rise and markets to adjust so that revenues will cover costs. Although the impact on any one firm cannot be specified in advance, nothing in the RTI study indicates that the cotton textile industry as a whole will be seriously threatened by the impact of the proposed standard for control of cotton dust exposure."...

The Court of Appeals found that the agency "explained the economic impact it projected for the textile industry," and that OSHA has "substantial support in the record for its ... findings of economic feasibility for the textile industry." On the basis of the whole record, we cannot conclude that the Court of Appeals "misapprehended or grossly misapplied" the substantial evidence test.

IV

The final Cotton Dust Standard places heavy reliance on the use of respirators to protect employees from exposure to cotton dust, particularly during the 4-year interim period necessary to install and implement feasible engineering controls. One part of the respirator provision requires the employer to give employees unable to wear a respirator the opportunity to transfer to another position, if available, where the dust level meets the standard's PEL. When such a transfer occurs, the employer must guarantee that the employee suffers no loss of earnings or other employment rights or benefits. Petitioners do not object to the transfer provision, but challenge OSHA's authority under the Act to require employers to guarantee employees' wage and employment benefits following the transfer. The Court of Appeals held that OSHA has such authority. We hold that, whether or not OSHA has this underlying authority, the agency has failed to make the necessary determination or statement of reasons that its wage guarantee requirement is related to the achievement of a safe and healthful work environment....

V

When Congress passed the Occupational Safety and Health Act in 1970, it chose to place pre-eminent value on assuring employees a safe and healthful working environment, limited only by the feasibility of achieving such an environment. We must measure the validity of the Secretary's actions against the requirements of that Act. For "[t]he judicial function does not extend to substantive revision of regulatory policy. That function lies elsewhere — in Congressional and Executive oversight or amendatory legislation." *Industrial Union Department* v. *American Petroleum Institute* (BURGER, C. J., concurring); see *Tennessee Valley Authority* v. *Hill,* (1978).

Accordingly, the judgment of the Court of Appeals is affirmed in all respects except to the extent of its approval of the Secretary's application of the wage guarantee provision of the Cotton Dust Standard. To that extent, the judgment of the Court of Appeals is vacated and the case remanded with directions to remand to the Secretary for further proceedings consistent with this opinion.

JUSTICE STEWART, dissenting.

Section 6 (b)(5) of the Occupational Safety and Health Act provides:

> "The Secretary, in promulgating standards dealing with toxic materials or harmful physical agents under this subsection, shall set the standard which most adequately assures, *to the extent feasible,* on the basis of the best available evidence, that no employee will suffer material impairment of health or functional capacity even if such employee has regular exposure to the hazard dealt with by such standard for the period of his working life.

Everybody agrees that under this statutory provision the Cotton Dust Standard must at least be *economically* feasible, and everybody would also agree, I suppose, that in order to determine whether or not something is economically feasible, one must have a fairly clear idea of how much it is going to cost. Because I believe that OSHA failed to justify its estimate of the cost of the Cotton Dust Standard on the basis of substantial evidence, I would reverse the judgment before us without reaching the question whether the Act requires that a standard, beyond being economically feasible, must meet the demands of a cost-benefit examination.

The simple truth about OSHA's assessment of the cost of the Cotton Dust Standard is that the agency never relied on any study or report purporting to predict the cost to industry of the Standard finally adopted by the agency. OSHA did have before it one cost analysis, that of the Research Triangle Institute, which attempted to predict the cost of the final Standard. However, as recognized by the Court, the agency flatly rejected that prediction as a gross over-estimate. The only other estimate OSHA had, the Hocutt-Thomas estimate prepared by industry researchers [Hovan Hocutt and Arthur Thomas, employees of dust control equipment manufacturers], was not designed to predict the cost of the final OSHA Standard. Rather, it assumed a far less stringent and inevitably far less costly standard for all phases of cotton production except roving. The agency examined the Hocutt-Thomas study, and concluded that it too was an over-estimate of the costs of the less stringent standard it was addressing. I am willing to defer to OSHA's determination that the Hocutt-Thomas study was such an over-estimate, conceding that such subtle financial and technical matters lie within the discretion and skill of the agency. But in a remarkable non sequitur, the agency decided that because the Hocutt-Thomas study was an over-estimate of the cost of a less stringent standard, it could be treated as a reliable estimate for the more costly final Standard actually promulgated, never rationally explaining how it came to this happy conclusion. This is not substantial evidence. It is unsupported speculation.

Of course, as the Court notes, this Court will reexamine a Court of Appeals' review of a question of substantial evidence "only in what ought to be the rare instance when the standard appears to have been misapprehended or grossly misapplied." *Universal Camera Corp.* v. *NLRB* [1951]. But I think this is one of those rare instances where an agency has categorically misconceived the nature of the evidence necessary to support a regulation, and where the Court of Appeals has failed to correct the agency's error. Of course, broad generalizations about the meaning of "substantial evidence" have limited value in deciding particular cases. But within the confines of a single statute, where the agency and reviewing courts have identified certain specific factual matters to be proved, we can establish practical general criteria for comprehending "substantial evidence."

Unlike the Court, I think it clear to the point of being obvious that, as a matter of law, OSHA's prediction of the cost of the Cotton Dust Standard lacks a basis in substantial evidence, since the agency did not rely on even a single estimate of the cost of the actual Standard it promulgated. Accordingly, I respectfully dissent.

JUSTICE REHNQUIST, with whom THE CHIEF JUSTICE joins, dissenting.

A year ago I stated my belief that Congress in enacting § 6 (b)(5) of the Occupational Safety and Health Act of 1970 unconstitutionally delegated to the Executive Branch the authority to make the "hard policy choices" properly the task of the legislature. *Industrial Union Department* v. *American Petroleum Institute* (1980) (concurring opinion). Because I continue to believe that the Act exceeds Congress' power to delegate legislative authority to nonelected officials, see *Hampton & Co.* v. *United States* (1928) and *Panama Oil Refining Co.* v. *Ryan* (1935), I dissent.

I will repeat only a little of what I said last Term. Section 6 (b)(5) provides in pertinent part:

> "The Secretary, in promulgating standards dealing with toxic materials or harmful physical agents under this subsection, shall set the standard which most adequately assures, *to the extent feasible,* on the basis of the best available evidence, that no employee will suffer material impairment of health or functional capacity even if such employee has regular exposure to the hazard dealt with by such standard for the period of his working life." (Emphasis added.)

As the Court correctly observes, the phrase "to the extent feasible" contains the critical language for the purpose of this case. We are presented with a remarkable range of interpretations of that language. Petitioners contend that the statute *requires* the Secretary to demonstrate that the benefits of its "Cotton Dust Standard," in terms of reducing health risks, bears a reasonable relationship to its costs. Respondents, including the Secretary of Labor at least until his postargument motion, counter that Congress itself balanced costs and benefits when it enacted the statute, and that the statute *prohibits* the Secretary from engaging in a cost-benefit type balancing. Their view is that the Act merely requires Secretary to promulgate standards that eliminate or reduce such risks "to the extent technologically or economically feasible." As I read the Court's opinion, it takes a different position. It concludes that, at least as to the "Cotton Dust Standard," the Act does not require the Secretary to engage in a cost-benefit analysis, which suggests of course that the Act *permits* the Secretary to undertake such an analysis if he so chooses.

Throughout its opinion, the Court refers to § 6 (b)(5) as adopting a "feasibility standard" or a "feasibility requirement." But as I attempted to point out last Term in *Industrial Union Department* v. *American Petroleum Institute,* the "feasibility standard" is no standard at all. Quite the contrary, I argued there that the insertion into § 6 (b)(5) of the words "to the extent feasible" rendered what had been had been a clear, if somewhat unrealistic, statute into one so vague and precatory as to be an unconstitutional delegation of legislative authority to the Executive Branch. Prior to the inclusion of the "feasibility" language, § 6 (b)(5) simply required the Secretary to "set the standard which most adequately assures, on the basis of the best available professional evidence, that no employee will suffer any impairment of health. . . ." Legislative History, Occupational Safety and Health Act of 1970, 92d Cong. 943 (hereinafter Legis. Hist.) Had that statute been enacted, it would undoubtedly support the result the Court reaches in this case and it would not have created an excessive delegation problem. The Secretary of Labor would quite clearly have been authorized to set exposure standards without regard to any kind of cost-benefit analysis.

But Congress did not enact the statute. . . . Congress simply said that the Secretary should set standards "to the extent feasible." Last year, JUSTICE POWELL reflected that "one might wish that Congress had spoken with greater clarity." *American Petroleum Institute,* (POWELL, J., concurring). I am convinced that the reason that Congress did not speak with greater "clarity" was because it could not. The words "to the extent feasible" were used to mask a fundamental policy disagreement in Congress. I have no doubt that if Congress had been required to choose whether to mandate, permit, or prohibit the Secretary from engaging in a cost-benefit analysis, there would have been no bill for the President to sign.

The Court seems to argue that Congress *did* make a policy choice when it enacted the "feasibility" language. Its view is that Congress required the Secretary to engage in something called "feasibility analysis." But those words mean nothing at all. They are a "legislative mirage, appearing to some members [of Congress] but not to others, and assuming any form desired by the beholder." *American Petroleum Institute.* Even the Court does not settle on a meaning. It first suggests that the language requires the Secretary to do what is "capable of being done." But, if that is all the language means, it is merely precatory and "no more than an admonition to the Secretary to do his duty. . . ." Legis. Hist. 367 (remarks of Sen. Dominick) [Peter H. Dominick, R-Colo.]. The Court then seems to adopt the Secretary's view that feasibility means "technological and economic feasibility." But there is nothing in the words of § 6 (b)(5), or their legislative history, to suggest why they should be so limited. One wonders why the "requirement" of § 6 (b)(5) could not include considerations of administrative or even political feasibility. As even the Court recognizes, when Congress has wanted to limit the concept of feasibility to technological and economic feasibility, it has said so. Thus the words "to the extent feasible" provide no meaningful guidance to those who will administer the law.

In believing that § 6 (b)(5) amounts to an unconstitutional delegation of legislative authority to the Executive Branch, I do not mean to suggest that Congress, in enacting a statute, must resolve all ambiguities or must "fill in all of the blanks." Even the neophyte student of government realizes that legislation is the art of compromise, and that an important, controversial bill is seldom enacted by Congress in the form in which it is first introduced. It is not unusual for the various factions supporting or opposing a proposal to accept some departure from the language they would prefer and to adopt substitute language agreeable to all. But that sort of compromise is a far cry from this case, where Congress simply abdicated its responsibility for the making of a fundamental and most difficult policy choice — whether and to what extent "the statistical possibility of future deaths should . . . be disregarded in light of the economic costs of preventing those deaths." *American Petroleum Institute.* That is a "quintessential legislative" choice and must be made by the elected representatives of the people, not by nonelected officials in the Executive Branch. As stated last term:

> In drafting § 6 (b)(5), Congress was faced with a clear, if difficult, choice between balancing statistical lives and industrial resources or authorizing the Secretary to elevate human life above all concerns save massive dislocation in an affected industry. That Congress recognized the difficulty of that choice is clear. . . . That Congress chose, intentionally or unintentionally, to pass this difficult choice on to the Secretary is evident from the special quality of the standard it selected.

In sum, the Court is quite correct in asserting that the phrase "to the extent feasible" is the critical language for the purposes of this case. But that language is critical, not because it establishes a general standard by which those charged with administering the statute may be guided, but because it has precisely the opposite effect: in failing to agree on whether the Secretary should be either mandated, permitted or prohibited from undertaking a cost-benefit analysis. Congress simply left the crucial policy choices in the hands of the Secretary of Labor. As I stated at greater length last Term, I believe that in so doing Congress unconstitutionally delegated its legislative responsibility to the Executive Branch.

AIR QUALITY COMMISSION REPORT

The National Commission on Air Quality, a 13-member bipartisan panel drawn from government and industry in 1977 when the Clean Air Act was revised, released its findings March 2, 1981, in a report entitled "To Breathe Clean Air." The report contained 433 findings and 109 recommendations on how Congress should amend the Act, which was scheduled for revision again in 1981. The most controversial recommendation was that Congress scrap the nationwide deadlines for cleaning up dirty-air cities. A proposed change in pollution control for clean-air cities was almost as controversial.

Following are excerpts from the commission's report and from the dissenting statement of Commissioner Richard E. Ayres, in which Commissioners Annemarie F. Crocetti and John J. Sheehan joined. Dissenters argued that members overreacted to complexities in the Act and chose to eliminate basic elements rather than improve them.

Introduction

A little more than a decade ago Congress passed the Clean Air Act, the first major substantive law designed to preserve the environment. Since that time the absolute level of improvement for the most widespread air pollutants has been significant. Between 1974 and 1978 there was an 18 percent reduction in the number of days during which air quality in 23 major metropolitan areas was classified as unhealthful. And nationwide, between 1973 and 1978, average annual concentrations of carbon monoxide decreased by 33 percent, sulfur dioxide by 20 percent, and suspended particulates by 7 percent.

More significant than the level of absolute reductions, however, is the difference between current pollution levels and those that would have occurred if major control efforts had not been required during the 1970s.

Prognosis for the 1980s

The prognosis for the 1980s reflects a need for the control of air pollution to be a continued national priority. During the 1980s millions of people will continue to live in areas exceeding healthful levels for ozone and suspended particulates. In at least one major urban area — Los Angeles — the ozone problem appears to be intractable and no reasonable level of effort is likely to result in attainment of the standard in that area.

The 1980s also will present new challenges that have begun to emerge during the past few years. These problems relate to toxic pollutants, indoor air pollution, acid rain, visibility degradation, and carbon dioxide buildup. In the past, attention has been focussed on the effects on public health of six pollutants over which there has been widespread concern because they are emitted by most mobile and stationary sources of pollution. The emerging problems are related to the protection of public welfare from some of these same pollutants and the protection of the health of a smaller number of persons from the effects of more toxic and potentially more harmful pollutants.

The need for continued substantial investments comes at a time when all Americans are concerned about economic problems of a magnitude experienced only a few other times in the history of the nation. Thus, it is incumbent upon policymakers to ensure that there is not only good air quality but also an appropriate balance among all of the nation's priorities. . . .

Economic Effects

While the public recognizes and continues to endorse the

national commitment to reduce the adverse effects of air pollution, the economic effects of programs developed to respond to this public concern have become a major focus of decisionmakers responsible for developing air pollution control policy. Congress has recognized since its enactment of the Clean Air Act in 1970 that a significant investment of economic resources would be necessary to accomplish the goal of providing good air quality throughout the country. Yet, as the U.S. economy has faltered in recent years and rates of inflation have reached levels previously believed possible only for countries with greater historical economic instability, concern has heightened about the effects on the economy of controlling air pollution. Studies show that this control in recent years has cost and may continue to cost $20 billion or more per year. Although these costs have had only minor effects on national indicators such as the consumer price index, gross national product, and unemployment rate, the amounts justify careful consideration of whether the nation's economic resources are being used wisely.

The small negative economic effects of air pollution controls would be minimized further if most of the benefits of control could be reflected in the statistics used in developing national economic indicators. Some studies suggest that economic benefits may even equal or exceed costs that have been borne by the nation's consumers. Because debate will continue about the validity of various studies as a result of inadequacies in available data and methodologies for calculating benefits, there will likely not be any consensus as to the relative levels of costs and benefits of the nation's air quality programs.

Concerns about economic effects are not limited to the desirability of making investments for controlling emissions. They relate also to effects on economic growth in general, and energy development in particular, and to complexities associated with locating new major facilities. Studies conducted for the Commission and others have found that there is virtually no evidence that approvals have been denied for new and expanded facilities wishing to locate in areas both meeting and not meeting the nation's air quality standards. Projections for the future indicate also that facilities can be sited even when assumptions of high levels of energy and other growth are made. Determining whether decisions have been made by corporate policymakers, however, not to seek approvals for industrial expansion presents myriad problems because of the difficulty of assessing the numerous factors important in making substantial capital investments.

Although it appears from Commission studies that energy and other economic expansion can proceed largely as planned under federal air quality laws, the conclusions reached also find that there are few projected benefits associated with parts of the nation's prevention of significant deterioration program. These findings do not relate to the parts of the program designed to protect clean air areas of major national significance, such as national parks. In addition, Commission studies demonstrate that complexities in other programs, particularly some associated with federal-state relationships, are yielding few benefits.

While any air pollution control program will be inherently complex because of the nature of air pollution and the methods for controlling it, each program must be carefully evaluated to determine whether the benefits justify the associated costs, including those related to complexity. Obviously, such complexity has its associated cost to industry and ultimately to consumers.

The Commission particularly emphasized studies to determine whether the nation's effort to reduce its reliance on imported oil through production of domestic energy resources such as coal would be impeded by current clean air programs. With isolated exceptions of little significance through 1990 and in the Southwest through 1995 the Commission found that even high levels of projected energy development could be accommodated. However, efforts on planning for certain energy facilities, particularly oil shale projects, could occur as early as the mid-1980s. Moreover, the projected development can proceed if appropriate controls are installed and other pollution control efforts are continued without exacerbating any problems associated with pollutants which have traditionally been controlled.

Climatic changes associated with carbon dioxide build-up, and possible emissions of toxic pollutants require, however, thoughtful planning of the nation's energy programs. They also vividly demonstrate that increased energy efficiency has substantially associated benefits which go far beyond lower energy costs to the public.

The Clean Air Act

The structure of the Clean Air Act — as it was enacted in 1970 and modified in 1977 — provided the framework for the Commission's research activities. While the cornerstone of the Act's requirements are the provisions providing for the establishment of national ambient air quality standards to protect public health and public welfare, the Act includes specific technology requirements that also must be met regardless of whether they are necessary to meet specific air quality standards. This structure reflects a decision by Congress to combine the two general approaches available for addressing pollution problems — a goals-oriented approach and a technology-based one, rather than rely on either one alone.

The goals of the Act are embodied in the separate ambient air quality standards that are to be established for the protection of public health with an adequate margin of safety (primary standards) and for the protection of public welfare (secondary standards). Congress did not specify in the Act criteria to be taken into consideration in determining appropriate primary and secondary standards, but included a procedure for the development of criteria documents which are to delineate the basis for standards established by EPA (Environmental Protection Agency).

The Act provided also for the establishment of technology-related emission standards to control pollutants that endanger Americans and their environment. The Environmental Protection Agency is to establish national emission standards for hazardous air pollutants to protect against risks of irreversible health effects and incapacitating reversible effects. Under the Act, these standards must be set so as to ensure an ample margin of safety. In the 1977 amendments, Congress authorized EPA to set design or equipment standards for these hazardous pollutants if it is unable to determine an appropriate level for setting an emission standard for a particular pollutant.

The most well-known of the emission standards are those for automobiles. Congress declared in 1970 that those standards should lead to the reduction of the three major transportation-related pollutants by 90 percent. Since that time, there have been extensions of the deadlines to meet the standards for two of the pollutants — hydrocarbons and carbon monoxide — and a relaxation and extension of the standard for the other pollutant — nitrogen oxides. Except for provision for waivers, the ultimate level of control from these standards will be achieved on all vehicles beginning in the 1981 model year. . . .

The Act directs that areas of the country be designated as attainment or nonattainment, depending upon whether they meet national ambient air quality standards. Attainment status determines which of two control programs apply to an area.

In areas not meeting an ambient standard, the nonattainment program requires adoption of all reasonable control measures, implementation of a permit program for new sources, and continuing progress toward meeting the standard by 1982 or, in some cases, 1987. . . .

In areas where air quality is better than required to meet national ambient standards, the Act limits the amount of additional pollution which will be permitted. In certain areas such as larger national parks, very little additional pollution is allowed, while in other areas limitations are less stringent. In no case may air quality exceed the level set by a national ambient standard. . . .

The Commission's recommendations reflect a general conclusion that the structure of the Clean Air Act is sound and needs refinement instead of fundamental changes. The changes proposed by the commission would acomplish this result by simplifying and strengthening the parts of the programs which have worked well, modifying or eliminating those which have not worked well, and adding new elements to address new problems. Taken as a whole, these recommendations would protect better the public health and welfare against air pollution; reduce unnecessary regulatory burdens; and ensure that we can meet our nation's economic, energy, and other important goals. . . .

Commission Findings

Public Health Standards

1. To protect public health, government must act to control potentially harmful pollutants despite scientific uncertainty about the precise harm they cause and the levels of exposure that cause that harm. On this principle, the Act requires EPA to set national primary air quality standards to protect against pollution levels that "endanger public health, allowing an adequate margin of safety." This statutory mandate, which does not include consideration of economic factors, and the legislative history describing populations Congress intends EPA to protect, give EPA authority of a broadly precautionary nature to protect people against the adverse health effects of air pollution in a context of scientific uncertainty. . . .

6. The costs of meeting primary air quality standards are best taken into account in determining what control programs should be implemented in specific areas of the country, not in establishing a national air quality standard to protect public health. Although the level of air pollution affecting public health generally does not vary in different locations, the costs of meeting any specific standard will vary substantially, depending upon the severity of existing pollution levels, from one area to another. Thus, if a national air quality standard were based in part on the costs of complying with it, the very high costs of meeting the standard in a few severely polluted areas would probably require that the standard be set at a less protective level than is achievable in a reasonable, economic fashion in most areas of the country. The most effective balance between the beneficial effects of good air quality on human health and the economic, social, energy, and other costs of meeting health-based standards will be achieved when conditions in particular areas can be considered in deciding when the standards should be met in the areas and what measures will be adopted to meet the standards.

7. Although not required by the Act to do so, EPA has conducted economic impact analyses as part of its process of revising the air quality standards for carbon monoxide, sulfur dioxide, ozone, and particulates. These analyses were required by an executive order issued in 1978 and superseded by an order issued February 17, 1981, that requires agencies to analyze and publish the possible economic consequences of proposed regulations that will have an estimated annual effect on the economy of at least $100 million. . . .

Nonattainment Program

47. . . . All state implementation plans as revised in 1979 and approved by EPA should remain in effect and be implemented on the schedule specified in the plans to the extent such plans are consistent with the Commission's recommendations. States should be required to continue to fulfill those responsibilities required by EPA in 1979 and 1980 conditional approvals that are consistent with the Commission's recommendations.

48. State plan revisions should continue to be required in 1982 for all areas determined to exceed air quality standards as of December 31, 1981. The revisions should be required to include requirements for the installation of reasonably available control technology on existing sources or measures that would lead to equivalent emission reductions, except in areas that EPA determines will meet the air quality standards by December 31, 1983, and requirements for the implementation of the offset policy. Transportation control measures in ozone and carbon monoxide plan revisions should no longer be mandatory.

49. Motor vehicle inspection and maintenance programs should be required only in urban areas with populations greater than 500,000 where peak 1981 air pollution levels (using existing EPA designation guidance) are 50 percent greater than either the ozone or the carbon monoxide ambient air quality standard, instead of in all areas exceeding the ozone or carbon monoxide air quality standard by December 31, 1982.

50. Areas exceeding the ozone or carbon monoxide air quality standard but not required to implement inspection and maintenance programs should be permitted to implement inspection and maintenance programs instead of the offset policy for ozone and carbon monoxide,

51. Every 3 years, all areas exceeding air quality standards should be required to implement additional reasonably available control technology identified by EPA or measures that would lead to equivalent reductions. States should be required to submit plan revisions that incorporate such technology requirements to EPA for review and approval.

52. The process for 3-year reviews described in the commission's recommendations should be substituted for the 1982 and 1987 deadlines for meeting air quality standards. This change does not affect approved dates of compliance for sources in state implementation plans. The states should continue to be required to meet air quality standards in all areas as expeditiously as practicable. The state should specify a date by which it intends to meet the standards. This date will not be subject to EPA and judicial review and will not be federally enforceable.

53. The Environmental Protection Agency should ensure that reasonably available control technology or offsets or other measures to achieve equivalent emission reductions are included in state plans where necessary to maintain air quality standards in areas meeting the standards.

54. As required by the Act, EPA should continue to be authorized to adopt requirements of reasonably available control technology in states not meeting air quality standards and failing to require that technology or equivalent measures.

55. The statutory system of withholding federal funds as sanctions in areas not meeting the Act's requirements for pollution controls in areas exceeding air quality standards should be replaced by a graduated system of sanctions. The sanctions should include those now mandated and authorized by the Act. EPA should be given discretionary authority to impose the sanctions based on the degree of failure to implement measures.

56. Existing sources that have been required to install equipment to control a particular pollutant should not be required during the next 10 years to install additional control equipment for that pollutant if the additional equipment would supplant the initial equipment. However, this exemption should not apply if new controls are needed to meet an air quality standard for a newly regulated pollutant or to comply with new regulations for a hazardous pollutant.

57. The Act's requirement that new sources in areas exceeding air quality standards install controls providing for the lowest achievable emission rate should be repealed and replaced by identical requirements for all new sources (in areas either violating or meeting standards), requiring best available control technology, the same type of technology now required in areas meeting air quality standards. The determination of best available control technology should be made on a case-by-case basis in accordance with the requirements under the Act's current definition of best available control technology with the following exceptions:

- A source that emits less than 500 tons of a pollutant per year and for which a new source performance standard has been established should be subject only to the new source performance standard; and
- A source that will emit 1,000 tons or more of a pollutant per year should be required to provide at least the same level of control that has been required in the same federal region for a source in the same category that emits 1,000 tons or more per year of the pollutant, unless the operator of the new source demonstrates that such previously determined control level will not provide sufficient air quality benefits to justify the incremental control over alternative best available control technology levels. In no case should emissions be allowed to exceed applicable new source performance standards. The Administrator would be authorized to modify the boundaries of a region, for the purposes of determining previously applicable best available control technology levels, to take into account regional air quality values.

58. New sources should not be required to install additional control equipment during the 10-year period after the source

started operations, unless new controls are needed to meet an air quality standard for a newly regulated pollutant or to comply with new regulations for a hazardous pollutant.

59. The emissions offset policy should be revised to allow a state to require a new source in an area violating air quality standards to pay a fee instead of securing offsets, if the state develops and agrees to implement a plan to use such fees to reduce other emissions of the same pollutant. The Environmental Protection Agency should set the fees on a national basis for each pollutant, based upon the emission control costs of new source performance standards.

60. If EPA sets an air quality standard for a new pollutant, states should have 3 years to adopt and implement reasonably available control technology in areas exceeding the standard.

61. The Environmental Protection Agency should determine by December 31, 1982, which areas of the country do not meet each air quality standard based on air quality information through December 31, 1981.

62. The Environmental Protection Agency should continue to issue, and should revise every 6 years, control technique guideline documents to help states determine reasonably available control technology for categories of sources contributing significantly to violations of air quality standards.

63. By January 30, 1984, and then at least once every 3 years, EPA should review each state's progress in meeting air quality standards. The Environmental Protection Agency should use this review after consultation with state officials, to determine whether an area continues to exceed an air quality standard, and if so, to provide necessary guidance to ensure that additional reasonably available control technologies and new revisions of the state's plans are adopted.

64. By July 30, 1984, and then every 3 years, EPA and appropriate state and local agencies should develop jointly a program plan for coordinated future federal, state, and local actions. The program plan should include additional reasonably available control technology necessary to meet and maintain standards, other necessary state procedural and administrative requirements, and an indication of state and federal funding and resource commitments. Funds for federal program grants should be made available upon completion of this program plan.

Prevention of Significant Deterioration

65. The preconstruction review requirements of the Act's prevention of significant deterioration (PSD) provisions should apply to all new major sources, as currently defined in the Act, and to modifications of existing major sources that increase net emissions from the source by more than *de minimis* levels. *De minimis* emission rates for nitrogen oxides, sulfur dioxide, particulate matter, and hydrocarbons should be increased to 100 tons.

66. Sources subject to preconstruction review should continue to be required to apply the best available control technology to control the emissions of any criteria or noncriteria pollutant that exceed *de minimis* levels after the application of pollution controls. The determination of best available control technology should be made on a case-by-case basis in accordance with the requirements under the Act's definitions, with the following exceptions:

- A source that emits less than 500 tons of a pollutant per year and for which a new source performance standard has been established should be subject only to the new source performance standard; and
- A source that will emit 1,000 tons or more of a pollutant per year should be required to provide at least the same level of control that has been required in the same federal region for a source in the same category that emits 1,000 tons or more per year of the pollutant, unless the operator of the new source demonstrates that such previously determined control level will not provide sufficient air quality benefits to justify the incremental control over alternative best available control technology levels. In no case should emissions be allowed to exceed applicable new source performance standards. The Administrator would be authorized to modify the boundaries of a region, for the purposes of determining previously applicable best available control technology levels, to take into account regional air quality values.

67. New sources should not be required to install additional control equipment during the 10-year period after the source started operations, unless new controls are needed to meet air quality standards for a newly regulated pollutant or to comply with new regulations for a hazardous pollutant.

68. The statutory requirement that proposed new sources submit air quality monitoring data gathered over a period of up to one calendar year should be eliminated. Instead, the reviewing agency should be given the discretion to require preconstruction monitoring for up to one year and postconstruction monitoring data. The Environmental Protection Agency should continue to publish guidelines for state use in determining the need for actual on-site monitoring. . . .

70. The Environmental Protection Agency should be required to publish a biannual list of best available control technology determinations, regional best available control technology determinations, and other control technology (for source categories that contribute significant amounts of pollution) that has been installed on various sources where such information is available. This information should include sufficient details to make it useful to reviewing agency personnel.

71. a. The existing Class I increment system should be retained without change. In addition, the federal land manager for each Class I area should be authorized to establish a monitoring network for detecting the effects of new pollution sources on air quality within the area. The federal land manager should be authorized to establish a baseline (for determining increments) if and when the federal land manager determines that new sources are likely to affect air quality-related values within the area. EPA, in consultation with the federal land manager, should publish guidelines adopted pursuant to public notice and comment procedures applicable to EPA, describing criteria for these determinations. In the absence of a determination by the federal land manager, the baseline should be determined according to the current provisions of the Act.

b. States and Indian governing bodies also should be authorized to establish a baseline under the same conditions as federal land managers, for Class I lands within their jurisdiction other than those federal lands for which the federal land manager has direct management responsibility. The Environmental Protection Agency, in consultation with the states and Indian governing bodies, should publish guidelines adopted pursuant to public notice and comment procedures applicable to EPA, describing criteria for these determinations. In the absence of a determination by a state or Indian governing body, the baseline should be determined according to the current provisions of the Act.

72. a. Class III should be eliminated.

b. Class II should be limited to (1) those areas that cannot be redesignated as Class III under the current Act; and (2) those clean air areas which states or Indian tribes choose to designate as Class II.

c. Tracking of short-term Class II increment consumption should be eliminated, but all major new and modified sources . . . subject to PSD review should still be required to demonstrate that the new source itself will not exceed short-term increments and that emissions from the major sources and other sources in the area will not cause or contribute to violation of annual increments.

73. The current visibility protection program, which is designed to protect visibility in Class I areas and in specified "integral vista" areas adjacent to some Class I areas, should be retained.

74. Surface mining of coal should be included in the list of sources subject to the visibility provisions of the Act. Congress should consider whether other types of surface mining should be included.

Mobile Source Controls

75. The statutory gasoline and diesel automobile hydrocarbon standard of 0.41 grams per mile should be retained.

76. The statutory nitrogen oxides standard of 1.0 grams per mile should be retained for gasoline automobiles. The Act should be amended to replace the waiver provision for light diesel automobiles through the 1984 model year with a 1.5 gram per mile standard through the 1984 model year. The existing provisions for exemptions from the nitrogen oxides standard for low volume manufacturers and innovative technology on automobiles should be retained.

77. The final statutory carbon monoxide automobile standard of 3.4 grams per mile should be changed to 7.0 grams per mile, to be effective as soon as practicable after enactment of amendments to the Act, and remain in effect through the 1986 model year. The Environmental Protection Agency should be given authority to continue the 7.0 grams per mile standard beyond model year 1986 or establish a standard between 3.4 and 7.0 grams per mile if it is found that protection of public health can be achieved as expeditiously and effectively with a 7.0 grams per mile or an intermediate standard as with the 3.4 grams per mile standard.

78. The Environmental Protection Agency should continue to evaluate the 0.2 gram per mile particulate standard for diesel automobiles and the 0.26 gram per mile standard for light diesel trucks currently scheduled to take effect in 1985, and report to Congress within 6 months of enactment of amendments to the Act.

79. The statutory carbon monoxide and hydrocarbon standards for heavy gasoline trucks, and the carbon monoxide and hydrocarbon standards established by EPA for light trucks, should be retained. The acceptable quality level for heavy gasoline trucks weighing 8,500 pounds and over should be revised to be consistent with those that apply to automobiles.

80. The Act's provisions on nitrogen oxides emission standards for light and heavy trucks should be retained, including the existing EPA authority to relax the standards from the presumed 75 percent reduction.

81. The current provisions of Sections 202 and 206 of the Act relating to motor vehicles at high altitude should be replaced by new provisions:

a. Affirming the 1982-1983 model year automobile and light truck high altitude standards adopted by the EPA, and establishing a similar requirement of proportional reduction at high altitude for 1984 and 1985 model year light trucks;

b. Requiring manufacturers to demonstrate that model year 1984 and later automobiles and 1986 and later light trucks sold in areas at least 4,000 feet above sea level will comply with the appropriate national emissions standards; EPA should be authorized to grant waivers from this requirement for those automobiles and light trucks for which EPA determines that compliance with the requirement would be unusually expensive or impractical, subject to a limit, to be determined by Congress, on the number of vehicles for which waivers may be granted to ensure that the waivers do not affect significantly air quality in high altitude areas;

c. Either requiring or explicitly authorizing EPA, after determining the air quality and other effects of doing so, to require manufacturers to demonstrate that heavy trucks at high altitude (1) will comply with the national emission standards, or (2) will reduce emissions at high altitude by the same percentage as the appropriate national emission standards represent for emissions at sea level;

d. Allowing EPA to use any appropriate means to review and approve the manufacturers' demonstration of compliance with the high altitude requirements in (a), (b), and (c); and

e. Requiring manufacturers to provide to appropriate dealers and service facilities in high altitude areas the specifications developed by the manufacturers, under Section 215 of the Act, for performance adjustments to vehicles that have not been designed or adjusted for use in high altitude areas....

Dissenting Statement

We must dissent from the Commission's report, which we feel falls short of providing an appropriate guide to Congress for its coming consideration of the Clean Air Act.

The Commission's report recommends fundamental alterations in two of the most basic programs of the Clean Air Act — the nonattainment program, designed to clean up unhealthy air, and the program to prevent deterioration of clean air. In these areas, the Commission's report has overreacted to acknowledged problems, eliminating necessary programs rather than correcting. These recommendations were adopted, and more modest alternatives rejected, by narrow margins (a tie vote in one case). Because we believe the Commission report's proposals would significantly weaken our nation's effort to cleanse dirty air and conserve clean air we cannot commend the entire report to Congress, even though we strongly agree with some of its recommendations....

Major Disagreements

We turn now to the areas where we must state our strong disagreement with the Commission's report — in particular its recommendations to eliminate deadlines for achieving health standards; to eliminate requiring new plants in polluted areas to meet "lowest achievable emission rate"; to allow automatic approval of even defective state programs if delay occurs in reviewing them, regardless of the reason; and to abandon the air quality management plan designed to limit significant deterioration of clean air outside national parklands and wilderness areas.

Deadlines

The Clean Air Act recognizes a basic right of the American people to air that is fit to breathe. To secure this right, the Act created a program with three essential parts:

—National air quality standards, set at the levels needed to protect people's health,

—Deadlines for meeting those standards, and

—State planning and implementation, under federal review, of the emission control measures needed to meet the standards by the deadline.

The program has brought about important progress. As the Commission has found, in the 1970's pollution levels in the nation's dirty areas dropped substantially. Vast areas of the country which exceeded the standards in 1970 now have met them. Scores of millions more people, who live in those areas, now enjoy healthful air. More than 13,000 premature deaths have been avoided every year. And if currently programmed pollution control efforts do not falter, by the Clean Air Act's 1987 deadline for meeting the last standards, most areas now failing to attain will meet the federal standards. This will provide healthful air quality for between 15 and 70 million more people, depending upon the pollutant.

Standards and deadlines, together, are responsible for these improvements. The plain fact is that the states and EPA would have adopted and implemented far weaker emission control measures than are in place without the pressure generated by deadlines. Without a specific time for attainment, standards become just laudable goals, much too easily deferred.

To be sure, some areas — especially Los Angeles, San Diego, the New York area, Houston, and Denver — suffer such severe pollution that they are not projected to meet the Act's 1987 attainment date. These areas and others with substantial particulate problems undeniably need more time. They need the opportunity, under extended deadlines, to plan and implement the long-term emission reductions needed to reach the standards there. But while they need more time, they also need the requirement of specific dates for attainment, to be able to defend the regulatory actions and other steps they will need to take to protect people's health in a timely manner.

Seriously overreacting, however, to these areas' problems with one specific date, the Commission report recommends abolishing deadlines altogether. What is more, the Commission does not limit this proposal to just those areas with genuine difficulty meeting the existing date. Rather, the report would eliminate deadlines for *all* areas, including those currently on track, in response to the 1987 date, to attaining healthful air quality....

Instead of a planning and implementation process to meet the standards by appropriate deadlines, the Commission would substitute a state and EPA review of control requirements every three years, to see what should be done in the next three years. Supposedly, the state air pollution control agency and EPA would negotiate a set of additional control measures for reducing existing pollution which are deemed "reasonably available." This involves requiring a greater degree of emission reduction from some categories of sources that have already been subject to some requirements. It also involves placing some control requirements for the first time on types of sources that have not been controlled at all.

We believe that without deadlines, the determination of what controls are "reasonably available" would slip inevitably toward justifying status quo controls, legitimizing a failure to do more, and achieving no progress towards healthful air.

What controls are "reasonably available" is a judgment made by the states and EPA balancing the need for prompt emission control and the costs of it. Industries that would be subject to control are extremely effective at stating — and often at exaggerating — the technical difficulties and economic costs they would face. The need to attain the air quality standards by a date certain is the foil to such arguments. Without the date certain, there will be nothing concrete to limit the weight given the industries' concerns in determining what is reasonable.

Congress considered abolishing the deadlines in 1977, and wisely decided against it. Explaining that decision to the full Senate, Senator Muskie quoted with approval the opinion of EPA that deadlines are the key to progress: "If the firm statutory deadlines are nullified, every air pollution control measure imposed by EPA or a State would be held hostage to legal challenges and possible reversals on grounds of judicially-perceived 'reasonableness.' The net effect could only be further delays in ever attaining the Act's health standards."...

We proposed to our fellow Commissioners a workable approach to deadlines that would have both the "action-forcing" quality needed to assure attainment, and the flexibility needed in the genuine problem areas. Deadlines are essential to let citizens know if public officials are doing their jobs.

First, retain the existing 1982 and 1987 deadlines for areas that can meet them.

Second, for areas the Commission has found will not meet them, establish a process that identifies what is necessary to come into attainment, and when it can be done. States would be required to revise their State Implementation Plans within two years. The revised SIP would have to (1) specify a new date for attaining the standards, and (2) state the emission reduction measures needed to meet those deadlines, and when they will be undertaken.

Third, require EPA to review the state's deadline choices and the means indicated to attain them. EPA would disapprove a SIP only if the emission control measures specified would not, in the Agency's judgment, succeed in meeting the state's chosen deadlines. EPA would also prepare a report for Congress covering areas that projected attainment after 1987, reviewing the deadlines and measures chosen by each state, whether the measures were realistic for meeting these deadlines, and whether the deadlines could be met sooner with controls the state had decided against or overlooked.

This approach would get the most polluted areas and EPA focussing on the long-term planning needed to eventually attain the health standards even in the severe trouble spots, while maintaining means for the public to push for rapid adoption of measures that can be put in place quickly. Focusing their attention on a more realistic long-term would also remove the incentives for exaggerating what to expect from a control measure, while keeping a deadline will assure continued pressure to achieve the standards. State Implementation Plans will become both more realistic and more effective....

Armed with the report prepared by EPA, Congress could judge the need for further enactments on deadlines. Congress would have a range of options. It could ratify the deadlines selected by the states. It could establish a range of attainment dates for different areas. It could set a single outside date by which all areas must meet the standards.

With this process of setting deadlines, the public would have the means to hold decisionmakers acountable for their control choices. While the Commission voted narrowly to abandon deadlines, we believe the Congress should consider the approach proposed here fully before repudiating the major device responsible for the progress achieved in the 1970s....

Prevention of Significant Deterioration

The Commission's report recommends the abandonment of the air quality management program designed to limit the pollution of clean air areas outside of our national parklands and wilderness areas.

The program Congress enacted in 1977 to protect clean air areas had as its central requirement the creation of a budget for additional pollution (called an "increment") which would limit the rate at which we spend or use up our nation's clean air resources. Congress' program established three budget levels for the country. It set a very tight budget (called Class I) for large national parks and wilderness areas, designed to restrain sharply additional pollution of those pristine areas. For the rest of the country Congress set a moderate budget (called Class II) that would allow substantial growth of well-controlled sources. To provide additional flexibility Congress set a third and larger budget (Class III) which a state could adopt for an area if it felt that the Class II budget might not provide enough room for growth.

The Commission's recommendation to drop the Class II/III program would eliminate the requirement of a moderate air pollution budget for all areas of the country outside of our national parklands and wilderness areas. Such a change would permit clean air areas in more than 90 percent of the nation to experience substantial and unnecessary pollution. This recommendation represents a major departure from a national policy of conservation of this valuable resource. We cannot support a drastic retrenchment.

The report's recommendation is not supported by its findings nor by the studies done for the Commission. The principal argument raised against the Class II/III program is that it is procedurally complex. The moderate remedy for complexity is to propose simplifying changes.... The report's recommendation chooses the extreme path of abolishing the program rather than attempting to fix it. Our nation's air resources are too important to be given away simply because the Commission did not make the effort to propose a simple and workable protection program.

The report's recommendation to eliminate Class II/III protection is by no means based on consensus. A proposal to continue Class II in a modified form failed in the Commission on a tie vote. Congress should consider this in weighing the recommendation included in the Commission's report....

CHROMOSOME REPORT ON LOVE CANAL RESIDENTS

A biomedical study suggesting that residents of Love Canal, a neighborhood near Niagara Falls, N.Y., had suffered chromosome damage from chemical wastes created a furor in 1980 and led to deepening concern over numerous other chemical dumps across the nation.

The study report, dated May 14, 1980, had been undertaken for two federal agencies, the Department of Justice and the Environmental Protection Agency (EPA). When accounts of the study appeared in newspapers, 710 families were evacuated from the vicinity of the Love Canal, at the expense of the federal government.

Carried out by the Biogenics Corp. of Houston, Texas, as a pilot project, the study showed that 11 of 36 Love Canal residents studied had chromosome aberrations and eight of the 11 had "supernumerary acentric fragments." That appeared to mean that the eight had more chromosomal material than they were born with. The EPA made it clear that the pilot study could not "be regarded as a complete and definitive scientific study." But chromosome damages as described in the report were suspected of being related to birth defects and, possibly, the future appearance of cancer.

Following are excerpts from Feb. 26, 1980, and May 5, 1980, statements on hazardous waste management regulations by Douglas M. Costle, then EPA administrator, and from the pilot cytogenetic study of Love Canal residents by Biogenics Corp.:

Feb. 26 Statement

The safe disposal of toxic chemical waste by industry is currently one of this country's most critical environmental problems.

Ever since the tragedy of Love Canal, the nation has been shocked by continuing discoveries of hazardous waste incidents which threaten public health and the environment.

We have seen the Valley of the Drums in Kentucky where barrels of chemicals hang from trees like Christmas ornaments.

We have seen miles of North Carolina roadside deadened by ditch dumping of PCB's.

We have seen entire mine shafts filled with chemical soup.

We have launched a major enforcement effort to identify these kinds of sites and to take legal action whenever the responsible party can be found.

But the eventual solution to the hazardous waste problem will require a transformation in the way that American industry handles its waste. And the size of the problem is staggering. Over 750,000 generators presently produce some 57 million tons of waste annually, of which 90 percent is disposed of by environmentally unsound methods.

As a nation, we paid too little attention to the byproducts of our chemical age. For decades, we dumped out the back door and into any vacant lot or inadequate landfill assuming that the wastes could be forgotten. Unfortunately, these wastes did not just go away. They have turned up, sometimes decades later, in people's drinking water supplies, in the nation's waterways, underneath housing developments and from there into people's homes. The toxic effects from these wastes cannot be underestimated.

Some of these wastes, byproducts from the production of pesticides, paints, industrial cleaners, solvents and other industrial chemicals, contain extremely dangerous substances.

What happened two years ago at Love Canal where hundreds of residents were displaced from their homes, some never to return, and where abnormal rates of miscarriages, birth defects and cancers have occurred, must never happen again.

We may continue to find abandoned waste sites from past decades of neglect. But the system I am announcing today is designed to prevent the creation of future Love Canals.

Today we are issuing three regulations which will give us a national roadmap of where waste is and where it is going. These regulations will:

—Create an inventory of all businesses in the nation which produce, transport, or dispose of hazardous waste.

—Establish a manifest system so that we will know at all times who is responsible for hazardous waste, where it is going, and whether it gets there safely.

The Manifest System

The manifest system is a central element in an emerging management system which will provide cradle-to-grave control over toxic chemical wastes. The manifest system is directed specifically at the midnight dumper who surreptitiously dumps wastes in sewers, in fields, or in the woods. It's designed to put the midnight dumper out of business.

Chris Beck, Assistant Administrator for Water and Hazardous Materials, will use the charts behind me to illustrate how the manifest system works.

—The generator of waste — here a chemical plant — must determine if his wastes are hazardous.

—If hazardous wastes are to be shipped, the generator must do several things:

•He must package and label the wastes in accordance with Department of Transportation shipping regulations.

•He must designate on the manifest the facility to which the wastes are to go. That facility must be permitted to handle his type of waste.

•He must prepare the manifest, which must contain
—the name of the generator,
—the name of all transporters,
—the name and address of the designated facility, and
—the description and quantity of the waste.

•Finally, he must give copies of that manifest to the transporter.

The transporter also has specified responsibilities:

•He must sign a copy of the manifest, acknowledging acceptance of the waste, and give it to the generator.

•He must deliver the waste to the designated facility, and receive from that facility a signed copy of the manifest.

•He must, in the case of a spill, take action to clean up that spill and contact the National Response Center and DOT.

—The facility, whether it be an incinerator, a treatment facility, or a disposal site, must sign a copy of the manifest and return it to the generator, thus closing the loop.

—The generator, when he receives the signed manifest, knows that his waste arrived safely. But if he does not receive a signed copy, he must

•Within 35 days, contact the transporter and the designated facility to find out the status of the waste.

•Within 45 days, submit a report to EPA.

Manifest systems are presently in operation in Europe and in several States. The system prevents illicit disposal and midnight dumping because responsibility is fixed, and evasion requires extensive collusion.

EPA and the Department of Transportation have worked closely together in developing the manifest regulations, and DOT will be revising its regulations to incorporate controls over shipments of hazardous waste.

Schedule for Implemenation

These three regulations — standards for generators and transporters, and requirements for notification — are key elements of the management system for hazardous wastes under the Resource Conservation and Recovery Act.

In April, EPA will define what wastes are hazardous and set forth operating standards for treatment, storage, and disposal facilities. We will also issue procedural regulations for permitting and state authorization.

By July, all businesses which handle hazardous waste must notify EPA, giving us for the first time a national inventory.

By October, all firms that store, treat, or dispose must apply for a permit. Those who notify and apply for a permit can obtain interim status to continue their operations.

Also in October, the program takes effect and goes into operation. The manifest system must be used for all waste shipments, and all sites with interim status must be in compliance with the interim operating standards.

Conclusion

We are the most highly industrialized society the world has ever known. Yet until now, no system has been institutionalized for properly disposing of our toxic wastes.

These regulations, and those that will be published in April, will create a new framework which will fundamentally change the ways in which industry manages its wastes.

We do not view these regulations as the final solution. No single stroke of a pen can quickly change old habits of waste mismanagement that industry has become accustomed to. But the new regulations are an essential first step towards preventing the creation of new Love Canals.

May 5 Announcement

Two weeks ago, on the 10th anniversary of Earth Day, the site where we intended to hold this news conference — the Chemical Control dumpsite in Elizabeth, N.J., — was transformed into a chemical inferno. It was a grim reminder on Earth Day that much remains to be done in protecting human health and the environment.

The regulations we are announcing today are designed to prevent the future creation of chemical dumps like the one in New Jersey. They establish a hazardous waste management system that provides cradle-to-grave control.

Two months ago EPA issued the first three regulations in this program. Those three regulations will give us a national roadmap of where waste is and where it is going. They will create an inventory of all businesses in the nation which produce, transport, or dispose of hazardous waste. They will establish a manifest system so that we will know at all times who is responsible for hazardous waste, where it is going, and whether it gets there safely.

Today, we are announcing the next installment of regulations to effectuate the hazardous waste program.

—These regulations identify and list the hazardous wastes which will be subject to control. They list 85 waste streams which are promulgated now, and an additional 25 waste streams which will be promulgated by May 30. They list 416 commercial products and chemicals which, if discarded, must be managed as hazardous waste. They also contain simple tests to be applied by generators to identify additional waste streams which may be ignitable, corrosive, reactive, or toxic.

—These regulations also set operating and technical standards for facilities which store, treat, or dispose of hazardous waste. In November, existing facilities will have to comply with these requirements. They will have to undertake regular inspections and provide security at their sites. They will have to train their employees properly and develop contingency plans to respond to accidents. They will have to begin to install groundwater monitoring systems. They will have to keep careful records of their operations and make regular reports. They will have to participate in the manifest system. And they will have to meet a series of technical standards regarding the storage, treatment, incineration or disposal of waste.

Let me predict now that the process we are starting will turn up information and situations which will shock our nation. We will find waste sites which are now unknown. We will document leaching of chemicals into aquifers which we have assumed were safe. We will gather hard data on a problem whose dimensions we now can only guess. But we will have begun the difficult transition from a time when wastes, once out-of-sight, were out-of-mind.

However, these regulations provide only one leg of a three-legged stool. It now is the law of the land that wastes must be managed properly. That is a critical first step. But two other conditions are necessary.

First, we must have a commitment of capital and expertise from firms willing to provide waste management. There is no reason why American technological genius, which produced these wastes, cannot provide the technological "know how" for disposing of it properly. We have tried to create a regulatory and financial climate in which responsible and capable companies step forward and take on this job.

Second, we must have sites at which good management can take place. Our citizens want the benefits to society that created those wastes. They must come to understand that all of us, in every state and locality, share responsibility for locating safe waste management sites.

Finally, let me turn to what is always the first question after EPA unveils new regulations — what will this program cost? We have studied 22 industrial sectors representing 29,000 generators responsible for gross sales of $350 billion. We estimate the cost of compliance to be $510 million — less than two-tenths of one percent of sales for these generators.

Significant Costs

These costs are significant. But they are also a bargain. For if we have learned nothing else since Love Canal, we have learned that an ounce of prevention in hazardous waste management is worth a pound of cure. At Love Canal, proper management of Hooker's wastes would have cost $3 million. Instead, the State of New York has already spent $36 million, EPA has filed four suits totaling $124 million, and over $14 billion in compensatory and punitive lawsuits are pending.

At another Hooker site near Muskegon, Michigan, chemical leachate has caused irreparable damage to local ground water supplies. Total clean-up could cost $30 million.

In Dover Township, New Jersey, improper disposal of 6,000 drums of chemical wastes has cost over $400,000 to clean up. Fourteen million dollars in lawsuits have been filed.

Velsicol Chemical Corporation's improper disposal of about 300,000 55-gallon drums of pesticide wastes near Toone, Tennessee, has contaminated local drinking water supplies. Estimates of remedial costs run from $6 million to $165 million. A class action suit for $2.5 billion has been filed against Velsicol.

Clearly, we could save ourselves broke by not dealing with these problems.

Today's regulations will not clean up past disasters such as those I just described. And there are others — Coventry, Rhode Island, Lowell, Massachusetts, Valley of the Drums, Kentucky. Each with stacks and stacks of deteriorating drums, many with unknown substances — a potential risk to health and environment, and limited funds, if any, to pay for cleanup.

Pilot Cytogenetic Study

Peripheral blood samples were obtained from the 36 individuals over a two day period. Samples from 19 individuals were obtained on day one, and samples from 17 individuals were obtained on day two. Five ml [milliliters] of blood was obtained via venipuncture from each individual. Blood was collected into a ten ml sterile, plastic syringe equipped with a sterile 21 gauge needle. The syringe had been pretreated with 500 units of preservative-free heparin (1000 units per ml). Samples were coded and immediately transferred to the tissue culture laboratory at the University of Buffalo and cultured according to the modification ... of the Moorhead technique....

Results

... 200 cells per individual were scored for the presence of chromatid breaks (deletions), chromatid intrachanges, chromatid interchanges, chromosome breaks (deletions), dicentric chromosomes, ring chromosomes, translocations, inversions, supernumerary acentric fragments, severely damaged cells, and total abnormal cells. Some of the slides from three individuals, B-29, B-31 and B-45, were broken while being transported, resulting in the reduction of the number of cells analyzed. Thus only 187 cells were analyzed for B-29, 131 for B-31, and 184 for B-45. The lower number of cells analyzed for these individuals can result only in an underestimate of the total number of aberrations present per individual.

Since a contemporary comparison group (control group) was not available for study, no unequivocal statement can be made concerning the cytogenetic results from the Love Canal residents. In the absence of a contemporary control group, we have compared our results with controls from a previous study ... historical controls. As seen ... 7102 cells were analyzed from 36 residents of Love Canal. There were 0.83% cells with chromatid breaks, 0.55% cells with chromosome breaks, 0.10% cells with marker chromosomes, 0.20% cells with supernumerary acentric chromosomes, 0 severely damaged cells and 1.10% abnormal cells. In a previous study ... on 44 non-exposed individuals, a total of 8,800 cells were examined. There were 1.1% cells with chromatid breaks, 0.35% cells with chromosome breaks, 0.06% cells with marker chromosomes, and 1.4% abnormal cells. Other types of aberrations were not reported. While there appears to be no difference in the percentage of chromatid breaks and total abnormal cells, there may be an increase in the percentage of cells with chromosome breaks (0.55% versus 0.35%) and in the percentage of cells with marker chromosomes (0.10% versus 0.06%) in the Love Canal residents.

Examination of the results of the Love Canal study on an individual basis rather than on a cellular basis . . . [shows] . . . the distribution of individuals with chromatid breaks, chromosome breaks, supernumerary acentric fragments and abnormal cells. . . . In the previously reported study . . . only the distribution of individuals related to chromosome breaks was presented. Comparison of these results with those from the Love Canal residents suggests an increase in the distribution of Love Canal residents with chromosome breaks, 17/36 (47.2%) versus 18/44 (40.9%). In addition, there appears to be a large increase in the distribution of Love Canal residents with supernumerary acentric fragments, 8/36 (22.2%). Since the distribution of individuals with supernumerary acentric fragments was not presented in the previously reported study. . ., we have estimated the distribution of individuals with supernumerary acentric fragments in the normal population to be approximately 1/100 (1.0%). We base this estimate upon our experience with the examination of over 6,000 individuals.

Examination of the distribution of individuals related to chromatid breaks and abnormal cells was unrevealing. . . .

Recommendations

We strongly recommend the genetic toxicological examination of as many of the Love Canal residents as possible. Specifically, three genetic toxicological tests can be performed directly in these residents: cytogenetics, body fluid analysis and fluorescent study of sperm. Such mutagenic studies have the following advantages: studies are performed in intact systems, results from studies need not be extrapolated as in animal investigations, and in general, one directly observes the mutational event. . . .

SUPREME COURT ON DANGEROUS WORKPLACES

In a unanimous ruling Feb. 26, 1980, the Supreme Court upheld a Department of Labor regulation giving workers the right to refuse dangerous work assignments. The decision in Whirlpool Corp. *v.* Marshall *upheld a regulation issued by Secretary of Labor F. Ray Marshall under provisions of the Occupational Safety and Health Act of 1970. The law prohibited employers from discriminating against workers who asserted any of the rights the act guaranteed.*

In June 1974 a maintenance worker at a plant of the Whirlpool Corp. in Marion, Ohio, fell to his death through a screen on which he was working. The screen had been erected to protect workers from objects that might fall from overhead conveyor belts.

The company, a manufacturer of household appliances, took a number of steps to remedy the situation that had led to the fatal accident. However, two plant maintenance men, Virgil Deemer and Thomas Cornwell, expressed to plant officials and to a regional representative of the Occupational Safety and Health Administration (OSHA) their continuing concern about their safety.

Deemer and Cornwell on July 10, 1974, refused to perform their regular duties cleaning the screen. They were sent home, not paid for their shift and officially reprimanded.

The Occupational Safety and Health Act itself did not guarantee a right to refuse to work in unsafe conditions. But Secretary Marshall's regulation did grant workers such a right when there was no available alternative way of dealing with hazardous conditions.

When Marshall sued the Whirlpool Corp. for discriminating against Deemer and Cornwell, the company challenged his regulation as inconsistent with the 1970 law. The justices, however, were not persuaded by Whirlpool's argument that Congress, in approving the Act, had rejected the right of workers to refuse a task because of a reasonable belief that injury or death might result.

Following are excerpts from the court's unanimous opinion, written by Justice Potter Stewart:

No. 78-1870

Whirlpool Corporation, Petitioner, *v.* Ray Marshall, Secretary of Labor.	On Writ of Certiorari to the United States Court of Appeals for the Sixth Circuit.

[February 26, 1980]

MR. JUSTICE STEWART delivered the opinion of the Court.

The Occupational Safety and Health Act of 1970 (Act) prohibits an employer from discharging or discriminating against any employee who exercises "any right afforded by" the Act. The Secretary of Labor (Secretary) has promulgated a regulation providing that, among the rights that the Act so protects, is the right of an employee to choose not to perform his assigned task because of a reasonable apprehension of death or serious injury coupled with a reasonable belief that no less drastic alternative is available. The question presented in the case before us is whether this regulation is consistent with the Act.

I

The petitioner company maintains a manufacturing plant in Marion, Ohio, for the production of household appliances. Overhead conveyors transport appliance components throughout the plant. To protect employees from objects that occasionally fall from these conveyors, the petitioner has installed a horizontal wire mesh guard screen approximately 20 feet above the plant floor. This mesh screen is welded to angle-iron frames suspended from the building's structural steel skeleton.

Maintenance employees of the petitioner spend several hours each week removing objects from the screen, replacing paper spread on the screen to catch grease drippings from the material on the conveyors, and performing occasional maintenance work on the conveyors themselves. To perform these duties, maintenance employees usually are able to stand on the iron frames, but sometimes find it necessary to step onto the steel mesh screen itself.

In 1973 the company began to install heavier wire in the screen because its safety had been drawn into question. Several employees had fallen partly through the old screen, and on one occasion an employee had fallen completely through to the plant floor below but had survived. A number of maintenance employees had reacted to these incidents by bringing the unsafe screen conditions to the attention of their foremen. The petitioner company's contemporaneous safety instructions admonished employees to step only on the angle-iron frames.

On June 28, 1974, a maintenance employee fell to his death through the guard screen in an area where the newer, stronger mesh had not yet been installed. Following this incident, the petitioner effectuated some repairs and issued an order strictly forbidding maintenance employees from stepping on either the screens or the angle-iron supporting structure. An alternative but somewhat more cumbersome and less satisfactory method was developed for removing objects from the screen. This procedure required employees to stand on power-raised mobile platforms and use hooks to recover the material.

On July 7, 1974, two of the petitioner's maintenance employees, Virgil Deemer and Thomas Cornwell, met with the plant maintenance superintendent to voice their concern about the safety of the screen. The superintendent disagreed with their view, but permitted the two men to inspect the screen with their foreman and to point out dangerous areas needing repair. Unsatisfied with the petitioner's response to the results of this inspection, Deemer and Cornwell met on July 9 with the plant safety director. At that meeting, they requested the name, address, and telephone number of a representative of the local office of the Occupational Safety and Health Administration (OSHA). Although the safety director told the men that they "had better stop and think about what [they] were doing," he furnished the men with the information they requested. Later that same day. Deemer contacted an official of the regional OSHA office and discussed the guard screen.

The next day, Deemer and Cornwell reported for the night shift at 10:45 p.m. Their foreman, after himself walking on some of the angle-iron frames, directed the two men to perform their usual maintenance duties on a section of the old screen. Claiming that the screen was unsafe, they refused to carry out this directive. The foreman then sent them to the personnel office, where they were ordered to punch out without working or being paid for the remaining six hours of the shift. The two men subsequently received written reprimands, which were placed in their employment files.

A little over a month later, the Secretary filed suit in the United States District Court for the Northern District of Ohio, alleging that the petitioner's actions against Deemer and Cornwell constituted discrimination in violation of ... [Occupational Safety and Health] Act. As relief, the complaint prayed, *inter alia,* that the petitioner be ordered to expunge from its personnel files all references to the reprimands issued to the two employees, and for a permanent injunction requiring the petitioner to compensate the two employees for the six hours of pay they had lost by reason of their disciplinary suspensions.

Following a bench trial, the District Court found that the regulation in question justified Deemer's and Cornwell's refusals to obey their foreman's order on July 10, 1974. The court found that the two employees had "refused to perform the cleaning operation because of a genuine fear of death or serious bodily harm," that the danger presented had been "real and not something which [had] existed only in the minds of the employees," that the employees had acted in good faith, and that no reasonable alternative had realistically been open to them other than to refuse to work. The District Court nevertheless denied relief, holding that the Secretary's regulation was inconsistent with the Act and therefore invalid. . . .

The Court of Appeals for the Sixth Circuit reversed the District Court's judgment. . . . Finding ample support in the record for the District Court's factual determination that the actions of Deemer and Cornwell had been justified under the Secretary's regulation ... the appellate court disagreed with the District Court's conclusion that the regulation is invalid. . . . It accordingly remanded the case to the District Court for further proceedings. . . . We granted certiorari ... because the decision of the Court of Appeals in this case conflicts with those of two other Courts of Appeals on the important question in issue. . . . That question, as stated at the outset of this opinion, is whether the Secretary's regulation authorizing employee "self-help" in some circumstances ... is permissible under the Act.

II

The Act itself creates an express mechanism for protecting workers from employment conditions believed to pose an emergent threat of death or serious injury. Upon receipt of an employee inspection request stating reasonable grounds to believe that an imminent danger is present in a workplace, OSHA must conduct an inspection. . . . In the event this inspection reveals workplace conditions or practices that "could reasonably be expected to cause death or serious physical harm immediately or before the imminence of such danger can be eliminated through the enforcement procedures otherwise provided by" the Act ... the OSHA inspector must inform the affected employees and the employer of the danger and notify them that he is recommending to the Secretary that injunctive relief be sought. . . . At this juncture, the Secretary can petition a federal court to restrain the conditions or practices giving rise to the imminent danger. By means of a temporary restraining order or preliminary injunction, the court may then require the employer to avoid, correct, or remove the danger or to prohibit employees from working in the area. . . .

To ensure that this process functions effectively, the Act expressly accords to every employee several rights, the exercise of which may not subject him to discharge or discrimination. An employee is given the right to inform OSHA of an imminently dangerous workplace condition or practice and request that OSHA inspect that condition or practice. . . . He is given a limited right to assist the OSHA inspector in inspecting the workplace ... and the right to aid a court in determining whether or not a risk of imminent danger in fact exists. . . . Finally, an affected employee is given the right to bring an action to compel the Secretary to seek injunctive relief if he believes the Secretary has wrongfully declined to do so. . . .

In the light of this detailed statutory scheme, the Secretary is obviously correct when he acknowledges in his regulation that, "as a general matter, there is no right afforded by the Act which would entitle employees to walk off the job because of potential unsafe conditions at the workplace." By providing for prompt notice to the employer of an inspector's intention to seek an injunction against an imminently dangerous condition, the legislation obviously contemplates that the employer will normally respond by voluntarily and speedily eliminating the danger. And in the few instances where this does not occur, the legislative provisions authorizing prompt judicial action are designed to give employees full protection in most situations from the risk of injury or death resulting from an imminently dangerous condition at the worksite.

As this case illustrates, however, circumstances may sometimes exist in which the employee justifiably believes that the express statutory arrangement does not sufficiently protect him from death or serious injury. Such circumstances will probably not often occur, but such a situation may arise when (1) the employee is ordered by his employer to work under conditions that the employee reasonably believes pose an imminent risk of death or serious bodily injury, and (2) the employee has reason to believe that there is not sufficient time or opportunity either to seek effective redress from his employer or to apprise OSHA of the danger.

Nothing in the Act suggests that those few employees who have to face this dilemma must rely exclusively on the remedies expressly set forth in the Act at the risk of their own safety. But nothing in the Act explicitly provides otherwise. Against this background of legislative silence, the Secretary has exercised his rulemaking power ... and has determined that, when an employee in good faith finds himself in such a predicament, he may refuse to expose himself to the dangerous condition, without being subjected to "subsequent discrimination" by the employer.

The question before us is whether this interpretative regulation constitutes a permissible gloss on the Act by the Secretary, in light of the Act's language, structure, and legislative history. Our inquiry is informed by an awareness that the regulation is entitled to deference unless it can be said not to be a reasoned and supportable interpretation of the Act. *Skidmore* v. *Swift & Co.* [1944].

A. The regulation clearly conforms to the fundamental objective of the Act — to prevent occupational deaths and serious injuries. The Act, in its preamble, declares that its purpose and policy is "to assure so far as possible every working man and woman in the Nation safe and healthful working conditions and to *preserve* our human resources. . . ."

To accomplish this basic purpose, the legislation's remedial orientation is prophylactic in nature. See *Atlas Roofing Co.* v. *Occupational Safety Comm'n* [1977]. The Act does not wait for an employee to die or become injured. It authorizes the promulgation of health and safety standards and the issuance of citations in the hope that these will act to prevent deaths or injuries from ever occurring. It would seem anomalous to construe an Act so directed and constructed as prohibiting an employee, with no other reasonable alternative, the freedom to withdraw from a workplace environment that he reasonably believes is highly dangerous.

Moreover, the Secretary's regulation can be viewed as an

appropriate aid to the full effectuation of the Act's "general duty" clause. That clause provides that "[e]ach employer ... shall furnish to each of his employees employment and a place of employment which are free from recognized hazards that are causing or are likely to cause death or serious physical harm to his employees." ... As the legislative history of this provision reflects, it was intended itself to deter the occurrence of occupational deaths and serious injuries by placing on employers a mandatory obligation independent of the specific health and safety standards to be promulgated by the Secretary. Since OSHA inspectors cannot be present around the clock in every workplace, the Secretary's regulation ensures that employees will in all circumstances enjoy the rights afforded them by the "general duty" clause.

The regulation thus on its face appears to further the overriding purpose of the Act, and rationally to complement its remedial scheme. In the absence of some contrary indication in the legislative history, the Secretary's regulation must, therefore, be upheld, particularly when it is remembered that safety legislation is to be liberally construed to effectuate the congressional purpose. *United States* v. *Bacto-Unidisk* [1969]; *Lilly* v. *Grand Trunk R. Co.* [1943].

B. In urging reversal of the judgment before us, the petitioner relies primarily on two aspects of the Act's legislative history.

1. ... The petitioner reads into this legislative history a congressional intent incompatible with an administrative interpretation of the Act such as is embodied in the regulation at issue in this case. The petitioner argues that Congress' overriding concern in rejecting the "strike with pay" provision was to avoid giving employees a unilateral authority to walk off the job which they might abuse in order to intimidate or harass their employer. Congress deliberately chose instead, the petitioner maintains, to grant employees the power to request immediate administrative inspections of the workplace which could in appropriate cases lead to coercive judicial remedies. As the petitioner views the regulation, therefore, it gives to workers precisely what Congress determined to withhold from them.

We read the legislative history differently. Congress rejected a provision that did not concern itself at all with conditions posing real and immediate threats of death or severe injury. The remedy which the rejected provision furnished employees could have been invoked only after 60 days had passed following HEW's inspection and notification that improperly high levels of toxic substances were present in the workplace. Had that inspection revealed employment conditions posing a threat of imminent and grave harm, the Secretary of Labor would presumably have requested, long before expiration of the 60-day period, a court injunction pursuant to other provisions of the Daniels bill. Consequently, in rejecting the Daniels bill's "strike with pay" provision, Congress was not rejecting a legislative provision dealing with the highly perilous and fast-moving situations covered by the regulation now before us.

It is also important to emphasize that what primarily troubled Congress about the Daniels bill's "strike with pay" provision was its requirement that employees be paid their regular salary after having properly invoked their right to refuse to work under the section. It is instructive that virtually every time the issue of an employee's right to absent himself from hazardous work was discussed in the legislative debates, it was in the context of the employee's right to continue to receive his usual compensation.

When it rejected the "strike with pay" concept, therefore, Congress very clearly meant to reject a law unconditionally imposing upon employers an obligation to continue to pay their employees their regular pay checks when they absented themselves from work for reasons of safety. But the regulation at issue here does not require employers to pay workers who refuse to perform their assigned tasks in the face of imminent danger. It simply provides that in such cases the employer may not "discriminate" against the employees involved. An employer "discriminates" against an employee only when he treats that employee less favorably than he treats others similarly situated.

2. The second aspect of the Act's legislative history upon which the petitioner relies is the rejection by Congress of provisions contained in both the Daniels and the Williams bills that would have given Labor Department officials, in imminent danger situations, the power temporarily to shut down all or part of an employer's plant. These provisions aroused considerable opposition in both Houses of Congress. The hostility engendered in the House of Representatives led Representative Daniels to delete his version of the provision in proposing amendments to his original bill. The Steiger bill that ultimately passed the House gave the Labor Department no such authority. The Williams bill, as approved by the Senate, did contain an administrative shutdown provision, but the conference committee rejected this aspect of the Senate bill.

The petitioner infers from these events a congressional will hostile to the regulation in question here. The regulation, the petitioner argues, provides employees with the very authority to shut down an employer's plant that was expressly denied a more expert and objective United States Department of Labor.

As we read the pertinent legislative history, however, the petitioner misconceives the thrust of Congress' concern. Those in Congress who prevented passage of the administrative shutdown provisions in the Daniels and Williams bills were opposed to the unilateral authority those provisions gave to federal officials, without any judicial safeguards, drastically to impair the operation of an employer's business. Congressional opponents also feared that the provisions might jeopardize the Government's otherwise neutral role in labor-management relations.

Neither of these congressional concerns is implicated by the regulation before us. The regulation accords no authority to government officials. It simply permits private employees of a private employer to avoid workplace conditions that they believe pose grave dangers to their own safety. The employees have no power under the regulation to order their employer to correct the hazardous condition or to clear the dangerous workplace of others. Moreover, any employee who acts in reliance on the regulation runs the risk of discharge or reprimand in the event a court subsequently finds that he acted unreasonably or in bad faith. The regulation, therefore, does not remotely resemble the legislation that Congress rejected.

C. For these reasons we conclude that ... [the regulation] was promulgated by the Secretary in the valid exercise of his authority under the Act. Accordingly, the judgment of the Court of Appeals is affirmed.

It is so ordered.

REPORT ON SMOKING BY WOMEN

In a report released Jan. 14, 1980, Dr. Julius B. Richmond, U.S. surgeon general, warned that lung cancer would overtake breast cancer as the leading cancer-related cause of death among women. "Within three years," the report stated, "the lung cancer death rate is expected to surpass that for breast cancer."

The 400-page report, entitled "The Health Consequences of Smoking for Women," was the 12th annual report to Congress on Smoking made by the Department of Health, Education and Welfare (now the Department of Health and Human Services). It said that women who smoked as men did incurred the same health risks. The surgeon general's report shattered the myth that women were not as susceptible as men to the health problems caused by smoking. It said that "is an illusion reflecting the fact that women lagged one-quarter century behind men in their widespread use of cigarettes." Following are excerpts from the surgeon general's report:

This report is more than a factual review of the health consequences of smoking for women. It is a document which challenges our society and, in particular, our medical and public health communities.

This report points out that the first signs of an epidemic of smoking-related disease among women are now appearing. Because women's cigarette use did not become widespread until the onset of World War II, those women with the greatest intensity of smoking are now only in their thirties, forties, and fifties. As these women grow older, and continue to smoke, their burden of smoking-related disease will grow larger. Cigarette smoking now contributes to one-fifth of the newly diagnosed cases of cancer and one-quarter of all cancer deaths among women — more cancer and more cancer deaths among women than can be atttributed to any other known agent. Within three years, the lung cancer death rate is expected to surpass that for breast cancer. A similar epidemic of chronic obstructive lung disease among women has also begun.

Four main themes emerge from this report to guide future public health efforts.

First, women are not immune to the damaging effects of smoking already documented for men. The apparently lower susceptibility to smoking related diseases among women smokers is an illusion reflecting the fact that women lagged one-quarter century behind men in their widespread use of cigarettes.

Second, cigarette smoking is a major threat to the outcome of pregnancy and well-being of the newborn baby.

Third, women may not start smoking, continue to smoke, quit smoking, or fail to quit smoking for precisely the same reasons as men. Unless future research clarifies these differences, we will find it difficult to prevent initiation or to promote cessation of cigarette smoking among women.

Fourth, the reduction of cigarette smoking is the keystone in our nation's long term strategy to promote a healthy lifestyle for women and men of all races and ethnic groups.

Women's Immunity?

All of the major prospective studies of smoking and mortality have reached consistent conclusions. Death rates from coronary heart disease, chronic lung disease, lung cancer, and overall mortality rates are significantly increased among both women and men smokers. These risks increase with the amount smoked, duration of smoking, depth of inhalation, and the "tar" and nicotine delivery of the cigarette smoked.

In these studies, conducted during the past three decades, relative mortality risks among female smokers appeared to be less than those of male smokers. It is now clear, however, that these studies were comparing the death rates of a generation of established, lifelong male smokers with a generation of women who had not yet taken up smoking with full intensity. Even those older women who reported smoking a large number of cigarettes per day had not smoked cigarettes in the same way as their male counterparts. Now that the cigarette smoking characteristics of women and men are becoming increasingly similar, their relative risks of smoking-related illness will become increasingly similar.

This fallacy of women's apparent immunity is clearly illustrated by differences in the timing of the growth in lung cancer among men and women in this century. Lung cancer deaths among males began to increase during the 1930s, as those men who had converted from other forms of tobacco to cigarette smoking before the turn of the century gradually accumulated decades of inhaled tobacco exposure. By the time of the first retrospective studies of smoking and lung cancer in 1950, two entire generations of men had already become lifelong cigarette smokers. Relatively few women from these generations smoked cigarettes, and even fewer had smoked cigarettes since their adolescence. Those young women who had taken up smoking intensively during World War II were only in their twenties and thirties. In 1950, women accounted for less than one in twelve deaths from lung cancer.

Thereafter, the age adjusted lung cancer death rate among women accelerated, and the male predominance in lung cancer declined. Lung cancer surpassed uterine cervical cancer as a cause of death in women. By 1968, as the findings of many large population prospective studies were being published, women accounted for one-sixth of all lung cancer deaths. These studies found that women cigarette smokers had 2.5 to 5 times greater death rates from lung cancer than women nonsmokers. By 1979, women accounted for fully one-fourth all lung cancer deaths. Over the next few years, women cigarette smokers' risk of lung cancer death will approach 8 to 12 times that of women nonsmokers, the same relative risk as that of men.

Lung cancer has four main histological types: epidermoid, small cell, adenocarcinoma, and large cell carcinoma. As several studies have shown, the incidence of each of these types of lung cancer displays a clear relationship to cigarette smoking among both men and women. Epidermoid and small cell lung cancer appear to be more prominent among men, while adenocarcinoma of the lung now appears to be more prominent among women.

The recent acceleration of lung cancer incidence among women has in fact been more rapid than the corresponding growth of lung cancer among men in the 1930s. Again, this difference in the initial rate of acceleration of lung cancer incidence does not refute the demonstrated causal relation between cigarette smoking and lung cancer among both sexes. Instead, differences in the rate of increase of lung cancer incidence may reflect changes in the carcinogenic properties of cigarette smoke, the style of cigarette smoking, or the interaction of cigarette smoking with other environmental hazards. It is noteworthy that those men who died of lung cancer in the 1930s came from a generation that had gradually converted to cigarettes from other, non-inhaled forms of tobacco. By contrast, the first regular tobacco users among women were almost exclusively cigarette smokers.

The 1979 Report on Smoking and Health documented numerous instances where cigarette smoking adds to the hazards of the workplace environment among men. Among women, this report reveals two such occupational exposures — asbestos and cotton dust — which have been clearly demonstrated to interact with cigarette smoking. The fact that evidence is limited among women does not imply that women are protected from the dangerous interactions of smoking and occupational exposures.

Health and Reproduction

Scientific studies encompassing various races and ethnic groups, cultures and countries, involving hundreds of thousands of pregnancies, have shown that cigarette smoking during pregnancy significantly affects the unborn fetus and the newborn baby. These damaging effects have been repeatedly shown to operate independently of all other factors which influence the outcome of pregnancy. The effects are increased by heavier smoking and are reduced if a woman stops smoking during pregnancy.

Numerous toxic substances in cigarette smoke, such as nicotine and hydrogen cyanide, cross the placenta to affect the fetus directly. The carbon monoxide from cigarette smoke is transported into the fetal blood and deprives the growing baby of oxygen. Fetal growth is directly retarded. The resulting reduction in fetal weight and size has many unfortunate consequences. Women who smoke cigarettes during pregnancy have more spontaneous abortions, and a greater incidence of bleeding during pregnancy, premature and prolonged rupture of amniotic membranes, abruptio placentae and placenta previa. Women who smoke cigarettes during pregnancy have more fetal and neonatal deaths than nonsmoking pregnant women. A relation between maternal smoking and Sudden Infant Death Syndrome has now been established.

Direct Harmful Effects

The direct harmful effects of smoking on the fetus have long term consequences. Children of mothers who smoked during pregnancy lag measurably in physical growth; there may also be effects on behavior and cognitive development. The extent of these deficiencies increases with the number of cigarettes smoked.

The damaging effects of maternal smoking on infants are not restricted to pregnancy. Nicotine, a known poison, is found in the breast milk of smoking mothers. Children whose parents smoke cigarettes have more respiratory infections and more hospitalizations in the first year of life.

Women who smoke cigarettes have more than three times the

risk of dying of stroke due to subarachnoid hemorrhage, and as much as two times the risk of dying of heart attack in comparison to nonsmoking women. The use of oral contraceptives in addition to smoking, however, causes a markedly increased risk, including a 22-fold increase in the risk of subarachnoid hemorrhagic stroke and a 20-fold increase in heart attack in heavy smokers.

Why Do Women Smoke?

Cigarette consumption in this country is now declining. Annual per capita consumption has decreased from 4,258 in 1965 to an estimated 3,900 in 1979. From 1965 to 1979, the proportion of adult male cigarette smokers declined from 51 to 37 percent. Not only have millions of men quit smoking, but the rate of initiation of smoking among adolescent males has now slowed.

From 1965 to 1976, the proportion of adult women cigarette smokers remained virtually unchanged at 32 to 33 percent. Since 1976, however, the proportion of adult women cigarette smokers appears to have declined to 28 percent. Although adult women are now beginning to quit smoking at rates comparable to adult men, the rate of initiation of smoking among younger women has not declined.

This report documents numerous differences by sex in the perceived role of cigarette smoking, in attitudes toward health and lifestyle, and in methods of coping with stress, anger, and boredom. Yet the significance of these differences, and their relation to differences in smoking patterns, remains poorly understood.

Although it is frequently observed that women in organized smoking cessation programs have more severe withdrawal symptoms and lower rates of successful quitting than men, these observations have not been systematically confirmed for the general population. In the past, women may have attempted to quit or succeeded in quitting smoking less frequently than men. The recent decline in the proportion of women smokers, however, suggests that women's attempted and successful quitting rates have now increased.

Although weight gain is a frequently cited consequence of quitting smoking, the association of weight gain with cessation of smoking has not been the subject of sufficient scrutiny. Controlled studies with careful measurement on representative populations of women do not exist. The impact of the fear of weight gain after quitting has not been adequately examined. If weight gain does result from cessation of smoking, its exact mechanism must be determined.

Even more problematic are marked differences by sex in the distribution of smoking prevalence by occupation. Men with advanced education and professional occupations have taken the lead in quitting smoking, but women in administrative and managerial positions have relatively high smoking prevalence rates. Although 20 percent or fewer male physicians smoke, the proportions of cigarette smokers among women health professionals, especially nurses and psychologists, remain disturbingly high.

Recent changes in smoking prevalence among black women and men have paralleled those of the general population. From 1965 to 1979, the proportion of black women cigarette smokers declined from 34 to 29 percent, while the proportion of black men smokers declined from 61 to 42 percent. However, differences by race in the onset, maintenance, and cessation of smoking have not been adequately explored. Little is known about cigarette smoking among other ethnic and minority groups.

Adolescent Smoking

The health consequences of smoking evolve over a lifetime. Evidence continues to accumulate, for example, that cigarette smoking produces measurable lung changes even in childhood and young adulthood. Young cigarette smokers of both sexes show more evidence of small airway dysfunction, and a higher prevalence of cough, wheezing, phlegm production, and other respiratory symptoms. The health damage due to cigarette smoking increases when an individual begins regular smoking earlier in life. Yet, as this report documents, the average age of onset of regular smoking among women has continuously declined during the last 50 years, and continues to decline.

According to a recent survey by the National Institute of Education, cigarette smoking among adolescent girls now exceeds that among adolescent boys. In the 17-19 year age group, there are almost 5 female cigarette smokers for every 4 male cigarette smokers. The causes of this inversion are far from clear. We do not yet understand the signal events in the initiation of smoking among young women. It is possible that parents set examples concerning lifestyle, health attitude, and risk-taking much earlier in childhood. The beginning of junior high school or entrance into the work force may be equally critical events. We do not know enough about an adolescent's sense of competence and self-mastery, and how these roles differ among women and men. Although smoking patterns among girls correlate with parental, peer and sibling smoking habits, educational level, type of school curriculum, academic performance, socioeconomic status, and other forms of substance abuse, the practical significance of these empirical correlations is unclear.

The Changing Cigarette

As this report documents, the proportion of men and women smokers using brands with lowered "tar" and nicotine continues to grow. Adolescents of both sexes have followed this trend, to the point where nonfilter cigarettes are relatively rare among young adults.

Although the preponderance of scientific evidence continues to suggest that cigarettes with lower "tar" and nicotine are less hazardous, four serious warnings are in order.

First, the reported "tar" and nicotine deliveries of cigarettes are standardized machine measurements. They do not necessarily represent the smoker's actual intake of these substances. Evidence is now mounting that individuals who switch to cigarettes with lowered "tar" and nicotine inhale more deeply, smoke a greater proportion of their cigarettes, and in some cases smoke more cigarettes.

Second, "tar" and nicotine are not the only dangerous chemical components of cigarette smoke. Many conventional filter cigarettes, in fact, may deliver more carbon monoxide than nonfilter cigarettes.

Third, it has not been established that lower "tar" and nicotine cigarettes have less harmful effects on the unborn fetus and baby; on women and men at high risk for developing coronary heart disease, such as those with elevated cholesterol or high blood pressure; or on workers with adverse occupational exposures. It has not been established that switching to a lower "tar" and nicotine cigarette has any salutary effect on individuals who already have smoking-related illnesses, such as coronary heart disease, chronic bronchitis, and emphysema.

Fourth, even the lowest yield cigarettes present health hazards for both women and men that are very much higher than smoking no cigarettes at all.

The single most effective way for both women and men smokers to reduce the hazards associated with cigarettes is to quit smoking.

As this report demonstrates, little is known about the effects of these product changes on the initiation, maintenance and cessation of smoking, particularly among women. It has not been determined whether the availability of cigarettes with lowered "tar" and nicotine has made it easier for young women to experiment with and become addicted to cigarettes. It is not known whether smokers of the lowest yield cigarettes are more or less likely to attempt to quit, or to succeed in quitting, than smokers of conventional filtertip or nonfilter cigarettes. The extent to which the act of switching to a lower "tar" cigarette may serve as a substitute for quitting may differ among women and men.

Public Health Responsibilities

This report . . . has confirmed in every way the judgement of the World Health Organization, that there can no longer be any doubt among informed people that cigarette smoking is a major and removable cause of ill health and premature death.

Each individual woman must make her own decision about this significant health issue. Secretary Harris has noted that the role of the Government, and all responsible health professionals, is to assure that this decision is an informed one. In issuing this report, we hope to help the public health community accomplish this purpose.

KEMENY COMMISSION: THREE MILE ISLAND CRISIS

Ending a six-month investigation, the President's Commission on the Accident at Three Mile Island issued its final report Oct. 30, 1979. It urged President Carter to abolish the Nuclear Regulatory Commission (NRC) and to create an executive agency charged with policing the nuclear power industry.

The 12-member commission, headed by John G. Kemeny, president of Dartmouth College, stopped short of recommending a halt to the construction of nuclear power plants. The report did say that fundamental changes were needed in the way reactors were built, operated and regulated to keep nuclear power risks "within tolerable limits."

Six commission members issued supplemental statements. Kemeny, the chairman, noted that eight different commission members had voted for at least one of three proposals recommending a moratorium, that is, a temporary halt to nuclear plant construction. But, Kemeny said, it was impossible for a majority of seven members to reach agreement on any one of the three moratorium proposals.

Following are excerpts from the report of the President's Commission on the Accident at Three Mile Island issued Oct. 30, 1979.

On March 28, 1979, the United States experienced the worst accident in the history of commercial nuclear power generation. Two weeks later, the President of the United States established a Presidential Commission. The President charged the 12-member Commission as follows:

"The purpose of the Commission is to conduct a comprehensive study and investigation of the recent accident involving the nuclear power facility on Three Mile Island in Pennsylvania. The Commission's study and investigation shall include:

(a) a technical assessment of the events and their causes; this assessment shall include, but shall not be limited to, an evaluation of the actual and potential impact of the events on the public health and safety and on the health and safety of workers;

(b) an analysis of the role of the managing utility;

(c) an assessment of the emergency preparedness and response of the Nuclear Regulatory Commission and other federal, state, and local authorities;

(d) An evaluation of the Nuclear Regulatory Commission's licensing, inspection, operation, and enforcement procedures as applied to this facility;

(e) an assessment of how the public's right to information concerning the events at TMI [Three Mile Island] was served and of the steps which should be taken during similar emergencies to provide the public with accurate, comprehensible, and timely information; and

(f) appropriate recommendations based upon the Commission's findings."

The Accident

At 4:00 a.m. on March 28, 1979, a serious accident occurred at the Three Mile Island 2 nuclear power plant near Middletown, Pennsylvania. The accident was initiated by mechanical malfunctions in the plant and made much worse by a combination of human errors in responding to it.... During the next 4 days, the extent and gravity of the accident was unclear to the managers of the plant, to federal and state officials, and to the general public. What is quite clear is that its impact, nationally and internationally, has raised serious concerns about the safety of nuclear power. This Commission was established in response to those concerns.

What We Did

The investigation of the Commission was carried out by our able and hard-working staff. We also had the help of a number of consultants and commissioned several studies. It is primarily due to the work of the staff that we accomplished the following.

We examined with great care the sequence of events that occurred during the accident, to determine what happened and why. We have attempted to evaluate the significance of various equipment failures as well as the importance of actions (or failures of actions) on the parts of individuals and organizations.

We analyzed the various radiation releases and came up with the best possible estimates of the health effects of the accident. In addition, we looked more broadly into how well the health and safety of the workers was protected during normal operating conditions, and how well their health and safety and that of the general public would have been protected in the case of a more serious accident.

We conducted an in-depth examination of the role played by the utility and its principal suppliers. We examined possible problems of organization, procedures, and practices that might have contributed to the accident. Since the major cause of the accident was due to inappropriate actions by those who were operating the plant and supervising that operation, we looked very carefully at the training programs that prepare operators and the procedures under which they operate.

As requested by the President, we examined the emergency plans that were in place at the time of the accident. We also probed the responses to the accident by the utility, by state and local governmental agencies in Pennsylvania, and by a variety of federal agencies. We looked for deficiencies in the plans and in their execution in order to be able to make recommendations for improvements for any future accident. In this process we had in mind how well the response would have worked if the danger to public health had been significantly greater.

We examined the coverage of the accident by the news media. This was a complex process in which we had to separate out whether errors in media accounts were due to ignorance or confusion on the part of the official sources, to the way they communicated this information to the media, or to mistakes committed by the reporters themselves. We examined what sources were most influential on the people who needed immediate information, and how well the public was served by the abundant coverage that was provided. We also attempted to evaluate whether the coverage tended to exaggerate the seriousness of the accident either by selectively using alarming quotes more than reassuring ones, or through purposeful sensationalism.

Finally, we spent a great deal of time on the agency that had a major role in all of the above: the Nuclear Regulatory Commission. The President gave us a very broad charge concerning this agency. We therefore tried to understand its complex structure and how well it functions, its role in licensing and rulemaking, how well it carries out its mission through its inspection and enforcement program, the role it plays in monitoring the training of operators, and its participation in the response to the emergency, including the part it played in providing information to the public.

We took more than 150 formal depositions and interviewed a significantly larger number of individuals. At our public hearings we heard testimony under oath from a wide variety of witnesses. We collected voluminous material that will fill about 300 feet of shelf-space in a library. All of this material will be placed into the National Archives. The most important information extracted from this in each of the areas will appear in a series of "Staff Reports to the Commission."

Based on all of this information, the Commission arrived at a number of major findings and conclusions. In turn, these findings led the Commission to a series of recommendations responsive to the President's charge.

At the beginning of this volume will be found an overview of our investigation, followed by those findings and recommendations which commanded a significant consensus among the members of the Commission. Each recommendation was approved by a majority of Commissioners.

What We Did Not Do

It is just as important for the reader to understand what the Commission did *not* do.

Our investigation centered on one accident at one nuclear power plant in the United States. While acting under the President's charge, we had to look at a large number of issues affecting many different organizations; there are vast related issues which were outside our charge, and which we could not possibly have examined in a 6-month investigation.

We did not examine the entire nuclear industry. (Although, through our investigation of the Nuclear Regulatory Commission, we have at least some idea of the standards being applied to it across the board.) We have not looked at the military applications of nuclear energy. We did not consider nuclear weapons proliferation. We have not dealt with the question of the disposal of radioactive waste or the dangers of the accumulation of waste fuel within nuclear power plants adjacent to the containment buildings. We made no attempt to examine the entire fuel cycle, starting with the mining of uranium. And, of course, we made no examination of the many other sources of radiation, both natural and manmade, that affect all of us.

We have not attempted to evaluate the relative risks involved in alternate sources of energy. We are aware of a number of studies that try to do this. We are also aware that some of these studies are subjects of continuing controversy.

We did not attempt to reach a conclusion as to whether, as a matter of public policy, the development of commercial nuclear power should be continued or should not be continued. That would require a much broader investigation, involving economic, environmental, and political considerations. We are aware that there are 72 operating reactors in the United States with a capacity of 52,000 megawatts of electric energy. An additional 92 plants have received construction permits and are in various stages of construction. If these are completed, they will roughly triple the present nuclear capacity to generate electricity. This would be a significant fraction of the total U.S. electrical generating capacity of some 600,000 megawatts. In addition, there are about 200 nuclear power plants in other countries throughout the world.

Therefore, the improvement of the safety of existing and planned nuclear power plants is a crucial issue. It is this issue that our report addresses, those changes that can and must be made as a result of the accident — the legacy of Three Mile Island.

Overview

In announcing the formation of the commission, the President of the United States said that the Commission "will make recommendations to enable us to prevent any future nuclear accidents." After a 6-month investigation of all factors surrounding the accident and contributing to it, the Commission has concluded that:

> *To prevent nuclear accidents as serious as Three Mile Island, fundamental changes will be necessary in the organization, procedures, and practices — and above all — in the attitudes of the Nuclear Regulatory Commission and, to the extent that the institutions we investigated are typical, of the nuclear industry.*

This conclusion speaks of *necessary* fundamental changes. We do not claim that our proposed recommendations are sufficient to assure the safety of nuclear power.

Given the nature of its Presidential mandate, its time limitations, and the complexity of both energy and comparative "risk-assessment" issues, this Commission has not undertaken to examine how safe is "safe enough" or the broader question of nuclear versus other forms of energy. The Commission's findings with respect to the accident and the regulation of the nuclear industry — particularly the current and potential state of public safety in the presence of nuclear power — have, we believe, implications that bear on the broad question of energy. But the ultimate resolution of the question involves the kind of economic, environmental, and foreign policy considerations that can only be evaluated through the political process.

Our findings do not, standing alone, require the conclusion that nuclear power is inherently too dangerous to permit it to continue and expand as a form of power generation. Neither do they suggest that the nation should move forward aggressively to develop additional commercial nuclear power. They simply state that if the country wishes, for larger reasons, to confront the risks that are inherently associated with nuclear power, fundamental changes are necessary if those risks are to be kept within tolerable limits.

We are very much aware that many other investigations into the accident are under way. There are several investigations by Congress, the NRC self-investigation, and a number of studies by the industry. Some will examine individual issues in much greater depth than we are able to do. And, no doubt, additional insights will emerge out of these various investigations. It is our hope that the results of our efforts may aid and accelerate the progress of the ongoing investigations, and help to bring about the required changes promptly.

Attitudes and Practices

Our investigation started out with an examination of the accident at Three Mile Island (TMI). This necessarily led us to look into the role played by the utility and its principal suppliers. With our in-depth investigation of the Nuclear Regulatory Commission (NRC), we gained a broader insight into the attitudes and practices that prevail in portions of the industry. However, we did not examine the industry in its totality.

Popular discussions of nuclear power plants tend to concentrate on questions of equipment safety. Equipment can and should be improved to add further safety to nuclear power plants, and some of our recommendations deal with this subject. But as the evidence accumulated, it became clear that the fundamental problems are people-related problems and not equipment problems.

When we say that the basic problems are people-related, we do not mean to limit this term to shortcomings of individual human beings — although those do exist. We mean more generally that our investigation has revealed problems with the "system" that manufactures, operates, and regulates nuclear power plants. There are structural problems in the various organizations, there are deficiencies in various processes, and there is a lack of communication among key individuals and groups.

We are convinced that if the only problems were equipment problems, this Presidential Commission would never have been created. The equipment was sufficiently good that, except for human failures, the major accident at Three Mile Island would have been a minor incident. But, wherever we looked, we found problems with the human beings who operate the plant, with the management that runs the key organization, and with the agency that is charged with assuring the safety of nuclear power plants.

In the testimony we received, one word occurred over and over again. That word is "mindset." At one of our public hearings, Roger Mattson, director of NRC's Division of Systems Safety, used that word five times within a span of 10 minutes. For example: "I think [the] mindset [was] that the operator was a force for good, that if you discounted him, it was a measure of conservatism." In other words, they concentrated on equipment, assuming that the presence of operators could only improve the situation — they would not be part of the problem.

After many years of operation of nuclear power plants, with no evidence that any member of the general public has been hurt, the belief that nuclear power plants are sufficiently safe grew into a conviction. One must recognize this to understand why many key steps that could have prevented the accident at Three Mile Island were not taken. The Commission is convinced that this attitude must be changed to one that says nuclear power is by its very nature potentially dangerous, and, therefore, one must continually question whether the safeguards already in place are sufficient to prevent major accidents. A comprehensive system is required in which equipment and human beings are treated with equal importance.

We note a preoccupation with regulations. It is, of course, the responsibility of the Nuclear Regulatory Commission to issue regulations to assure the safety of nuclear power plants. However, we are convinced that regulations alone cannot assure safety. Indeed, once regulations become as voluminous and complex as those regulations now in place, they can serve as a negative factor in nuclear safety. The regulations are so complex that immense efforts are required by the utility, by its suppliers, and by the NRC to assure that regulations are complied with. The satisfaction of regulatory requirements is equated with safety. This Commission believes that it is an absorbing concern with safety that will bring about safety — not just the meeting of narrowly prescribed and complex regulations.

We find a fundamental fault even with the existing body of regulations. While scientists and engineers have worried for decades about the safety of nuclear equipment, we find that the approach to nuclear safety had a major flaw. It was natural for the regulators and the industry to ask: "What is the worst kind of equipment failure that can occur?" Some potentially serious scenarios, such as the break of a huge pipe that carries the water cooling the nuclear reactor, were studied extensively and diligently, and were used as a basis for the design of plants. A preoccupation developed with such large-break accidents as did the attitude that if they could be controlled, we need not worry about the analysis of "less important" accidents.

Large-break accidents require extremely fast reaction, which therefore must be automatically performed by the equipment. Lesser accidents may develop much more slowly and their control may be dependent on the appropriate actions of human beings. This was the tragedy of Three Mile Island, where the equipment failures in the accident were significantly less dramatic than those that had been thoroughly analyzed, but where the results confused those who managed the accident. A potentially insignificant incident grew into the TMI accident, with severe damage to the reactor. Since such combinations of minor equipment failures are likely to occur much more often than the huge accidents, they deserve extensive and thorough study. In addition, they require operators and supervisors who have a thorough understanding of the functioning of the plant and who can respond to combinations of small equipment failures.

The most serious "mindset" is the preoccupation of everyone with the safety of equipment, resulting in the down-playing of the importance of the human element in nuclear power generation. We are tempted to say that while an enormous effort was expended to assure that safety-related equipment functioned as well as possible, and that there was backup equipment in depth, what the NRC and the industry have failed to recognize sufficiently is that the human beings who manage and operate the plants constitute an important safety system.

Causes of the Accident

Other investigations have concluded that, while equipment failures initiated the event, the fundamental cause of the accident was "operator error." It is pointed out that if the operators (or those who supervised them) had kept the emergency cooling systems on through the early stages of the accident, Three Mile Island would have been limited to a relatively insignificant incident. While we agree that this statement is true, we also feel that it does not speak to the fundamental causes of the accident.

Let us consider some of the factors that significantly contributed to operator confusion.

First of all, it is our conclusion that the training of TMI operators was greatly deficient. While training may have been adequate for the operation of a plant under normal circumstances, insufficient attention was paid to possible serious accidents. And the depth of understanding, even of senior reactor operators, left them unprepared to deal with something as confusing as the circumstances in which they found themselves.

Second, we found that the specific operating procedures, which were applicable to this accident, are at least very confusing and could be read in such a way as to lead the operators to take the incorrect actions they did.

Third, the lessons from previous accidents did not result in new, clear instructions being passed on to the operators. Both points are illustrated in the following case history.

A senior engineer of the Babcock & Wilcox [B&W] Company (suppliers of the nuclear steam system) noted in an earlier accident, bearing strong similarities to the one at Three Mile Island, that operators had mistakenly turned off the emergency cooling system. He pointed out that we were lucky that the circumstances under which this error was committed did not lead to a serious accident and warned that under other circumstances (like those that would later exist at Three Mile Island), a very serious accident could result. He urged, in the strongest terms, that clear instructions be passed on to the operators. This memorandum was written 13 months before the accident at Three Mile Island, but no new instructions resulted from it. The Commission's investigation of this incident, and other similar incidents within B&W and the NRC, indicates that the lack of understanding that led the operators to incorrect action existed both within the Nuclear Regulatory Commission and within the utility and its suppliers.

We find that there is a lack of "closure" in the system — that is, important safety issues are frequently raised and may be studied to some degree of depth, but are not carried through to resolution; and the lessons learned from these studies do not reach those individuals and agencies that most need to know about them. This was true in the B&W incident described above, it was true about various warnings within NRC that inappropriate operator actions could result in the case of certain small-break accidents, and it was true in several examples of questions raised in connection with licensing procedures that were not followed to their conclusion by the NRC staff.

There are many other examples mentioned in our report that indicate the lack of attention to the human factor in nuclear safety. We note only one more (a fourth) example. The control room, through which the operation of the TMI-2 plant is carried out, is lacking in many ways. The control panel is huge, with hundreds of alarms, and there are some key indicators placed in locations where the operators cannot see them. There is little evidence of the impact of modern information technology within the control room. In spite of this, this control room might be adequate for the normal operation of nuclear power plants.

However, it is seriously deficient under accident conditions. During the first few minutes of the accident, more than 100 alarms went off, and there was no system for suppressing the unimportant signals so that operators could concentrate on the significant alarms. Information was not presented in a clear and sufficiently understandable form; for example, although the pressure and temperature within the reactor coolant system were shown, there was no direct indication that the combination of pressure and temperature meant that the cooling water was turning into steam. Overall, little attention had been paid to the interaction between human beings and machines under the rapidly changing and confusing circumstances of an accident. Perhaps these design failures were due to a concentration on the large-break accidents — which do not allow time for significant operator action — and the design ignored the needs of operators during a slowly developing small-break (TMI-type) accident. While some of us may favor a complete modernization of control rooms, we are all agreed that a relatively few and not very expensive improvements in the control room could have significantly facilitated the management of the accident.

In conclusion, while the major factor that turned this incident into a serious accident was inappropriate operator action, many factors contributed to the action of the operators, such as deficiencies in their training, lack of clarity in their operating procedures, failure of organizations to learn the proper lessons from previous incidents, and deficiencies in the design of the control room. These shortcomings are attributable to the utility, to suppliers of equipment, and to the federal commission that regulates nuclear power. Therefore — whether or not operator error "explains" this particular case — given all the above deficiencies, we are convinced that an accident like Three Mile Island was eventually inevitable.

Severity of the Accident

Just how serious was the accident? Based on our investigation of the health effects of the accident, we conclude that in spite of serious damage to the plant, most of the radiation was contained and the actual release will have a negligible effect on the physical health of individuals. The major health effect of the accident was found to be mental stress.

The amount of radiation received by any one individual outside the plant was very low. However, even low levels of radiation may result in the later development of cancer, genetic defects, or birth defects among children who are exposed in the womb. Since there is no direct way of measuring the danger of low-level radiation to health, the degree of danger must be estimated indirectly. Different scientists make different assumptions about how this estimate should be made and, therefore, estimates vary. Fortunately, in this case the radiation doses were so low that we conclude that the overall health effects will be minimal. There will either be no case of cancer or the number of cases will be so small that it will never be possible to detect them. The same conclusion applies to the other possible health effects. The reasons for these conclusions are as follows.

An example of a projection derived for the total number of radiation-induced cancers among the population affected by the accident at TMI was 0.7. This number is an estimate of an average, such as the one that appears in the statement: "The average American family has 2.3 children."

In the case of TMI, what it really means is that each of some 2 million individuals living within 50 miles has a miniscule [*sic*] additional chance of dying of cancer, and when all of these minute probabilities are added up, they total 0.7. In such a situation, a mathematical law known as a Poisson distribution (named after a famous French mathematician) applies. If the estimated average is 0.7, then the actual probabilities for cancer deaths due to the accident work out as follows: There is a roughly 50 percent chance that there will be no additional cancer deaths, a 35 percent chance that one individual will die of cancer, a 12 percent chance that two people will die of cancer, and it is practically certain that there will not be as many as five cancer deaths.

Similar probabilities can be calculated for our various estimates. All of them have in common the following: It is entirely possible that not a single extra cancer death will result. And for all our estimates, it is practically certain that the additional number of cancer deaths will be less than 10.

Since a cancer caused by nuclear radiation is no different from any other cancer, additional cancers can only be determined statistically. We know from statistics on cancer deaths that among the more than 2 million people living within 50 miles of TMI, eventually some 325,000 people will die of cancer, for reasons having nothing to do with the nuclear power plant. Again, this number is only an estimate, and the actual figure could be as much as 1,000 higher or 1,000 lower. Therefore, there is no conceivable statistical method by which fewer than 10 additional deaths would ever be detected. Therefore, the accident may result in *no* additional cancer deaths or, if there were any, they would be so few that they could not be detected.

We found that the mental stress to which those living within the vicinity of Three Mile Island were subjected was quite severe. There were several factors that contributed to this stress. Throughout the first week of the accident, there was extensive speculation on just how serious the accident might turn out to be. At various times, senior officials of the NRC and the state government were considering the possibility of a major evacuation. There were a number of advisories recommending steps short of a full evacuation. Some significant fraction of the population in the immediate vicinity voluntarily left the region. NRC officials contributed to the raising of anxiety in the period from Friday to Sunday (March 30-April 1). On Friday, a mistaken interpretation of the release of a burst of radiation led some NRC officials to recommend immediate evacuation. And on Friday Governor Thornburgh advised pregnant women and preschool aged children within 5 miles of TMI to leave the area. On Saturday and Sunday, other NRC officials mistakenly believed that there was an imminent danger of an explosion of a hydrogen bubble within the reactor vessel, and evacuation was again a major subject of discussion.

We conclude that the most serious health effect of the accident was severe mental stress, which was short-lived. The highest levels of distress were found among those living within 5 miles of TMI and in families with preschool children.

There was very extensive damage to the plant. While the reactor itself has been brought to a "cold shutdown," there are vast amounts of radioactive material trapped within the containment and auxiliary buildings. The utility is therefore faced with a massive cleanup process that carries its own potential dangers to public health. The ongoing cleanup operation at TMI demonstrates that the plant was inadequately designed to cope with the cleanup of a damaged plant. The direct financial cost of the accident is enormous. Our best estimate puts it in a range of $1 to $2 billion, even if TMI-2 can be put back into operation. (The largest portion of this is for replacement power estimated for the next few years.) And since it may not be possible to put it back into operation, the cost could even be much larger.

The accident raised concerns all over the world and led to a lowering of public confidence in the nuclear industry and in the NRC.

From the beginning, we felt it important to determine not only how serious the actual impact of the accident was on public health, but whether we came close to a catastrophic accident in which a large number of people would have died. Issues that had to be examined were whether a chemical (hydrogen) or steam explosion could have ruptured the reactor vessel and containment building, and whether extremely hot molten fuel could have caused severe damage to the containment. The danger was never — and could *not* have been — that of a *nuclear* explosion (bomb).

We have made a conscientious effort to get an answer to this difficult question. Since the accident was due to a complex combination of minor equipment failures and major inappropriate human actions, we have asked the question: "What if one more thing had gone wrong?"

We explored each of several different scenarios representing a change in the sequence of events that actually took place. The greatest concern during the accident was that significant amounts of radioactive material (especially radioactive iodine) trapped within the plant might be released. Therefore, in each case, we asked whether the amount released would have been smaller or greater, and whether large amounts could have been released.

Some of these scenarios lead to a more favorable outcome than what actually happened. Several other scenarios lead to increases in the amount of radioactive iodine released, but still at levels that would not have presented a danger to public health. But we have also explored two or three scenarios whose precise consequences are much more difficult to calculate. They lead to more severe damage to the core, with additional melting of fuel in the hottest regions. These consequences are, surprisingly, independent of the age of the fuel.

Because of the uncertain physical condition of the fuel, cladding, and core, we have explored certain special and severe conditions that would, unequivocally, lead to a fuel-melting accident. In this sequence of events fuel melts, falls to the bottom of the vessel, melts through the steel reactor vessel, and finally, some fuel reaches the floor of the containment building below the reactor vessel where there is enough water to cover the molten fuel and remove some of the decay heat. To contain such an accident, it is necessary to continue removing decay heat for a period of many months.

At this stage we approach the limits of our engineering knowledge of the interactions of molten fuel, concrete, steel, and water, and even the best available calculations have a degree of uncertainty associated with them. Our calculations show that even if a meltdown occurred, there is a high probability that the containment building and the hard rock on which the TMI-2 containment building is built would have been able to prevent the escape of a large amount of radioactivity. These results derive from very careful calculations, which hold only insofar as our assumptions are valid. We cannot be absolutely certain of these results.

Some of the limits of this investigation were: (1) We have not examined possible consequences of operator error during or after the fuel melting process which might compromise the effectiveness of containment; (2) We have not examined the vulnerability of the various electrical and plumbing penetrations through the walls or the doorways for people and equipment; (3) The analysis was specific to the TMI-2 design and location (for example, the bedrock under the plant); (4) We recognize that we have only explored a limited number of alternatives to the question "What if...?" and, others may come up with a plausible scenario whose results would have been even more serious.

We strongly urge that research be carried out promptly to identify and analyze the possible consequences of accidents leading to severe core damage. Such knowledge is essential for coping with results of future accidents. It may also indicate weaknesses in present designs, whose correction would be important for the prevention of serious accidents.

These uncertainties have not prevented us from reaching an overwhelming consensus on corrective measures. Our reasoning is as follows: Whether in this particular case we came close to a catastrophic accident or not, this accident was too serious. Accidents as serious as TMI should not be allowed to occur in the future.

The accident got sufficiently out of hand so that those attempting to control it were operating somewhat in the dark. While today the causes are well understood, 6 months after the accident it is still difficult to know the precise state of the core and what the conditions are inside the reactor building. Once an accident reaches this stage, one that goes beyond well-understood principles, and puts those controlling the accident into an experimental mode (this happened during the first day), the uncertainty of whether an accident could result in major releases of radioactivity is too high. Adding to this the enormous damage to the plant, the expensive and potentially dangerous cleanup process that remains, and the great cost of the accident, we must conclude that — whatever worse could have happened — the accident had already gone too far to make it tolerable.

While throughout this entire document we emphasize that fundamental changes are necessary to prevent accidents as serious as TMI, we must not assume that an accident of this or greater seriousness cannot happen again, even if the changes we recommend are made. Therefore, in addition to doing everything to prevent such accidents, we must be fully prepared to minimize the potential impact of such an accident on public health and safety, should one occur in the future.

Handling of the Emergency

Another area of our investigation dealt with the questions of whether various agencies made adequate preparations for an emergency and whether their responses to the emergency were satisfactory. Our finding is negative on both questions.

We are disturbed both by the highly uneven quality of emergency plans and by the problems created by multiple jurisdictions in the case of a radiation emergency. Most emergency plans rely on prompt action at the local level to initiate a needed evacuation or to take other protective action. We found an almost total lack of detailed plans in the local communities around Three Mile Island. It is one of the many ironies of this event that the most relevant planning by local authorities took place during the accident. In an accident in which prompt defensive steps are necessary within a matter of hours, insufficient advance planning could prove extremely dangerous.

We favor the centralization of emergency planning and response in a single agency at the federal level with close coordination between it and state and local agencies. Such agencies would need expert input from many other organizations, but there should be a single agency that has the responsibility both for assuring that adequate planning takes place and for taking charge of the response to the emergency. This will require organizational changes, since the agencies now best organized to deal with emergencies tend to have most of their experience with such events as floods and storms, rather than with radiological events. And, insofar as radiological events require steps that go beyond those in a normal emergency, careful additional planning is needed.

A central concept in the current siting policy of the NRC is that reactors should be located in a "low population zone" (LPZ), an area around the plant in which appropriate protective action could be taken for the residents in the event of an accident. However, this concept is implemented in a strange, unnatural, and round-about manner. To determine the size of the LPZ, the utility calculates the amount of radiation released in a *very serious* hypothetical accident. Using geographical and meteorological data, the utility then calculates that area within which an individual would receive 25,000 millirems or more to the whole body, during the entire course of the accident. This area is the LPZ. The 25,000-millirem standard is an extremely large dose, many times more serious than that received by any individual during the entire TMI incident.

The LPZ approach has serious shortcomings. First, because of the extremely large dose by which its size is determined, the LPZs for many nuclear power plants are relatively small areas, 2 miles in the case of TMI. Second, if an accident as serious as the one used to calculate the LPZ were actually to occur, it is evident that many people living outside the LPZ would receive smaller, but still massive doses of radiation. Third, the TMI accident shows that the LPZ has little relevance to the protection of the public — the NRC itself was considering evacuation distances as far as 20 miles, even though the accident was far less serious than those postulated during siting. We have therefore concluded that the entire concept is flawed.

We recommend that the LPZ concept be abandoned in siting and in emergency planning. A variation of possible accidents should be considered during siting, particularly "smaller" accidents which have a higher probability of occurring. For each such accident, one should calculate probable levels of radiation releases at a variety of distances to decide the kinds of protective action that are necessary and feasible. Such protective actions may range from evacuation of an area near the plant, to the distribution of potassium iodide to protect the thyroid gland from radioactive iodine, to a simple instruction to people several miles from the plant to stay indoors for a specified period of time. Only such an analysis can predict the true consequences of a radiological incident and determine whether a particular site is suitable for a nuclear power plant. Similarly, emergency plans should have built into them a variety of responses to a variety of possible kinds of accidents. State and local agencies must be prepared with the appropriate response once information is available on the nature of an accident and its likely levels of release.

The response to the emergency was dominated by an atmosphere of almost total confusion. There was lack of communication at all levels. Many key recommendations were made by individuals who were not in possession of accurate information, and those who managed the accident were slow to realize the significance and implications of the events that had taken place. While we have attempted to address these shortcomings in our recommendations, it is important to reiterate the fundamental philosophy we stated above: One must do everything possible to prevent accidents of this seriousness, but at the same time assume that such an accident may occur and be prepared for response to the resulting emergency. The fact that too many individuals and organizations were not aware of the dimensions of serious accidents at nuclear power plants accounts for a great deal of the lack of preparedness and the poor quality of the response.

Public and Worker Health and Safety

We have identified a number of inadequacies with respect to procedures and programs to prevent or minimize hazards to health from radiation exposure from the operations of nuclear power plants. In setting standards for permissible levels of worker exposure to radioactivity, in plant siting decisions, and in other areas related to health, the NRC is not required to, and does not regularly seek, advice or review of its health-related guidelines and regulations from other federal agencies with radiation-related responsibilities in the area of health, for example the Department of Health, Education, and Welfare (HEW) or the Environmental Protection Agency (EPA). There is inadequate knowledge of the effects of low levels of ionizing radiation, and of other areas relating to regulation setting to protect worker and public health. In preparation for a possible emergency such as the accident at TMI-2, various federal agencies (NRC, Department of Energy, HEW, and EPA) have assigned responsibilities, but planning prior to the accident was so poor that ad hoc arrangements among these federal agencies had to be made to involve them and coordinate their activities.

The Commonwealth of Pennsylvania, its Bureau of Radiation Protection and Department of Health — agencies with responsibilities for public health — did not have adequate resources for dealing with radiation health programs related to the operation of TMI. The utility was not required to, and did not, keep a record on workers of the total work-related plus non-work-related (for example, medical or dental) radiation exposure.

We make recommendations with respect to improving the coordination and collaboration among federal and state agencies with radiation-related responsibilities in the health area. We believe more emphasis is required on research on the health effects of radiation to provide a sounder basis for guidelines and regulations related to worker and public health and safety. We believe that both the state and the utility have an opportunity and an obligation to establish more rigorous programs for informing workers and the public on radiation health-related issues and procedures to prevent adverse health effects of radiation. . . .

The Nuclear Regulatory Commission

We had a broad mandate from the President to investigate the Nuclear Regulatory Commission. When NRC was split off from the old Atomic Energy Commission, the purpose of the split was to separate the regulators from those who were promoting the peaceful uses of atomic energy. We recognize that the NRC has an assignment that would be difficult under any circumstances. But, we have seen evidence that some of the old promotional philosophy still influences the regulatory practices of the NRC. While some compromises between the needs of safety and the needs of an industry are inevitable, the evidence suggests that the NRC has sometimes erred on the side of the industry's inconvenience rather than carrying out its primary mission of assuring safety.

Two of the most important activities of NRC are its licensing function and its inspection and enforcement (I&E) activities. We found serious inadequacies in both.

In the licensing process, applications are only *required* to analyze "single-failure" accidents. They are not required to analyze what happens when two systems fail independently of each other, such as the event that took place at TMI. There is a sharp delineation between those components in systems that are "safety-related" and those that are not. Strict reviews and requirements apply to the former; the latter are exempt from most requirements — even though they can have an effect on the safety of the plant. We feel that this sharp either/or definition is inappropriate. Instead, there should be a system of priorities as to how significant various components and systems are for the overall safety of the plant. There seems to be a persistent assumption that plants can be made sufficiently safe to be "people-proof." Thus, not enough attention is paid to the training of operating personnel and operator procedures in the licensing process. And, finally, plants can receive an operating license with several safety issues still unresolved. This places such a plant into a regulatory "limbo" with jurisdiction divided between two different offices within NRC. TMI-2 was in this status at the time of the accident, 13 months after it received its operating license.

NRC's primary focus is on licensing and insufficient attention has been paid to the ongoing process of assuring nuclear safety. An important example of this is the case of "generic problems," that is, problems that apply to a number of different nuclear power plants. Once an issue is labeled "generic," the individual plant being licensed is not responsible for resolving the issue prior to licensing. That, in itself, would be acceptable, if there were a strict procedure within NRC to assure the timely resolution of generic problems, either by its own research staff, or by the utility and its suppliers. However, the evidence indicates that labeling of a problem as "generic" may provide a convenient way of postponing decision on a difficult question.

The old AEC attitude is also evident in reluctance to apply new safety standards to previously licensed plants. While we would accept a need for reasonable timetables for "backfitting," we did not find evidence that the need for improvement of older plants was systematically considered prior to Three Mile Island.

The existence of a vast body of regulations by NRC tends to focus industry attention narrowly on the meeting of regulations rather than on a systematic concern for safety. Furthermore, the nature of some of the regulations, in combination with the way rate bases are established for utilities, may in some instances have served as a deterrent for utilities or their suppliers to take the initiative in proposing measures for improved safety.

Previous studies of I&E have criticized this branch severely. Inspectors frequently fail to make independent evaluations or inspections. The manual according to which inspectors are supposed to operate is so voluminous that many inspectors do not understand precisely what they are supposed to do. There have been a number of incidents in which inspectors have had difficulty in getting their superiors to concentrate on serious safety issues. The analysis of reported incidents by licensees has tended to concentrate on equipment malfunction, and serious operator errors have not been focused on. Finally, while the statutory authority to impose fines is fairly limited, a previous study shows that I&E has made minimal use of even this authority.

Since in many cases NRC does not have the first-hand information necessary to enforce its regulations, it must rely heavily on the industry's own records for its inspection and enforcement activities. NRC accumulates vast amounts of information on the operating experience of plants. However, prior to the accident there was no *systematic* method of evaluating these experiences, and no systematic attempt to look for patterns that could serve as a warning of a basic problem.

NRC is vulnerable to the charge that it is heavily equipment-oriented, rather than people-oriented. Evidence for this exists in the weak and understaffed branch of NRC that monitors operator training, in the fact that inspectors who investigate accidents concentrate on what went wrong with the equipment and not on what operators may have done incorrectly, in the lack of attention to the quality of procedures provided for operators, and in an almost total lack of attention to the interaction between human beings and machines.

In addition to all the other problems with the NRC, we are extremely critical of the role the organization played in the response to the accident. There was a serious lack of communication among the commissioners, those who were attempting to make the decisions about the accident in Bethesda, the field offices, and those actually on site. This lack of communication contributed to the confusion of the accident. We are also skeptical whether the collegial mode of the five commissioners makes them a suitable body for the management of an emergency, and of the agency itself.

We found serious managerial problems within the organization. These problems start at the very top. It is not clear to us what the precise role of the five NRC commissioners is, and we have evidence that they themselves are not clear on what their role should be. The huge bureaucracy under the commissioners is highly compartmentalized with insufficient communication among the major offices. We do not see evidence of effective managerial guidance from the top, and we do not see evidence of some of the old AEC promotional philosophy in key officers below the top. The management problems have been made much harder by adoption of strict rules that prohibit the commissioners from talking with some of their key staff on issues involved in the licensing process; we believe that these rules have been applied in an unnecessarily severe form within this particular agency. The geographic spread, which places top management in Washington and most of the staff in Bethesda and Silver Spring, Maryland (and in other parts of the country), also inhibits the easy exchange of ideas.

We therefore conclude that there is no well-thought-out, integrated system for the assurance of nuclear safety within the current NRC.

We have found evidence of repeated in-depth studies and criticisms both from within the agency and from without, but we found very little evidence that these studies have resulted in significant improvement. This fact gives us particular concern for the future of the present NRC.

For all these reasons we recommend a total restructuring of the NRC. We recommend that it be an independent agency within the executive branch, headed by a single administrator, who is in every sense chief executive officer, to be chosen from outside NRC. The new administrator must be provided with the freedom to reorganize and to bring new blood into the restructured NRC's staff. This new blood could result in the change of attitudes that is vital for the solution of the problems of the nuclear industry.

We have also recommended a number of other organizational and procedural changes designed to make the new agency truly effective in assuring the safety of nuclear power plants. Included in these are an oversight committee to monitor the performance of the restructured NRC and mandatory review by HEW of radiation-related health issues.

The Utility

When the decision was made to make nuclear power available for the commercial generation of energy, it was placed into the hands of the existing electric utilities. Nuclear power requires management qualifications and attitudes of a very special character as well as an extensive support system of scientists and engineers. We feel that insufficient attention was paid to this by the General Public Utilities Corporation (GPU).

There is a divided system of decision-making within GPU and its subsidiaries. While the utility has legal responsibility for a wide range of fundamental decisions, from plant design to operator training, some utilities have to rely heavily on the expertise of their suppliers and on the Nuclear Regulatory Commission. Our report contains a number of examples where this divided responsibility, in the case of TMI, may have led to less than optimal design and operating practices. For example, we have received contradictory testimony on how the criteria under which the containment building isolates were selected. Similarly, the design of the control room seems to have been a compromise among of [*sic*] the utility, its parent company, the architect-engineer, and the nuclear steam system supplier (with very little attention from the NRC). But the clearest example of the shortcomings of divided responsibility is the area of operator training.

The legal responsibility for training operators and supervisors for safe operation of nuclear power plants rests with the utility. However, Met Ed [Metropolitan Edison], the GPU subsidiary which operates TMI, did not have sufficient expertise to carry out this training program without outside help. They, therefore, contracted with Babcock & Wilcox, supplier of the nuclear steam system, for various portions of this training program. While B&W has substantial expertise, they had no responsibility for the quality of the *total* training program, only for carrying out the contracted portion. And coordination between the training programs of the two companies was extremely loose. For example, the B&W instructors were not aware of the precise operating procedures in effect at the plant.

A key tool in the B&W training is a "simulator," which is a mock control console that can reproduce realistically events that happen within a power plant. The simulator differs in certain significant ways from the actual control console. Also, the simulator was not programmed, prior to March 28, to reproduce the conditions that confronted the operators during the accident.

We found that at both companies, those most knowledgeable about the workings of the nuclear power plant have little communication with those responsible for operator training, and therefore, the content of the instructional program does not lead to sufficient understanding of reactor systems.

It is our conclusion that the role that the NRC plays in monitoring operator training contributes little and may actually aggravate the problem. NRC has a limited staff for supervising operator licensing, and many of these do not have actual experience in power plants. Therefore, NRC activities are limited to the administration of fairly routine licensing examinations and the spotchecking of requalification exams and training programs. In evaluating the training of operators to carry out emergency procedures, NRC failed to recognize basic faults in the procedures in existence at TMI. Since the utility has the tendency of equating the passing of an NRC examination with the satisfactory training of operators, NRC may be perpetuating a level of mediocrity.

The way that NRC evaluates the safety of proposed plants during the licensing process has a most unfortunate impact on the way operators are trained. Since during the licensing process applicants for licenses concentrate on the consequences of single failures, there is no attempt in the training program to prepare operators for accidents in which two systems fail independently of each other.

There were significant deficiencies in the management of the TMI-2 plant. Shift foremen were burdened with paper work not relevant to supervision and could not adequately fulfill their supervisory roles. There was no systematic check on the status of the plant and the line-up of valves when shifts changed. Surveillance procedures were not adequately supervised. And there were weaknesses in the program of quality assurance and control.

We agree that the utility that operates a nuclear power plant must be held legally responsible for the fundamental design and procedures that assure nuclear safety. However, the analysis of this particular accident raises the serious question of whether all electric utilities automatically have the necessary technical expertise and managerial capabilities for administering such a dangerous high-technology plant. We, therefore, recommend the development of higher standards of organization and management that a company must meet before it is granted a license to operate a nuclear power plant.

The Transition

We recognize that even with the most expeditious process for implementation, recommendations as sweeping as ours will take a significant amount of time to implement. Therefore, the Commission had to face the issue of what should be done in the interim with plants that are currently operating and those that are going through the licensing process.

The Commission unanimously voted:

> Because safety measures to afford better protection for the affected population can be drawn from the high standards for plant safety recommended in this report, the NRC or its successor should, on a case-by-case basis, before issuing a new construction permit or operating license: (a) assess the need to introduce new safety improvements recommended in this report, and in NRC and industry studies; (b) review, considering the recommendations set forth in this report, the competency of the prospective operating licensee to manage the plant and the adequacy of its training program for operating personnel; and (c) condition licensing upon review and approval of the state and local emergency plans.

A Warning

During the time that our Commission conducted its investigation, a number of other reports appeared with recommendations for improved safety in nuclear power plants. While we are generally aware of the nature of these recommendations, we have not attempted a systematic analysis of them. Insofar as other agencies may have reached similar conclusions and proposed similar remedies, several groups arriving at the same conclusions should reinforce the weight of these conclusions.

But we have an overwhelming concern about some of the reports we have seen so far. While many of the proposed "fixes" seem totally appropriate, they do not come to grips with what we consider to be the basic problem. We have stated that fundamental changes must occur in organizations, procedures, and, above all, in the attitudes of people. No amount of technical "fixes" will cure this underlying problem. There have been many previous recommendations for greater safety for nuclear power plants, which have limited impact. What we consider crucial is whether the proposed improvements are carried out by the same organizations (unchanged), with the same kinds of practices and the same attitudes that were prevalent prior to the accident. As long as proposed improvements are carried out in a "business as usual" atmosphere, the fundamental changes necessitated by the accident at Three Mile Island cannot be realized.

We believe that we have conscientiously carried out the mandate of the President of the United States, within our limits as human beings and within the limitations of the time allowed us. We have not found a magic formula that would guarantee that there will be no serious future nuclear accidents. Nor have we come up with a detailed blueprint for nuclear safety. And our recommendations will require great efforts by others to translate them into effective plans.

Nevertheless, we feel that our findings and recommendations are of vital importance for the future of nuclear power. We are convinced that, unless portions of the industry and its regulatory agency undergo fundamental changes, they will over time totally destroy public confidence and, hence, *they* will be responsible for the elimination of nuclear power as a viable source of energy.

Commission Recommendations

The Commission found a number of inadequacies in the NRC and, therefore, proposes a restructuring of the agency. Because there is insufficient direction in the present statute, the President and Congress should consider incorporating many of the following measures in statutory form.

Agency Organization and Management. The Commission believes that as presently constituted, the NRC does not possess the organizational and management capabilities necessary for the effective pursuit of safety goals. The Commission recommends:

1. The Nuclear Regulatory Commission should be restructured as a new independent agency in the executive branch.

a. The present five-member commission should be abolished.

b. The new agency should be headed by a single administrator appointed by the President, subject to the advice and consent of the Senate, to serve a substantial term (not coterminous with that of the President) in order to provide an expectation of continuity, but at the pleasure of the President to allow removal when the President deems it necessary. The administrator should be a person from outside the present agency.

c. The administrator should have substantial discretionary authority over the internal organization and management of the new agency, and over personnel transfers from the existing NRC. Unlike the present NRC arrangement, the administrator and major staff components should be located in the same building or group of buildings.

d. A major role of the administrator should be assuring that offices within the agency communicate sufficiently so that research, operating experience, and inspection and enforcement affect the overall performance of the agency.

2. An oversight committee on nuclear reactor safety should be established. Its purpose would be to examine, on a continuing basis, the performance of the agency and of the nuclear industry in addressing and resolving important public safety issues associated with the construction and operation of nuclear power plants, and in exploring the overall risks of nuclear power.

a. The members of the committee, not to exceed 15 in number, should be appointed by the President and should include: persons conversant with public health, environmental protection, emergency planning, energy technology and policy, nuclear power generation, and nuclear safety; one or more state governors; and members of the general public.

b. The committee, assisted by its own staff, should report to the President and to Congress at least annually.

3. The Advisory Committee on Reactor Safeguards (ACRS) should be retained, in a strengthened role, to continue providing an independent technical check on safety matters. The members of the committee should continue to be part-time appointees; the Commission believes that the independence and high quality of the members might be compromised by making them full-time federal employees. The Commission recommends the following changes:

a. The staff of ACRS should be strengthened to provide increased capacity for independent analysis. Special consideration should be given to improving ACRS' capabilities in the field of public health.

b. The ACRS should not be required to review each license application. When ACRS chooses to review a license application, it should have the statutory right to intervene in hearings as a party. In particular, ACRS should be authorized to raise any safety issue in licensing proceedings, to give reasons and arguments for its views, and to require formal response by the agency to any submission it makes. Any member of ACRS should be authorized to appear and testify in hearings, but should be exempt from subpoena in any proceedings in which he has not previously appeared voluntarily or made an individual written submission.

c. ACRS should have similar rights in rulemaking proceedings. In particular, it should have the power to initiate a rulemaking proceeding before the agency to resolve any generic safety issue it identifies.

The Agency's Substantive Mandate. The new agency's primary statutory mission and first operating priority must be the assurance of safety in the generation of nuclear power, including safeguards of nuclear materials from theft, diversion, or loss. Accordingly, the Commission recommends the following:

4. Included in the agency's general substantive charge should be the requirement to establish and explain safety-cost trade-offs; where additional safety improvements are not clearly outweighed by cost considerations, there should be a presumption in favor of the safety change. Transfers of statutory jurisdiction from the NRC should be preceded by a review to identify and remove any unnecessary responsibilities that are not germane to safety. There should also be emphasis on the relationship of the new agency's safety activities to related activities of other agencies. . . .

a. The agency should be directed to upgrade its operator and supervisor licensing functions. These should include the accreditation of training institutions from which candidates for a license must graduate. Such institutions should be required to employ qualified instructors, to perform emergency and simulator training, and to include instruction in basic principles of reactor science, reactor safety, and the hazards of radiation. The agency should also set criteria for operator qualifications and background investigations, and strictly test license candidates for the particular power plant they will operate. The agency should periodically review and reaccredit all training programs and relicense individuals on the basis of current information on experience in reactor operations. . . .

b. The agency should be directed to employ a broader definition of matters relating to safety that considers thoroughly the full range of safety matters, including, but not limited to, those now identified as "safety-related" items, which currently receive special attention.

c. Other safety emphases should include:

(i) a systems engineering examination of overall plant design and performance, including interaction among major systems and increased attention to the possibility of multiple failures;

(ii) review and approval of control room design; the agency should consider the need for additional instrumentation and for changes in overall design to aid understanding of plant status, particularly for response to emergencies. . .

(iii) an increased safety research capacity with a broadly defined scope that includes issues relevant to public health. It is particularly necessary to coordinate research with the regulatory process in an effort to assure the maximum application of scientific knowledge in the nuclear power industry.

5. Responsibility and accountability for safe power plant operations, including the management of a plant during an accident, should be placed on the licensee in all circumstances. It is therefore necessary to assure that licensees are competent to discharge this responsibility. To assure this competency, and in light of our findings regarding Metropolitan Edison, we recommend that the agency establish and enforce higher organizational and manage-

ment standards for licensees. Particular attention should be given to such matters as the following: integration of decision-making in any organization licensed to construct or operate a plant; kinds of expertise that must be within the organization; financial capability; quality assurance programs; operator and supervisor practices and their periodic reevaluation; plant surveillance and maintenance practices; and requirements for the analysis and reporting of unusual events.

6. In order to provide an added contribution to safety, the agency should be required, to the maximum extent feasible, to locate new power plants in areas remote from concentrations of population. Siting determinations should be based on technical assessments of various classes of accidents that can take place, including those involving releases of low doses of radiation. . . .

7. The agency should be directed to include, as part of its licensing requirements, plans for the mitigation of the consequences of accidents, including the cleanup and recovery of the contaminated plant. The agency should be directed to review existing licenses and to set deadlines for accomplishing any necessary modifications. . . .

8. Because safety measures to afford better protection for the affected population can be drawn from the high standards for plant safety recommended in this report, the NRC or its successor should, on a case-by-case basis, before issuing a new construction permit or operating license:

a. assess the need to introduce new safety improvements recommended in this report, and in NRC and industry studies;

b. review, considering the recommendations set forth in this report, the competency of the prospective operating licensee to manage the plant and the adequacy of its training program for operating personnel; and

c. condition licensing upon review and approval of the state and local emergency plans.

Agency Procedures. The Commission believes that the agency must improve on prior performance in resolving generic and specific safety issues. Generic safety issues are considered in rulemaking proceedings that formulate new standards for categories of plants. Specific safety issues are considered in adjudicative proceedings that determine whether a particular plant should receive a license. Both kinds of safety issues are then dealt with in inspection and enforcement processes. The Commission believes that all of these agency functions need improvement, and accordingly recommends the following measures:

9. The agency's authorization to make general rules affecting safety should:

a. require the development of a public agenda according to which rules will be formulated;

b. require the agency to set deadlines for resolving generic safety issues;

c. require a periodic and systematic reevaluation of the agency's existing rules; and

d. define rulemaking procedures designed to create a process that provides a meaningful opportunity for participation by interested persons, that ensures careful consideration and explanation of rules adopted by the agency, and that includes appropriate provision for the application of new rules to existing plants. In particular, the agency should: accompany newly proposed rules with an analysis of the issues they raise and provide an indication of the technical materials that are relevant; provide a sufficient opportunity for interested persons to evaluate and rebut materials relied on by the agency or submitted by others; explain its final rules fully, including responses to principal comments by the public, the ACRS, and other agencies on proposed rules; impose when necessary special interim safeguards for operating plants affected by generic safety rulemaking; and conduct systematic reviews of operating plants to assess the need for retroactive application of new safety requirements.

10. Licensing procedures should foster early and meaningful resolution of safety issues before major financial commitments in construction can occur. In order to ensure that safety receives primary emphasis in licensing, and to eliminate repetitive consideration of some issues in that process, the Commission recommends the following:

a. Duplicative consideration of issues in several stages of one plant's licensing should, wherever possible, be reduced by allocating particular issues (such as the need for power) to a single stage of the proceedings.

b. Issues that recur in many licensings should be resolved by rulemaking.

c. The agency should be authorized to conduct a combined construction permit and operating license hearing whenever plans can be made sufficiently complete at the construction permit stage.

d. There should be provision for the initial adjudication of license applications and for appeal to a board whose decisions would not be subject to further appeal to the administrator. Both initial adjudicators and appeal boards should have a clear mandate to pursue any safety issue, whether or not it is raised by a party.

e. An Office of Hearing Counsel should be established in the agency. This office would not engage in the informal negotiations between other staff and applicants that typically precede formal hearings on construction permits. Instead, it would participate in the formal hearings as an objective party, seeking to assure that vital safety issues are addressed and resolved. The office should report directly to the administrator and should be empowered to appeal any adverse licensing board determination to the appeal board.

f. Any specific safety issue left open in licensing proceedings should be resolved by a deadline.

11. The agency's inspection and enforcement functions must receive increased emphasis and improved management, including the following elements:

a. There should be an improved program for the systematic safety evaluation of currently operating plants, in order to assess compliance with current requirements, to assess the need to make new requirements retroactive to older plants, and to identify new safety issues.

b. There should be a program for the systematic assessment of experience in operating reactors, with special emphasis on discovering patterns in abnormal occurrences. An overall quality assurance measurement and reporting system based on this systematic assessment shall be developed to provide: 1) a measure of the overall improvement or decline in safety, and 2) a base for specific programs aimed at curing deficiencies and improving safety. Licensees must receive clear instructions on reporting requirements and clear communications summarizing the lessons of experience at other reactors.

c. The agency should be authorized and directed to assess substantial penalties for licensee failure to report new "safety-related" information or for violations of rules defining practices or conditions already known to be unsafe.

d. The agency should be directed to require its enforcement personnel to perform improved inspection and auditing of licensee compliance with regulations and to conduct major and unannounced on-site inspections of particular plants.

e. Each operating licensee should be subject periodically to intensive and open review of its performance according to the requirements of its license and applicable regulations.

f. The agency should be directed to adopt criteria for revocation of licenses, sanctions short of revocation such as probationary status, and kinds of safety violations requiring immediate plant shutdown or other operational safeguards.

The Utility and Its Suppliers

1. To the extent that the industrial institutions we have examined are representative of the nuclear industry, the nuclear industry must dramatically change its attitudes toward safety and regulations. The Commission has recommended that the new regulatory agency prescribe strict standards. At the same time, the Commission recognizes that merely meeting the requirements of a government regulation does not guarantee safety. Therefore, the industry must also set and police its own standards of excellence to ensure the effective management and safe operation of nuclear power plants.

a. The industry should establish a program that specifies appropriate safety standards including those for management, quality assurance, and operating procedures and practices, and that conducts independent evaluations. The recently created Institute of Nuclear Power Operations, or some similar organization, may be an appropriate vehicle for establishing and implementing this program.

b. There must be a systematic gathering, review, and analysis of operating experience at all nuclear power plants coupled with an industry-wide international communications network to facilitate the speedy flow of this information to affected parties. If such experiences indicate the need for modifications in design or operation, such changes should be implemented according to realistic deadlines.

2. Although the Commission considers the responsibility for safety to be with the total organization of the plant, we recommend that each nuclear power plant company have a separate safety group that reports to high-level management. Its assignment would be to evaluate regularly procedures and general plant operations from a safety perspective; to assess quality assurance programs; and to develop continuing safety programs.

3. Integration of management responsibility at all levels must be achieved consistently throughout this industry. Although there may not be a single optimal management structure for nuclear power plant operation, there must be a single accountable organization with the requisite expertise to take responsibility for the integrated management of the design, construction, operation, and emergency response functions, and the organizational entities that carry them out. Without such demonstrated competence, a power plant operating company should not qualify to receive an operating license.

a. These goals may be obtained at the design stage by 1) contracting for a "turn-key" plant in which the vendor or architect-engineer contracts to supply a fully operational plant and supervises all planning, construction, and modification; or 2) assembling expertise capable of integrating the design process. In either case, it is critical that the knowledge and expertise gained during design and construction of the plant be effectively transferred to those responsible for operating the plant.

b. Clearly defined roles and responsibilities for operating procedures and practices must be established to ensure accountability and smooth communication.

c. Since, under our recommendations, accountability for operations during an emergency would rest on the licensee, the licensee must prepare clear procedures defining management roles and responsibilities in the event of a crisis.

4. It is important to attract highly qualified candidates for the positions of senior operator and operator supervisor. Pay scales should be high enough to attract such candidates.

5. Substantially more attention and care must be devoted to the writing, reviewing, and monitoring of plant procedures.

a. The wording of procedures must be clear and concise.

b. The content of procedures must reflect both engineering thinking and operating practicalities.

c. The format of procedures, particularly those that deal with abnormal conditions and emergencies, must be especially clear, including clear diagnostic instructions for identifying the particular abnormal conditions confronting the operators.

d. Management of both utilities and suppliers must insist on the early diagnosis and resolution of safety questions that arise in plant operations. They must also establish deadlines, impose sanctions for the failure to observe such deadlines, and make certain that the results of the diagnoses and any proposed procedural changes based on them are disseminated to those who need to know them.

6. Utility rate-making agencies should recognize that implementation of new safety measures can be inhibited by delay or failure to include the costs of such measures in the utility rate base. The Commission, therefore, recommends that state rate-making agencies give explicit attention to the safety implications of rate-making when they consider costs based on "safety-related" changes.

Training of Operating Personnel

1. The Commission recommends the establishment of agency-accredited training institutions for operators and immediate supervisors of operators. These institutions should have highly qualified instructors, who will maintain high standards, stress understanding of the fundamentals of nuclear power plants and the possible health effects of nuclear power, and who will train operators to respond to emergencies. . . .

a. These institutions could be national, regional, or specific to individual nuclear steam systems.

b. Reactor operators should be required to graduate from an accredited training institution. Exemption should be made only in cases where there is clear, documentary evidence that the candidate already has the equivalent training.

c. The training institutions should be subject to periodic review and reaccreditation by the restructured NRC.

d. Candidates for the training institute must meet entrance requirements geared to the curriculum.

2. Individual utilities should be responsible for training operators who are graduates of accredited institutions in the specifics of operating a particular plant. These operators should be examined and licensed by the restructured NRC, both at their initial licensing and at the relicensing stage. In order to be licensed, operators must pass every portion of the examination. Supervisors of operators, at a minimum, should have the same training as operators.

3. Training should not end when operators are given their licenses.

a. Comprehensive ongoing training must be given on a regular basis to maintain operators' level of knowledge.

b. Such training must be continuously integrated with operating experience.

c. Emphasis must be placed on diagnosing and controlling complex transients and on the fundamental understanding of reactor safety.

d. Each utility should have ready access to a control room simulator. Operators and supervisors should be required to train regularly on the simulator. The holding of operator licenses should be contingent on performance on the simulator.

4. Research and development should be carried out on improving simulation and simulation systems: 1) to establish and sustain a higher level of realism in the training of operators, including dealing with transients; and b) to improve the diagnostics and general knowledge of nuclear power plant systems.

Technical Assessment

1. Equipment should be reviewed from the point of view of providing information to operators to help them prevent accidents and to cope with accidents when they occur. Included might be instruments that can provide proper warning and diagnostic information; for example, the measurement of the full range of temperatures within the reactor vessel under normal and abnormal conditions, and indication of the actual position of valves. Computer technology should be used for the clear display for operators and shift supervisors of key measurements relevant to accident conditions, together with diagnostic warnings of conditions.

In the interim, consideration should be given to requiring, at TMI and similar plants, the grouping of these key measurements, including distinct warning signals on a single panel available to a specified operator and the providing of a duplicate panel of these key measurements and warnings in the shift supervisor's office.

2. Equipment design and maintenance inadequacies noted at TMI should be reviewed from the point of view of mitigating the consequences of accidents. Inadequacies noted in the following should be corrected: iodine filters, the hydrogen recombiner, the vent gas system, containment isolation, reading of water levels in the containment isolation, reading of water levels in the containment area, radiation monitoring in the containment building, and the capability to take and quickly analyze samples of containment atmosphere and water in various places. . . .

3. Monitoring instruments and recording equipment should be

provided to record continuously all critical plant measurements and conditions.

4. The Commission recommends that continuing in-depth studies should be initiated on the probabilities and consequences (on-site and off-site) of nuclear power plant accidents, including the consequences of meltdown.

a. These studies should include a variety of small-break loss-of-coolant accidents and multiple-failure accidents, with particular attention to human failures.

b. Results of these studies should be used to help plan for recovery and cleanup following a major accident.

c. From these studies may emerge desirable modifications in the design of plants that will help prevent accidents and mitigate their consequences. For example:

(i) Consideration should be given to equipment that would facilitate the controlled safe venting of hydrogen gas from the reactor cooling system.

(ii) Consideration should be given to overall gas-tight enclosure of the let-down/make-up system with the option of returning gases to the containment building.

d. Such studies should be conducted by the industry and other qualified organizations and may be sponsored by the restructured NRC and other federal agencies.

5. A study should be made of the chemical behavior and the extensive retention of radioactive iodine in water, which resulted in the very low release of radioiodine to the atmosphere in the TMI-2 accident. This information should be taken into account in the studies of the consequences of other small-break accidents.

6. Since there are still health hazards associated with the cleanup and disposal process, which is being carried out for the first time in a commercial nuclear power plant, the Commission recommends close monitoring of the cleanup process at TMI and of the transportation and disposal of the large amount of radioactive material. As much data as possible should be preserved and recorded about the conditions within the containment building so that these may be used for future safety analyses.

7. The Commission recommends that as a part of the formal safety assurance program, every accident or every new abnormal event be carefully screened, and where appropriate be rigorously investigated, to assess its implications for the existing system design, computer models of the system, equipment design and quality, operations, operator training, operator training simulators, plant procedures, safety systems, emergency measures, management, and regulatory requirements.

Worker and Public Health and Safety

1. The Commission recommends the establishment of expanded and better coordinated health-related radiation effects research. This research should include, but not be limited to:

a. biological effects of low levels of ionizing radiation;

b. acceptable levels of exposure to ionizing radiation for the general population and for workers;

c. development of methods of monitoring and surveillance, including epidemiologic surveillance to monitor and determine the consequences of exposure to radiation of various population groups, including workers;

d. development of approaches to mitigate adverse health effects of exposure to ionizing radiation; and

e. genetic or environmental factors that predispose individuals to increased susceptibility to adverse effects.

This effort should be coordinated under the National Institutes of Health — with an interagency committee of relevant federal agencies to establish the agenda for research efforts — including the commitment of a portion of the research budget to meet the specific needs of the restructured NRC.

2. To ensure the best available review of radiation-related health issues, including reactor siting issues, policy statements or regulations in that area of the restructured NRC should be subject to mandatory review and comment by the Secretary of the Department of Health and Human Services. A time limit for the review should be established to assure such review is performed in an expeditious manner.

3. The Commission recommends, as a state and local responsibility, an increased program for educating health professionals and emergency response personnel in the vicinity of nuclear power plants.

4. Utilities must make sufficient advance preparation for the mitigation of emergencies:

a. Radiation monitors should be available for monitoring of routine operations as well as accident levels.

b. The emergency control center for health-physics operations and the analytical laboratory to be used in emergencies should be located in a well-shielded area supplied with uncontaminated air.

c. There must be a sufficient health-related supply of instruments, respirators, and other necessary equipment for both routine and emergency conditions.

d. There should be an adequate maintenance program for all such health-related equipment.

5. An adequate supply of the radiation protective (thyroid blocking) agent, potassium iodide for human use, should be available regionally for distribution to the general population and workers affected by a radiological emergency.

Emergency Planning and Response

1. Emergency plans must detail clearly and consistently the actions public officials and utilities should take in the event of off-site radiation doses resulting from the release of radioactivity. Therefore the Commission recommends that:

a. Before a utility is granted an operating license for a new nuclear power plant, the state within which that plant is to be sited must have an emergency response plan reviewed and approved by the Federal Emergency Management Agency (FEMA). The agency should assess the criteria and procedures now used for evaluating state and local government plans and for determining their ability to activate the plans. FEMA must assure adequate provision, where necessary, for multi-state planning.

b. The responsibility at the federal level for radiological emergency planning, including planning for coping with radiological releases, should rest with FEMA. In this process, FEMA should consult with other agencies, including the restructured NRC and the appropriate health and environmental agencies. . .

c. The state must effectively coordinate its planning with the utility and with local officials in the area where the plant is to be located.

d. States with plants already operating must upgrade their plans to the requirements to be set by FEMA. Strict deadlines must be established to accomplish this goal.

2. Plans for protecting the public in the event of off-site radiation releases should be based on technical assessment of various classes of accidents that can take place at a given plant.

a. No single plan based on a fixed set of distances and a fixed set of responses can be adequate. Planning should involve the identification of several different kinds of accidents with different possible radiation consequences. For each scenario, there should be clearly identified criteria for the appropriate responses at various distances, including instructing individuals to stay indoors for a period of time, providing special medication, or ordering an evacuation.

b. Similarly, response plans should be keyed to various possible scenarios and activated when the nature and potential hazard of a given accident has been identified.

c. Plans should exist for protecting the public at radiation levels lower than those currently used in NRC-prescribed plans.

d. All local communities should have funds and technical support adequate for preparing the kinds of plans described above.

3. Research should be expanded on medical means of protecting the public against various levels and types of radiation. This research should include exploration of appropriate medications that can protect against or counteract radiation.

4. State emergency plans should include provision for creation of local broadcast media networks for emergencies that will supply timely and accurate information. Arrangements should be made to make available knowledgeable briefers to go on the air to clear up rumors and explain conditions at the plant. Communications between state officials, the utility, and the network should be prearranged to handle the possibility of an evacuation announcement.

5. The Commission recommends that the public in the vicinity of a nuclear power plant be routinely informed of local radiation measurements that depart appreciably from normal background radiation, whether from normal or abnormal operation of the nuclear power plant, from a radioactivity cleanup operation such as that at TMI-2, or from other sources.

4. If emergency planning and response to a radiation-related emergency is to be effective, the public must be better informed about nuclear power. The Commission recommends a program to educate the public on how nuclear power plants operate, on radiation and its health effects, and on protective actions against radiation. Those who would be affected by such emergency planning must have clear information on actions they would be required to take in an emergency.

5. Commission studies suggest that decision-makers may have over-estimated the human costs, in injury and loss of life, in many mass evacuation situations. The Commission recommends study into the human costs of radiation-related mass evacuation and the extent, if any, to which the risks in radiation-related evacuations differ from other types of evacuations. Such studies should take into account the effects of improving emergency planning, public awareness of such planning, and costs involved in mass evacuations.

6. Plans for providing federal technical support, such as radiological monitoring, should clearly specify the responsibilities of the various support agencies and the procedures by which those agencies provide assistance. Existing plans for the provision of federal assistance, particularly the Radiological Assistance Plan and the various memoranda of understanding among the agencies, should be reexamined and revised by the appropriate federal authorities in the light of the experience of the TMI accident, to provide for better coordination and more efficient federal support capability.

The Public's Right to Information

1. Federal and state agencies, as well as the utility, should make adequate preparation for a systematic public information program so that in time of a radiation-related emergency, they can provide timely and accurate information to the news media and the public in a form that is understandable. There should be sufficient division of briefing responsibilities as well as availability of informed sources to reduce confused and inaccurate information. The Commission therefore recommends:

a. Since the utility must be responsible for the management of the accident, it should also be primarily responsible for providing information on the status of the plant to the news media and to the public; but the restructured NRC should also play a supporting role and be available to provide background information and technical briefings.

b. Since the state government is responsible for decisions concerning protective actions, including evacuations, a designated state agency should be charged with issuing all information on this subject. This agency is also charged with the development of and dissemination of accurate and timely information on off-site radiation doses resulting from appropriate sources.... This agency should also set up the machinery to keep local officials fully informed of developments and to coordinate briefings to discuss any federal involvement in evacuation matters.

2. The provision of accurate and timely information places special responsibilties on the official sources of this information. The effort must meet the needs of the news media for information but without compromising the ability of operating personnel to manage the accident. The Commission therefore recommends that:

a. Those who brief the news media must have direct access to informed sources of information.

b. Technical liaison people should be designated to inform the briefers and to serve as a resource for the news media.

c. The primary official news sources should have plans for the prompt establishment of press centers reasonably close to the site. These must be properly equipped, have appropriate visual aids and reference materials, and be staffed with individuals who are knowledgeable in dealing with the news media. These press centers must be operational promptly upon the declaration of a general emergency or its equivalent.

3. The coverage of nuclear emergencies places special responsibilities on the news media to provide accurate and timely information. The Commission therefore recommends that:

a. All major media outlets (wire services, broadcast networks, news magazines, and metropolitan daily newspapers) hire and train specialists who have more than a passing familiarity with reactors and the language of radiation. All other news media, regardless of their size, located near nuclear power plants should attempt to acquire similar knowledge or make plans to secure it during an emergency.

b. Reporters discipline themselves to place complex information in a context that is understandable to the public and that allows members of the public to make decisions regarding their health and safety.

c. Reporters educate themselves to understand the pitfalls in interpreting answers to "what if" questions. Those covering an accident should have the ability to understand uncertainties expressed by sources of information and probabilities assigned to various possible dangers.

Bibliography

Books

American Chemical Society. *Cleaning Our Environment, The Chemical Basis For Action.* Washington, D.C., 1969.

Ashford, Nicholas. *Crisis in the Workplace: Occupational Disease and Injury.* Cambridge, Mass.: MIT Press, 1976.

Axelrod, Regina S., ed. *Environment, Energy, Public Policy: Toward a Rational Future.* Lexington, Mass.: Lexington Books, 1981.

Breuer, Georg. *Air In Danger: Ecological Perspectives of the Atmosphere.* New York: Cambridge University Press, 1980.

Brown, Michael H. *Laying Waste: The Poisoning of America by Toxic Chemicals.* New York: Pantheon, 1980.

Calabrese, Edward J. *Nutrition and Environmental Health: The Influence of Nutritional Status on Pollutant Toxicity and Carcinogenicity.* New York: John Wiley, 1981.

Carson, Rachel. *Silent Spring.* Greenwich, Conn.: Fawcett Publications, 1962.

Coates, Gary J. *Resettling America: Energy, Ecology and the Community.* Andover, Mass.: Brick House Publishing, 1981.

Congressional Quarterly Inc. *Health Policy, The Legislative Agenda.* Washington, D.C., 1980.

Cordia, Louis F. *OSHA and Environmental Health.* Washington, D.C.: The Heritage Foundation, 1980.

Courrier, Kathleen. *Life After '80: Environmental Choices We Can Live With.* Andover, Mass.: Brick House Publishing, 1980.

Dubos, René. *The Wooing of Earth: New Perspectives on Man's Use of Nature.* New York: Charles Scribner's, 1981.

Duffus, John H. *Environmental Toxicology.* New York: John Wiley, 1980.

Eckholm, Erik P. *The Picture of Health: Environmental Sources of Disease.* New York: W. W. Norton, 1977.

Editorial Research Reports. *Earth, Energy and Environment.* Washington, D.C.: Congressional Quarterly Inc., 1977.

Editorial Research Reports. *National Health Issues.* Washington, D.C.: Congressional Quarterly Inc., 1977.

Egginton, Joyce. *The Poisoning of Michigan.* New York: W.W. Norton, 1980.

Epstein, Samuel S. *The Politics of Cancer.* San Francisco: Sierra Club Books, 1978.

FitzPatrick, Malcolm S. *Environmental Health Planning: Community Development Based on Environmental and Health Precepts.* Cambridge, Mass.: Ballinger, 1978.

Fuller, John G. *The Poison That Fell From the Sky.* New York: Random House, 1977.

Keough, Carol. *Water Fit To Drink.* Emmaus, Pa.: Rodale Press, 1980.

Glasstone, Samuel and Jordan, Walter H. *Nuclear Power and Its Environmental Effects.* La Grange Park, Ill.: American Nuclear Society, 1980.

Makower, Joel. *Office Hazards: How Your Job Can Make You Sick.* Washington, D.C.: Tilden Press, 1981.

Marcus, Alfred A. *Promise and Performance: Choosing and Implementing An Environmental Policy.* Westport, Conn.: Greenwood Press, 1980.

Nader, Ralph and Brownstein, Ronald. *Who's Poisoning America: Corporate Polluters In the Chemical Age.* San Francisco, Calif.: Sierra Club, 1981.

Pelham, Ann. *Energy Policy.* Washington, D.C.: Congressional Quarterly Inc., 1981.

Pennsylvania Governor's Committee on Three Mile Island. *Report, February 26, 1980.* Harrisburg, Pa., 1980.

Pilat, J. F. *Ecological Politics: The Rise of the Green Movement.* Beverly Hills, Calif.: Sage Publications, 1980.

Ridker, Ronald G. and Watson, William D. *To Choose a Future: Resources and Environment Consequences of Alternative Growth Paths.* Baltimore, Md.: Johns Hopkins, 1980.

Sandbach, Francis. *Environment, Ideology and Policy.* Montclair, N.J.: Allanheld, Osmun, 1980.

Sell, Nancy J. *Industrial Pollution Control: Issues and Techniques.* New York: Van Nostrand Reinhold, 1981.

Siebert, Horst, *Economics of the Environment.* Lexington, Mass.: Lexington Books, 1981.

Stephens, Mark. *Three Mile Island.* New York: Random House, 1981.

Stever, Donald W. Jr. *Seabrook and the Nuclear Regulatory Commission: The Licensing of a Nuclear Plant.* Hanover, N.H.: University Press of New England, 1980.

Turner, James S. *The Chemical Feast.* New York: Grossman, 1970.

Union of Concerned Scientists. *The Nuclear Fuel Cycle.* Cambridge, Mass.: MIT Press, 1975.

Verrett, Jacqueline and Carper, Jean. *Eating May Be Hazardous To Your Health.* New York: Anchor Press, 1975.

Whiteside, Thomas. *The Pendulum and The Toxic Cloud: The Course of Dioxin Contamination.* New Haven, Conn.: Yale University Press, 1979.

Wilson, Richard and others. *Health Effects of Fossil Fuel Burning: Assessment and Mitigation.* Cambridge, Mass.: Ballinger, 1980.

Articles

Ackerman, Bruce A. and Hassler, William T. "Beyond the New Deal: Coal and the Clean Air Act." *Yale Law Review,* July 1980, pp. 1466-1571.

"Agent Orange: A Problem of Exposure." *Science News,* January 26, 1980, p. 55.

Alexander, Tom. "The Hazardous-Waste Nightmare." *Fortune,* April 21, 1980, pp. 52-54.

Alexander, Tom. "A Simpler Path to a Cleaner Environment." *Fortune,* May 1981, pp. 234-236.

"Allocating the Cost of Hazardous Waste Disposal." *Harvard Law Review,* January 1981, pp. 584-604.

"Anger At Love Canal." *America,* June 7, 1980, p. 472.

Beck, E. C. "Coping With Ground Water Contamination." *USA Today,* March 1981, pp. 44-47.

Beecher, J. L. and Fossa, A. S. "Problem With Toxic Wastes," *Conservationist,* March/April 1980, pp. 28-31.

Beyea, Jan. "Emergency Planning for Reactor Accidents." *Bulletin of the Atomic Scientists,* December 1980, pp. 40-45.

Boraiko, A. A. "Pesticide Dilemma." *National Geographic,* February 1980, pp. 144-183.

Broad, William J. "Export of Hazardous Goods Raises Congressional Ire." *Science,* March 27, 1981, pp. 1401-1405.

Brown, Michael. "Drums of Death." *Audubon,* July 1980, pp. 120-133.

Cahan, Vicky. "Overhaul That Could Give OSHA Life Under Reagan." *Business Week,* January 19, 1981, pp. 88-89.

Campbell, William A. "The 1977 Clean Air Act Amendments: Their Potential Impact on Economic Growth." *Popular Government,* Spring 1980, pp. 21-25.

Carter, Luther J. "Global 2000 Report: Vision of a Gloomy World." *Science,* August 1, 1980, pp. 575-576.

Carter, Luther J. "New Call For Abolishing the NRC." *Science,* February 8, 1980, p. 634.

Chapin, Georganne and Wasserstrom, Robert. "Bitter Harvest." *Progressive,* March 1980, pp. 31-34.

Del Duca, Patrick. "The Clean Air Act: A Realistic Assessment of Cost-Effectiveness." *Harvard Environmental Law Review,* No. 1, 1981, pp. 184-203.

Doughlass, E. "DOE's Hazardous Waste." *Nation,* December 27, 1980, p. 689.

"Earth's Endangered Ozone." *Futurist,* February 1980, pp. 74-75.

Eaton, Scott F. "Legal Consequences In New Hampshire from Asbestos Contamination of Drinking Water by Asbestos Cement Pipe." *IDEA,* No. 2, 1980.

Fine, John C. "Toxic Waste Dangers." *Water Spectrum,* Winter 80/81, pp. 23-30.

Ford, Daniel. "Reporter At Large: Three Mile Island." *The New Yorker,* April 6 and 13, 1981, pp. 49-50 and 46-48.

Frankel, David R. "Nuclear Waste Management." *Ecology Law Quarterly,* No. 4, 1980, pp. 790-800.

Friedland, Steven I. "The New Hazardous Waste Management System: Regulation of Wastes or Wasted Regulations?" *Harvard Environmental Law Review,* No. 1, 1981, pp. 89-129.

Gilmour, John. "Hazardous and Toxic Waste Disposal." *University of Virginia Newsletter,* September 1980, pp. 1-4.

Golay, M. W. "How Prometheus Came to be Bound: Nuclear Regulation In America." *Technology Review,* June/July 1980, pp. 28-34.

Grugiel, Fred S. and Zarillo, Anthony J. "Three Mile Island: The New Jersey Regulatory Response." *Public Utilities Fortnightly,* December 18, 1980, pp. 23-28.

"Have Three Mile Island's Lessons Been Learned?" *Economist,* February 2, 1980, pp. 79-80.

Hirsch, Allan. "The Impact of Ocean Pollution." *EPA,* March 1981, pp. 16-19.

Holden, Constance. "Love Canal Residents Under Stress." *Science,* June 13, 1980, pp. 1242-1244.

Holdren, John P. "Environmental Liabilities of Nuclear Power." *Bulletin of the Atomic Scientists,* January 1980, pp. 31-32.

Hughey, Ann. "Cleaning the Air." *Forbes,* November 10, 1980, pp. 45-46.

Jackson, Benjamin. "Auto Pollution: The Remaining Job." *EPA,* June 1980, pp. 22-23.

Janerich, Dwight T. and others. "Cancer Incidences In the Love Canal Area." *Science,* June 19, 1981, pp. 1404-1407.

Kerr, Richard A. "Is all Acid Rain Polluted?" *Science,* May 29, 1981, p. 1014.

Kerr, Richard A. "There's More to Acid Rain Than Rain." *Science,* February 13, 1981, pp. 692-693.

Kesnikoff, M. "Nuclear Wastes, the Myths and the Realities." *Sierra,* July/August 1980, pp. 30-34.

Krugman, Hartmut and Von Hippel, Frank. "Radioactive Waste: The Problem of Plutonium." *Science,* October 17, 1980, pp. 319-321.

Lehman, Andrew T. "Implications of the Resource Conservation and Recovery Act of 1976, Public Law 94-580." *Environmental Comment,* September 1980, pp. 4-7.

Lewis, Harold. "Safety of Fission Reactors." *Scientific American,* March 1980, pp. 53-65.

"Love Canal: A Federal Emergency." *Science News,* May 31, 1980, p. 340.

Luoma, Jon R. "Troubled Skies, Troubled Waters." *Audubon,* November 1980, pp. 88-111.

Mendeloff, J. "Reducing Occupational Health Risks: Uncertain Effects and Unstated Benefits." *Technology Review,* May 1980, pp. 66-68.

"More Evidence on Three Mile Island." *Consumers Research Magazine,* July 1980, pp. 15-16.

Moss, Ralph W. "Look What's Back In Our Hotdogs." *Nation,* February 17, 1981, pp. 139-141.

Nader, Ralph and Brownstein, Ronald. "Beyond Love Canal." *Progressive,* May 1980, pp. 28-31.

Navarro, Peter. "The Politics of Air Pollution." *Public Interest,* Spring 1980, pp. 36-44.

"New Age of Coal: A Health Problem for the '80s?" *Current Health,* April 1980, pp. 20-21.

"Nuclear Accidents: The 10-Minute Myth." *Science News,* July 19, 1980, p. 37.

O'Connell, S. M. "Shooting Arrows Into the Air Act." *International Wildlife,* March/April 1981, p. 28.

O'Donnell, Francis J. "Turbulence Ahead for the Clean Air Act; But Its Skies Have Never Been Clear." *Progressive,* May 1981, pp. 29-31.

"Oil Spills and Cleanup Bills: Federal Recovery of Oil Spill Cleanup Costs." *Harvard Law Review,* June 1980, pp. 1761-1785.

Ostrander, Judy L. and Masters, Lorelie S. "Nuclear Waste Management: The Need for Immediate Legislative Reform." *Journal of Legislation,* 1980, pp. 78-92.

"Other Pollution: Noise." *Current Health,* January 1980, pp. 4-15.

Perlam, Christine. "EPA's Role At Three Mile Island." *EPA,* October 1980, pp. 18-20.

Piller, C. "Toxic Time Bombs In the Factory." *Nation,* April 4, 1981, pp. 395-398.

Pratt, John S. "Catastrophic Nuclear Power Reactor Accidents: An Issue of Safety, A Question of Record." *Georgia Law Review,* Winter 1980, pp. 265-298.

Quinlan, Martin. "The Way Towards Clean Seas." *Petroleum Economist,* February 1980, pp. 55-57.

Randal, Judith. "Going After Nuclear Offenders." *Change,* February/March 1980, pp. 52-53.

Reinhardt, W. G. "Nuclear Wastes: Where Do They Go?" *Sciquest,* May/June 1980, pp. 12-17.

Rosbe, William L. "RCRA and Regulation of Hazardous and Nonhazardous Solid Wastes: Closing the Circle of Environmental Control." *Business Lawyer,* July 1980, pp. 1519-1543.

Shaw, Jane S. and Canape, Charlene. "Is the EPA Saddled With More Than It Can Handle?" *Business Week,* May 26, 1980, p. 148.

Simon, Anne W. "Spill of Missed Opportunity." *Nation,* July 19-26, 1980, pp. 68-69.

Smith, R. Jeffrey. "The Fight Over the Clean Air Begins." *Science,* March 20, 1981, pp. 1328-1330.

Smith, R. Jeffrey. "OSHA Shifts Direction on Health Standards." *Science,* June 26, 1981, pp. 1482-1483.

Solomon, Norman. "Nuclear Big Brother." *Progressive,* January 1980, pp. 14-21.

Solomon, Norman. "Nuclear Burial Ground: An Industry Suffocating In Its Garbage." *Progressive,* April 1979, pp. 33-39.

Speth, Gus. "Our Nation's Water." *Current,* October 1980, pp. 20-23.

Starr, Roger. "Three Mile Shadow." *Commentary,* October 1980, pp. 15-16.

Stief, William. "Agent Orange Disaster." *Progressive,* February 1980, p. 8.

Stoffel, Jennifer. "Acid Rain Clouds Coal's Future." *State Government News,* June 1980, pp. 3-4.
Stoler, P. "Is Clean Water a Thing of the Past?" *Sierra,* March/April 1981, pp. 14-15.
Sun, Marjorie. "White Sands, Warm Winds, and Toxic Wastes?" *Science,* January 23, 1981, p. 367.
Sweet, William. "Air Pollution Control: Progress and Prospects." *Editorial Research Reports,* November 21, 1980, pp. 843-862.
Trauberman, J. "Superfund." *Environment,* March 1981, pp. 25-29.
Tucker, William. "Marketing Pollution." *Harper's,* May 1981, pp. 31-34.
Walker, Richard and Storper, Michael. "Erosion of the Clean Air Act of 1970: A Study in the Failure of Government Regulation and Planning." *Boston College Environmental Affairs Law Review,* No. 2, 1978, pp. 189-257.
Walton, S. "Noise Pollution: Environmental Battle of the 1980s." *Bioscience,* March 1980, pp. 205-207.
Wiegner, Kathleen K. "Beyond Asbestos." *Forbes,* May 12, 1980, pp. 122-127.
Weir, David and Shapiro, Mark. "Circle of Poison." *Nation,* November 25, 1980, p. 497.
Wolf, Sidney M. "Public Opposition to Hazardous Waste Sites." *Boston College Environmental Affairs Law Review,* No. 3, 1980, pp. 463-540.
Zacovic, B. "Deadly Spray." *Progressive,* August 1980, pp. 31-33.

Documents

Council on Environmental Quality 11th Annual Report to Congress. Washington, D.C.: Government Printing Office, 1981.
Council on Environmental Quality and the Department of State. *Global Future: Time to Act: Report to the President on Global Resources, Environment and Population.* Washington, D.C.: Government Printing Office, 1981.
Council On Environmental Quality and the Department of State. *The Global 2000 Report to the President: Entering the Twenty-First Century.* Washington, D.C.: Government Printing Office, 1980.
Council on Environmental Quality. *Contamination of Ground Water by Toxic Organic Chemicals.* Washington, D.C.: Government Printing Office, 1981.
National Commission on Air Quality. *To Breathe Clean Air.* Washington, D.C.: Government Printing Office, 1981.
President's Commission, a National Agenda for the Eighties. *Energy, Natural Resources and the Environment in the Eighties.* Washington, D.C.: Government Printing Office, 1980.
U. S. Congress. House. Committee on Interstate and Foreign Commerce. Subcommittee on Health and the Environment. *Clean Air Act Oversight-1980: Hearings, June 16, 1980.* 96th Cong., 2d sess. Washington, D.C.: Government Printing Office, 1980.
U. S. Congress. House. Committee on Interstate and Foreign Commerce. Subcommittee on Oversight and Investigations. *Acid Rain: Hearings, February 26, 27, 1980.* 96th Cong., 2d sess. Washington, D.C.: Government Printing Office, 1980.
U. S. Congress. House. Committee on Interstate and Foreign Commerce. Subcommittee on Oversight and Investigations. *Hazardous Waste Disposal: Hearings, March 21, 22, April 5, 10, May 16, 23, 30; June 1, 4, 5, 15, 18, 19, 1979.* 96th Cong., 1st sess. Washington, D.C.: Government Printing Office, 1980.
U. S. Congress. House. Committee on Interstate and Foreign Commerce. *Hazardous Waste Disposal: Our Number One Environmental Problem: Hearings June 9, 1980.* 96th Cong., 2d sess. Washington, D.C.: Government Printing Office, 1981.
U. S. Congress. House. Committee on Interstate and Foreign Commerce. Subcommittee on Oversight and Investigations. *Love Canal: Health Studies and Relocation: Hearings, May 22, 1980.* 96th Cong. 2d sess. Washington, D.C.: Government Printing Office, 1980.
U. S. Congress. House. Committee on Public Works and Transportation. Subcommittee on Surface Transportation. *Transportation of Hazardous Materials Through City Streets: Hearings, May 27, 1980.* 96th Cong., 2d sess. Washington, D.C.: Government Printing Office, 1981.
U. S. Congress. House. Committee on Public Works and Transportation. Subcommittee on Water Resources. *Hazardous Chemicals Under the Federal Water Pollution Control Act: Hearings, April 15-17, 1980.* 96th Cong., 2d sess. Washington, D.C.: Government Printing Office, 1981.
U. S. Congress. House. Committee on Science and Technology. Subcommittee on Energy Research and Production. *Nuclear Power Plant Safety After Three Mile Island: Report, March 1980.* 96th Cong. 2d sess. Washington, D.C.: Government Printing Office, 1980.
U. S. Congress. House. Committee on Science and Technology. Subcommittee on Natural Resources and Environment. *Three Mile Island Nuclear Plant Accident: Hearings, June 2, 1979.* 96th Cong., 1st sess. Washington, D.C.: Government Printing Office, 1980.
U. S. Congress. Joint Economic Committee. *Averting Catastrophe: The Global Challenge. Report, October 10, 1980.* 96th Cong., 2d sess. Washington, D.C.: Government Printing Office, 1980.
U. S. Congress. Senate. Committee on Energy and Natural Resources. Subcommittee on Energy Conservation and Supply. *Effects of Acid Rain: Hearings, June 21, 1980.* 96th Cong., 2d sess. Washington, D.C.: Government Printing Office, 1980.
U. S. Congress. Senate. Committee on Energy and Natural Resources. Subcommittee on Energy Regulation. *Nuclear Waste and Facility Siting Policy: Hearings, August 26, 1980.* 96th Cong., 2d sess. Washington, D.C.: Government Printing Office, 1980.
U.S. Congress. Senate. Committee on Environment and Public Works. *Health Effects of Toxic Pollution: A Report from the Surgeon General and a Brief Review of Selected Environmental Contamination Incidents With a Potential for Health Effects, August 1980.* 96th Cong., 2d sess. Washington, D.C.: Government Printing Office, 1980.
U. S. Congress. Senate. Committee on Environment and Public Works. *Nuclear Accident and Recovery At Three Mile Island: A Special Report, June 1980.* 96th Cong., 2d sess. Washington, D.C.: Government Printing Office, 1980.
U. S. Congress. Senate. Committee on Environment and Public Works. Subcommittee on Nuclear Regulation. *Nuclear Waste Disposal: Hearings, September 11, 1979; January 24, 1980.* 96th Cong., 1st and 2d sess. Washington, D.C.: Government Printing Office, 1980.
U. S. Congress. Senate. Committee on Governmental Affairs. *Benefits of Environmental, Health, and Safety Regulations.* 96th Cong., 2d sess. Washington, D.C.: Government Printing Office, 1980.
U. S. Congress. Senate. Committee on Governmental Affairs. Subcommittee on Oversight of Government Management. *Oversight of Hazardous Waste Management and the Resource Conservation and Recovery Act; Hearings July 19, August 1, 1979.* 96th Cong., 1st sess. Washington, D.C.: Government Printing Office, 1979.
U. S. Congress. Senate. Committee on Government Affairs. Subcommittee on Oversight of Government Management. *Report on Hazardous Waste Management and the Implementation of the Resource Conservation and Recovery Act.* 96th Cong., 2d sess. Washington, D.C.: Government Printing Office, 1980.
U. S. Congress. Senate. Select Committee on Small Business. *Economic Impact of Acid Rain; Hearings, September 23, 1980.* 96th Cong., 2d sess. Washington, D.C.: Government Printing Office, 1981.
U. S. General Accounting Office. *Environmental Protection Issues in the 1980s.* Washington, D.C.: 1980.
U.S. General Accounting Office. *The Problem of Disposing of Nuclear Low-Level Waste: Where Do We Go From Here? Report to the Congress by the Comptroller General of the United States.* Washington, D.C., 1980.
U.S. Department of Health and Human Services. *Healthy People, The Surgeon General's Report on Health Promotion and Disease Prevention.* Washington, D.C., 1979.

Index

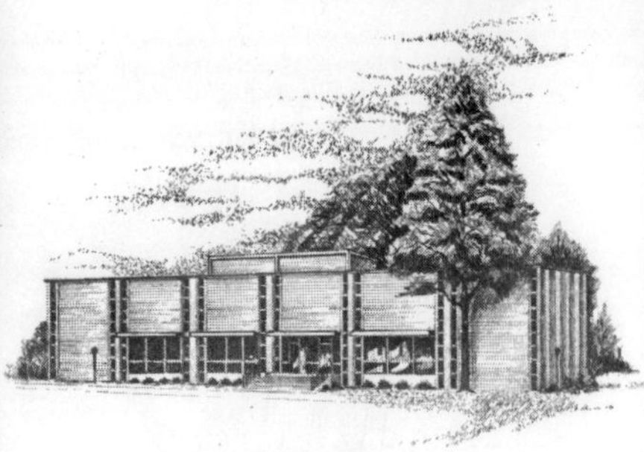

FUNDERBURG LIBRARY
MANCHESTER COLLEGE